INSIDE *the*
OUTBREAKS

Books by MARK PENDERGRAST

For God, Country and Coca-Cola

Victims of Memory

Uncommon Grounds

Mirror Mirror

Inside the Outbreaks

INSIDE *the*
OUTBREAKS

The Elite
Medical Detectives
of the Epidemic
Intelligence Service

MARK PENDERGRAST

MARINER BOOKS HOUGHTON MIFFLIN HARCOURT
BOSTON • NEW YORK

First Mariner Books edition 2011

Copyright © 2010 by Mark Pendergrast

www.hmhbooks.com

Library of Congress Cataloging-in-Publication Data
Pendergrast, Mark.
    Inside the outbreaks : the elite medical detectives of the Epidemic Intelligence Service / Mark Pendergrast.
        p. cm.
    Includes bibliographical references.
    ISBN 978-0-15-101120-9
    ISBN 978-0-547-52030-8 (pbk.)
    1. Centers for Disease Control (U.S.). Epidemic Intelligence Service — Popular works. 2. Epidemiology — Popular works. 3. Epidemiologists — United States — Popular works. I. Title. [DNLM: 1. Centers for Disease Control (U.S.). Epidemic Intelligence Service. 2. Communicable Disease Control — history — United States. 3. Epidemiology — history — United States. 4. History, 20th Century — United States. 5. United States Government Agencies — United States. WA 11 AA1 P397i 2010]
    RA653.P46 2010
    614.4 — dc22   2009029871

Book design by Linda Lockowitz

Printed in the United States of America

DOC 10 9 8 7 6 5 4 3 2 1

*This book is dedicated to all who
work to protect the public health, and
to the memory of my friend Liz Lasser,
who died of malaria in 2003
at the age of forty-nine.*

CONTENTS

II

THE GOLDEN AGE OF EPI
(1970–1982)

III

COMPLEX CHALLENGES
(1982–PRESENT)

THE PARABLE OF THE CLINICIAN
AND THE EPIDEMIOLOGIST

THE BROWN RIVER usually flows lazily through the middle of town. But today it is a torrent carrying human bodies. Some, still alive, are gasping for air and thrashing the water.

Approaching the river to enjoy lunch on its banks, two doctors, horrified by what they see, begin to haul people out of the water. There are no signs of violence, but the victims' eyes are glazed, their weak pulses racing.

The doctors cannot keep up with the flow of bodies. They save a few and watch helplessly as the others drift beyond them.

Suddenly, one of the doctors lowers an old man to the ground and starts to run. "What are you doing?" yells the other doctor. "For God's sake, help me save these people!"

Without stopping, she yells back over her shoulder, "I'm going upstream to find out why they're falling in."

INTRODUCTION

SINCE ITS FOUNDING IN 1951 by Alexander Langmuir as a service/ training program, the Epidemic Intelligence Service, working out of the CDC* in Atlanta, Georgia, has sent out more than three thousand officers to combat every imaginable human (and sometimes animal) ailment.

These young people — doctors, veterinarians, dentists, statisticians, nurses, microbiologists, academic epidemiologists, sociologists, anthropologists, and now even lawyers — call themselves "shoe-leather epidemiologists." EIS officers have ventured over the globe in search of diseases, sometimes in airplanes or jeeps, on bicycles, aboard fragile boats, on dogsleds, atop elephants and camels.

EIS officers generally have performed their tasks without fanfare or notice. They have saved uncountable lives, preventing uncontrolled spread of disease and diagnosing problems before they escalated. They even may have saved your life, though you were probably unaware of it.

Inside the Outbreaks follows Epidemic Intelligence Service officers in their efforts to solve medical mysteries. Through their stories, read-

---

*CDC originally stood for Communicable Disease Center. Over time the name changed several times and is now called the Centers for Disease Control and Prevention.

ers will learn about the causes of epidemics, the threat of bioterrorism, environmental hazards, and chronic diseases, as well as about societal problems such as violence, malnutrition, and overpopulation.

The first EIS officers were mostly young white male U.S. physicians avoiding the military draft. Today about 15 percent of each class comes from other countries, and over half are female. Many arrive in the EIS with extensive experience and education in public health, and others come with Ph.D.s or other non-M.D. training. The average age of the EIS recruit has increased from twenty-seven to thirty-four.

The EIS has carried on the tradition of field epidemiology begun in the mid-nineteenth century by John Snow, among others. By going door-to-door in London, mapping cases during an 1854 cholera outbreak, Snow noted that infections in one area centered around the Broad Street pump and that employees at a nearby brewing company, which had its own springwater (and sanitary beer), remained well. Snow concluded that an infectious agent must be in the public water supply. On his advice authorities removed the pump handle and the epidemic ceased. As Alexander Langmuir put it, such "direct field observations, orderly arraying of evidence, and incisive inductive reasoning have set a pattern for all epidemiologists to emulate today."

Early EIS officers, like Snow, employed simple descriptive epidemiology, looking for the frequency and pattern of an outbreak by examining a particular time period in a well-defined place and population. Over time, the EIS methodology has become more sophisticated, employing case-control studies, computing odds ratios, and utilizing other complex statistical analyses.

Even today, though, epidemiology is a science of probability, not proof. If everyone who drinks the water from a particular source gets sick, and no one else does, it is a good bet that there is something harmful in the water. But only when the same pathogenic strain is found in victims' stools and in the water will the case be proved. EIS officers must constantly be on guard against confounding factors, i.e., everyone who drank the water did so because they had eaten hot Tex-Mex food, and the food was at fault. Correlation does not necessarily equal causation.

In the 1950s and 1960s there was widespread optimism that infectious diseases could be defeated with proper antibiotic use, vaccines, and sometimes quarantine, but pathogens developed resistance to antibiotics. Disease carriers such as mosquitoes were difficult to control. Not all diseases had effective vaccines, and immunization sometimes caused its own problems. The infrastructure to deliver vaccines to every child was difficult to build, even in the United States, while posing a huge challenge in the developing world. Also, as humans have invaded every ecosystem, and as modern technology has changed our way of life, emerging diseases have appeared.

The focus of the original EIS was primarily domestic, but as the program evolved, EIS officers ventured overseas with increasing frequency in the belief that if the disease burden is reduced elsewhere, it is less likely to be imported to the United States. But most EIS officers and CDC employees believe that humanitarian concerns alone justify international work. Indeed, diseases such as malaria, smallpox, AIDS, and cholera disproportionately ravage the developing world and appear throughout the history of the EIS.

The book is divided into three sections. Part I, "The Grand Adventures of Dr. Langmuir's Boys," covers the beginning years 1951 through 1970. Part II, "The Golden Age of Epi," takes the story through 1982, encompassing a period when field epidemiology came of age. Part III, "Complex Challenges," brings the saga to the present.

While in general I chose epidemics that highlighted successful disease detectives, not all EIS investigations have solved medical mysteries. I have also included a few diseases whose etiologies still remain unknown, as well as some pseudoepidemics.

A note on bureaucratic structure: The EIS is a service/training program of the CDC, which is part of the U.S. Public Health Service in the Department of Health and Human Services. Many EIS officers enter the USPHS Commissioned Corps, a uniformed service originally connected with the U.S. Navy. Others become federal civil servants. After their two years in the EIS, alums often remain at the CDC, but they are under no obligation to do so.

No organization is without flaws or failures, and this, of course, includes the EIS and the CDC. The overarching take-home lesson from this history, though, is that dollars spent on public health surveillance and prevention programs are cost-effective. In the United States, we tend to react to health problems and seek heroic individual clinical resolutions, spending most of our health budget on extreme measures. Because public health efforts like those of the EIS are largely invisible — few people know they are being protected — they are both undervalued and underfunded, despite their efficiency.

Enough introductory remarks. Prepare to enter the world of the Epidemic Intelligence Service.

I

THE GRAND ADVENTURES
OF DR. LANGMUIR'S BOYS
(1951–1970)

1

COLD WAR, HOT PATHOGENS

IN FEBRUARY 1951 Alexander Langmuir, the epidemiologist for the Communicable Disease Center (CDC) in Atlanta, Georgia, delivered a lecture at the Kansas City Medical Center. "Many pathogenic agents may be grown in almost limitless quantities and may be dispersed into the air as single cells," he said. Langmuir bent his six-foot-two-inch frame over the lectern, his booming baritone filling the hall. "The purposeful creation of such clouds is biological warfare." He described how atomizers could spray dangerous microbes in crowded enclosed spaces and how bombs could create smoglike pathogens that would hang over a city for hours. He spoke of contaminated water systems and of food infected at a banquet. "The planning of appropriate defensive measures must not be delayed," Langmuir advised.

The press had warned of biological warfare since 1946. But with the start of the Korean War in June 1950, fear and rhetoric escalated. By early 1951 Langmuir had convinced the federal government to support a ready-response team at the CDC. In June 1951 American soldiers in Korea began dying of a mysterious infection that started with high fever, aches, nausea, and vomiting. Then victims' blood vessels burst, causing internal and often external bleeding. The infection, dubbed Korean hemorrhagic fever, affected twenty-five thousand

United Nations (mostly American) troops, killing nearly three thousand of them during the course of the conflict. Fear of this new epidemic disease solidified funding for Langmuir's trainees.*

The program was named the Epidemic Intelligence Service (EIS), deliberately employing a military term and implying a comparison with the recently created Central Intelligence Agency. The two-year EIS experience in the U.S. Public Health Service Commissioned Corps would satisfy the new obligation for doctors to perform military service. Langmuir suddenly had bright young physicians who did not want to go to war begging to join the CDC.

A Shoe-Leather Epidemiologist

Born in 1910 in Santa Monica, California, and raised in Englewood, New Jersey, Alexander Langmuir graduated from Harvard and went to Cornell University Medical College. After finishing his internship, he began a career in public health. Before the war, he practiced what he called "shoe-leather epidemiology" in New York State, going into the field to investigate epidemics of polio, tuberculosis, pneumonia, and other diseases. During World War II he was tapped by the army to serve on the Commission on Acute Respiratory Diseases based at Fort Bragg, North Carolina. The commission feared another massive influenza epidemic such as the one that had killed so many in 1918. No such pandemic materialized, but the soldiers, packed in crowded barracks, provided ideal subjects for Langmuir's studies of acute respiratory disease epidemics.

Armed with a high-security clearance, Langmuir was also admitted into the top-secret confines of Camp Detrick (renamed Fort Detrick in 1956), in Frederick, Maryland, where military scientists experimented with infectious agents, trying to develop strategies to combat biological warfare if the enemy unleashed it, as well as preparing to inflict retaliatory epidemics.

---

*Korean hemorrhagic fever was a hantavirus (named after the Han River in South Korea, and finally isolated in 1976). It was spread by rodents, not Communists.

A Happy Hunting Ground

The CDC was three years old when Langmuir arrived there in 1949, lured from an associate professorship in epidemiology at Johns Hopkins. His friends lamented his commitment to this "dying field," since antibiotics and vaccines presumably would solve everything. Langmuir countered, "I firmly believe that in the field of infectious diseases there is a happy hunting ground for major discoveries and contributions," and the CDC's broad mandate impressed him. "The range of opportunity, the potential was obvious," he said later, "and with my considerable self-confidence, I had no trouble going."

"Considerable self-confidence" was an understatement. "People knew when he entered a room," Langmuir's daughter Lynn recalled. "He tipped the boat. You had to scramble to keep your equilibrium."

An EIS alum spoke of others quailing before "the peals of Langmuirian thunder." His successor as the head of the program described Langmuir after his death as "visionary, clairvoyant, tenacious, well-prepared, scientifically honest, and optimistic." Others used adjectives such as "loud, intimidating, pompous, bombastic, aggressive, and domineering." Yet most agree that without Alexander Langmuir's strong leadership and vision, the EIS program would never have endured.

Epidemic Twists and Curves

In tracing epidemics, Langmuir espoused what came to be called a cohort study of a carefully defined group of people (*Who attended the church supper?*), comparing their behavior (*What did they eat? Where did they go? Who did they associate with?*) and looking for key differences between those who had become ill and those who had not. Sometimes through such comparisons, the cause of an epidemic became obvious. *It was the potato salad!*

Langmuir stressed the importance of long division to find the rate of a given disease in a particular population — the number of ill over a defined period of time as a numerator and the population at risk as a denominator. "Stripped to its basics," he said, "epidemiology is simply a process of obtaining the appropriate numerator and denominator, determining a rate, and interpreting that rate." Thus, the three essential elements were time (when were people exposed and when did they become ill?), person (who was affected in what defined population?), and place (where did the epidemic take place?).

But how do you know that an epidemic is occurring? First, you establish the "normal" rate of disease for that area. Langmuir talked about the importance of routine disease surveillance to establish baseline data and to look for anomalous blips.

Traced on a time line that tracks the number of accumulating daily cases, most epidemics form a classic bell-shaped epidemic curve. In the simplest version, an outbreak begins in a particular community with an index case, spreads to others, reaches a peak, and then gradually burns itself out, as susceptibles either survive and become immune or die. Looking at this epi-curve, the disease detective could deduce a fair amount. A common source epidemic, such as bad potato salad at a picnic, would have a sudden onset, sharp peak, and rapid resolution among a limited population, whereas an ongoing problem such as a contaminated water supply might affect an entire community for a longer time. Once a likely moment of exposure was determined, i.e., the time of the picnic, the epi-curve also revealed the average incubation period, the time between infection and disease onset.

Tiny Parasites, Unwilling Hosts

Fossilized bacteria have been found in rocks over 3 billion years old. These single-cell organisms reproduce by dividing by fission — often in less than twenty minutes. Some bacteria are helpful, such as those that help us digest food, while others release chemicals that poison our tissues. To fight off infections, our bodies developed an elaborate immune system that creates specific antibodies for specific microbes. There are at least 10 million known species of bacteria.

Also ancient, a virus is a protein shell surrounding a strand of nucleic acid, either DNA or RNA. It cannot reproduce on its own but must invade a living cell, which it takes over, commanding the cell to reproduce the virus at an incredible rate. There are millions of different types of viruses.

Then there are the one-celled parasites, such as those that cause malaria, whose vector (delivery system) is the mosquito; larger bacteria called *Rickettsia*, usually inserted into humans by ticks or fleas; and fungi whose spores float from the air into the lungs or onto pre-existing skin lesions. There are also chemical toxins produced by bacteria and other quick-acting poisons that, while not infectious, can kill people.

Microbes have evolved mechanisms to proliferate — for example, measles and influenza victims cough, spraying virus into the air; *Shigella* causes diarrhea in order to spread bacteria. Man against microbes is a fight for survival.

The Hazards of Improved Sanitation

Langmuir's epidemiological techniques led to two important discoveries even before the creation of the EIS. When he arrived at the CDC, a $7 million budget was still devoted to fighting malaria because Southern doctors continued to report thousands of malaria cases when there was no other obvious cause of the fever. Langmuir's first surveillance effort sent out teams to conduct surveys about the frequency of attacks, symptoms, treatment, and patient travels, and to collect blood samples. Investigations unearthed only nineteen positive cases of indigenous malaria and these were not in the significant clusters that would indicate a potential epidemic. Malaria had been virtually eliminated from the United States, but no one in the medical field had realized it.

In 1950 Langmuir sent twenty-six-year-old Ira Myers, one of the few doctors he was able to recruit before the "doctor draft" of 1951, to Charleston, West Virginia, to determine if flies transmitted poliomyelitis, the viral crippler that terrified postwar America. Myers discovered that there was a much higher rate of paralytic polio in upscale Kanawha City, a suburb of Charleston, West Virginia, than in Chandler Branch, a poor area where cesspools dumped into the drinking water supply. By the time they were six months old, most babies in Chandler Branch had developed mild infections and were immune to polio. Poor sanitation had provided the Chandler Branch children with a surprising advantage over the kids in the more sanitary Kanawha City.

2
THROWING THEM OVERBOARD

MAYBE IT'S THE HONEY buckets, Donald Schliessmann thought. Fresh from the first EIS immersion course, the thirty-four-year-old sanitary engineer watched as several men defecated explosively atop a fifty-five-gallon drum that had been cut in half lengthwise, with rough wooden seats installed on top. These so-called honey buckets were emptied every evening into the ocean surrounding Koje-do, a mountainous island off the coast of Korea. The rice paddies in the valleys of the island had been turned into prisoner-of-war compounds for more than 150,000 captured North Korean and Chinese soldiers.

Could be, but there must be more to it, Schliessmann concluded. As primitive as the toilets were, they were relatively well-maintained, flushed with water daily, the seats soaped down, and the latrine areas sprayed with DDT.

Schliessmann had arrived on the island in mid-August 1951 as part of the Joint Dysentery Unit, formed to respond to a massive diarrhea epidemic among the POWs. In the crowded conditions of a makeshift camp near the mainland town of Pusan, the epidemic had spread swiftly in the fall of 1950, and by the time Schliessmann arrived, nearly two thousand POWs had died.

When the prisoners were moved to Koje-do in February 1951, the death rate declined and then halted, primarily due to the use of new antibiotics, which American drug companies tested on the worst POW cases. But the epidemic continued. Schliessmann sought to learn how the primary infectious agent, *Shigella* bacillus, was being spread.

Shigella dysenteriae causes intestinal ulcerations and abscesses, characteristically producing a bloody diarrhea, along with fever, nausea, and vomiting. Untreated, it can kill as intestinal wounds turn septic.

Shigellosis (dysentery) is spread by the fecal-oral route, the EIS officer knew, and the unwashed human hand usually transports the microbe from anus to mouth. So Schliessmann performed an experiment. "In one of the compounds," he recalled, "I made all of the prisoners who frequented the latrine wash their hands when they emerged. They used soapy, dirty water that was thrown out after every tenth person and replaced with polluted water, but at least it had soap in it." After three weeks there was a substantial decrease in the number from that compound reporting for sick call and admission to the camp hospital. The experiment's conclusion: "With a more adequate supply of water for personal hygiene, the incidence of enteric infections declined."

Learning to Swim in an Epidemic

Langmuir usually sent out only one or two EIS officers at a time. "We'll get them on an epidemic as fast as we can," he said. "Throw them overboard. See if they can swim, and if they can't, throw them a life ring, pull them out and throw them in again."

Schliessmann's early temporary international assignment was unusual. Most EIS officers were assigned around the United States, in carefully selected state and city health departments, research universities and hospitals, the CDC headquarters in Atlanta, or in a CDC branch, but all of them were on call twenty-four hours a day.

Langmuir could not dispatch an EIS officer to a state unless the state health department issued an invitation. Because many states resented federal bureaucrats, they frequently didn't ask for help, or called only when an epidemic had done its worst already. Langmuir eased this problem by lending EIS officers to states for their two-year assignment, where the officers became part of the local structure, though they could be snatched at any moment for an emergency else-where.

The members of the first EIS class spread across the country, often driving on back roads and flying into storms. They dealt with encephalitis, diarrhea, hepatitis, conjunctivitis, histoplasmosis, botulism, typhoid fever, leptospirosis, polio, psittacosis, and tetanus, among other diseases.

Mystery in Tuba City

On New Year's Day 1952, twenty-seven-year-old EIS officer Charles "Mickey" LeMaistre held on as the Piper Cub landed on an isolated, snow-covered airstrip. When LeMaistre got out, the pilot immediately took off, leaving him completely alone. "I was a dot on a white landscape," he recalled. Finally a truck with two teachers from Tuba City, Arizona, arrived to take him to a remote Navajo boarding school, where most of the students were ill.

The epidemic had begun the last week of November 1951, peaking three weeks later. Two children had died, and the teachers believed that 417 others were ill or had been ill. When the EIS officer performed quick autopsies, he found that the children had died from infectious hepatitis, now called hepatitis A.

The local twenty-five-bed hospital was already filled with critically ill Native American tuberculosis patients, as it usually was. So LeMaistre asked the teachers to close the school and organize makeshift wards there, isolating the sick children. He called Atlanta for medical supplies and New York Hospital of Cornell, where he was based, asking for consultants to fly in.

Once medical care was in place, LeMaistre tried to find the source of the hepatitis. Hepatitis A is spread by the fecal-oral route, so once it hit the crowded school, it had moved quickly. He learned that the school's vegetables were stored in local caves and that one of the men who went into the caves had hepatitis, but LeMaistre was unable to connect him with the children or to prove that the vegetables had been contaminated. Fortunately, with proper care, the surviving children recovered.

Though he was not able to find the source of the hepatitis, Le-Maistre nevertheless took steps to improve public health in the area. He secured a supply of isoniazid, a new drug that would revolutionize the care of tuberculosis and thus reduce the burden on the local hospital. An outpatient program was set up, working closely with the Navajo and incorporating some of their tribal medicine.

Confined Guinea Pigs

In the early 1950s very little was known about hepatitis. Yellow fever vaccine given to U.S. troops in North Africa during World War II had been contaminated with what came to be called serum hepatitis (hepatitis B). The resulting epidemic, which affected nearly a quarter of the troops, called attention to this bloodborne form of the disease.

Twenty-seven-year-old EIS officer Jerry Barondess was assigned to the Children's Hospital of Philadelphia, where he worked both in the laboratory and in the field. "We went hammer and tongs, going after a vaccine for both types of hepatitis," Barondess recalled. To test the vaccine, he went to several New Jersey prisons, a home for mentally disabled children, and a hospital for the criminally insane. In each place, using various combinations for controls and cases, he injected both hepatitis A and B virus and/or vaccine into inmates and children to study the disease and to determine if the vaccine worked. Such human experimentation was accepted practice in the early 1950s.*

"The prison volunteers were eager to get off work details to be inoculated," Barondess reported. "My job was to inoculate them, then examine them once a week to see who got sick and who didn't, to take blood samples, and to make sure they eventually got well. The danger was not thought to be very great. Most people with hepatitis A don't even know they've got it, don't turn jaundiced. They just get what they call flu for a few days."

Yet hepatitis B can cause chronic liver disease that leads to cirrho-

---

*A few years later, in 1955, medical researcher Saul Krugman began similar studies in the Willowbrook State School for retarded children in New York State, which led to the discovery of the agent for hepatitis B, but also contributed to the creation of ethical review boards to prevent abuse of human subjects.

sis. "We didn't know it was a big bad disease at the time," Barondess said. "We were just trying to learn about its transmissibility." The vaccine didn't work very well. No one followed up to see whether any of the experimental subjects suffered from long-term effects. The ethics of experimentation on humans would evolve along with the EIS.

Rare and Invariably Fatal

As a resident at the University of Chicago Medical School, Tom Grayston examined a hospitalized Indiana farmer who had a fever and bad cough. The farmer's chest X-rays were startling, dotted with lesions across his lungs. Grayston and his supervisor finally diagnosed his ailment as histoplasmosis, a fungal infection. "We knew nothing about it," Grayston recalled, "so we looked it up in textbooks, which said that histoplasmosis was extremely rare and invariably fatal."

Yet the farmer didn't appear to be terribly sick. "In talking to him, we learned that he and his children had recently cleaned out an old silo. So we went out to his farm, collected some dirt from the silo floor, and examined the family members." The daughter and son had had a brief flu-like illness, and X-rays revealed that they, too, had disseminated lesions in their lungs. The silo soil contained *Histoplasma capsulatum*. It appeared that histoplasmosis might be more common and less deadly than previously believed.

Alex Langmuir was excited when he heard Grayston present a paper on the case. "Alex felt this was field epidemiology," Grayston said. Facing the doctor draft, he was happy to be recruited for the Epidemic Intelligence Service in 1951, and he was sent to the CDC's Kansas City field station.

Over the next two years Grayston became a leading authority on histoplasmosis. Tramping all over the Midwest, working both retrospectively and keeping an eye out for current cases, he identified thirteen histoplasmosis outbreaks, accounting for two hundred cases. The emerging pattern was clear: Histoplasmosis grew best in moist, decayed bird droppings. The hardy spores survived for years and, if disturbed in dry conditions, could be aerosolized and inhaled. The incubation period for the disease was generally one to two weeks.

In addition, he performed skin tests on schoolchildren in various areas of the Midwest, which appeared to be the histo belt, demonstrating that 80 percent of the eighteen-year-olds were histoplasmin reactors. Histoplasmosis was neither rare nor invariably fatal. Once exposed to the fungus, people appeared to develop at least a partial immunity.

Inflamed Brains, Mosquitoes, and Earthquakes

In the summer of 1952 an epidemic of western equine encephalitis (WEE), mixed with some cases of St. Louis encephalitis, hit California's Central Valley. By July 31, when the CDC was called, seventy-six people had been diagnosed and three hundred more were suspected victims. Symptoms are generally mild fever and headache, but cases of coma and death can occur.

Violating his own rule of sending only one or two EIS officers to an epidemic, Langmuir dispatched eleven EIS officers plus engineers, entomologists, and veterinarians, all expected to report there by August 2. Grayston flew to Bakersfield, California, where he discovered one reason for the epidemic. A major earthquake had recently hit the area. Afraid to sleep indoors, people were more vulnerable to getting bitten by mosquitoes outdoors.

Encephalitis, an inflammation of the brain, can be caused by different organisms, but the culprit in this case was a virus carried by a mosquito, the *Culex tarsalis*. Grayston and others urged people to sleep indoors and use repellent.

Another EIS officer, Henry Shinefield, helped set up clinics up and down the California Central Valley. "I visited one pregnant woman who had contracted the disease. She delivered twins who had WEE at birth." No one had previously known that the virus could be passed in the womb.

The Classic Church Supper

Twenty-six-year-old Harold Nitowsky was in remote Trinidad, Colorado, in the summer of 1952, investigating a typhoid epidemic. A variant of the *Salmonella* bacterium, typhoid was rare in the United States, and carriers like the infamous "Typhoid Mary" Mallon had to register with state health departments. The disease is spread by fecal-oral contact, and unless their hands are washed very thoroughly, typhoid carriers can contaminate the food they prepare. If not countered by antibiotics or a vaccine, typhoid causes a rash, tender spleen, high fever, slow pulse, nausea, and diarrhea—the symptoms of six people who had eaten at a church potluck supper in Trinidad.

Nitowsky contacted everyone who had attended the dinner, asking them to recall what they had eaten. He made a chart with the different food and drink items running down a page on the left, and two columns marked ILL and NOT ILL at the top. Basically, this was a modified form of what epidemiologists call a 2 x 2 table, where two opposite conditions for each food item (or whatever variable is being examined) are listed on two sides of a four-part square: ATE — DIDN'T EAT on the left side and ILL — NOT ILL across the top. There are four possible permutations: 1) People ate a particular item and got ill. 2) They ate it and did not get ill. 3) They didn't eat it but got ill anyway. 4) They didn't eat it and didn't get ill. From the results, the epidemiologist can ascertain how strong an association the illness has with a particular food item.

The carrot salad, made by a church volunteer, had a very high food-specific attack rate.* When her stool sample was tested, the woman turned out to be an unrecognized typhoid carrier. "She was very upset," Nitowsky recalled. "She had to be registered and had to avoid serving food to others. And I cautioned her to be very careful washing her hands."

During his second EIS year, Nitowsky studied a mysterious disease called sarcoidosis, which mostly seemed to afflict black World War II veterans living in rural areas of the southeastern United States. Sarcoidosis is an inflammation that produces tiny lumps in various

---

*The food-specific attack rate is a percentage derived by dividing the number of those who ate carrot salad and got sick by the total number of people who ate the salad.

organs of the body, usually beginning in the lungs. Early symptoms can be a dry cough or enlarged lymph nodes. In mild cases, the symptoms can disappear over time, although in more severe cases it can affect other organs, including the eyes, heart, and brain.

"It was a complete mystery what caused sarcoidosis," Nitowsky said. He looked at every conceivable variable — eating habits, lifestyle, contact with plant and animal life, a previously unidentified bacterium or fungus — but couldn't find anything. To this day, no one knows what causes the disease. Like a number of investigations, it was filed under "Suspected Agent: Unknown." Then as now, EIS officers could not solve every case.

Creating Traditions

After its first six months, the EIS program earned the stamp of approval of Leonard Scheele, the U.S. surgeon general. In May 1952 Langmuir gathered his new class, numbering seventeen, for a conference in Atlanta, at which he established a tradition. An EIS officer was given ten minutes to present an outbreak investigation including results and action recommendations. Then he had to field audience questions for another ten minutes.

The introductory course for the second class of EIS officers began in July and lasted six weeks. During the first 1951 session, Langmuir had lectured along with guest speakers from Johns Hopkins, using the case-study method in the afternoons to present sample outbreaks. In 1952 he established the precedent of using second-year EIS officers to lead the afternoon sessions. These barely seasoned instructors were enthusiastic mentors for the new recruits.

An esprit de corps was born. Because Langmuir stressed shoe-leather epidemiology, one of the officers created a logo featuring the sole of a shoe, a prominent hole worn through the bottom, superimposed over the Earth. Irreverent humor became an early class tradition. Sung to the tune of "Old MacDonald Had a Farm," one effort began, "Alex Langmuir has a branch called EI-EIS, / And in this branch he has some docs, EI-EIS. With a quack quack here and a quack quack there ..."

Modern Poisons

No sooner had the fledgling EIS created its first traditions than one of its members broke new ground. On his first day at the Chicago City Health Department in mid-August 1952, EIS officer Bob Mellins rushed to Children's Memorial Hospital, where patients were said to be dying of St. Louis encephalitis. "I knew pretty quickly that it was lead poisoning. I had studied medicine at Johns Hopkins in Baltimore, where I had seen a lot of lead poisoning among inner-city kids in the summer." Why that season? Increased sunlight mobilizes calcium and other heavy metals from the bones into the bloodstream.

"I pulled up to the home of the first dead child in the slums. I looked up, and there was a toddler eating paint chips from the windowsill." He made a half dozen home visits that day and found more lead-paint chips. Mellins asked to be reassigned to study unintentional poisoning in children, becoming the first EIS officer to specialize in a noninfectious disease. He discovered that many children died after ingesting kerosene, insecticides, rodenticides, liniments, aspirin, laxatives, bleach, Lysol, and turpentine, among other household items. As a result, in 1953 he started the first poison control program in the United States, in Chicago.

Choking to Death in Ohio

Reimert Ravenholt was assigned to the Ohio State Health Department when a five-year-old died of diphtheria in the Ohio State Hospital. A rare disease because of an effective vaccine, diphtheria is a bacterium exuding a toxin that can create a membrane to block the throat, causing victims to choke to death. Antibiotics and a specific antitoxin can help if not given too late — which was unfortunately the case for this unvaccinated child.

EIS officer Ravenholt drove to the deceased child's home, learning that his seven-year-old sister also had had a sore throat. "This led me to the victim's second-grade class, where the teacher said, yes, there had been a number of sore throats in her children." Eleven children tested positive for diphtheria. Ravenholt swabbed the throats of the entire school population, and set up for mass immunization, since these rural children had not been vaccinated. The outbreak was contained.

A few months later Ravenholt returned to the school for a follow-up visit. The principal mentioned that some children had been coughing up blood. "I got chest X-rays that clearly showed a pneumonic process. I took blood specimens. The first tip-off was an increase in eosinophils, a type of white blood cell." That indicates an allergic state that can be caused by parasitic worms.

By this time, school had let out, so Ravenholt tracked the children down in their homes in poverty-stricken hollows. "I remember one home vividly, where Will, an eighth-grade boy, showed pneumonia in his chest X-ray. I got his medical history from the mother, who was nursing her ninth child. The unemployed father sat on the sofa. They told me that a cousin had a similar illness last year and had died of it, and they had found a quart of worms in his intestines."

He asked where they got their water. "A spring out back" was the response, but Ravenholt discovered a concrete basin holding stagnant water, halfway between the house and the outhouse. "I left stool specimen containers. As I finished up, the mother invited me to stay for lunch, but I declined.

"If you're a doctor just in a hospital, you see sick kids, but now I could see where it all came from. And yes, we found roundworms in the stool samples." Ravenholt contacted a local doctor, who prescribed medication to flush out the worms.

Parrot Fever and the Parakeet Craze

The problem began in Florida, where EIS officer Martin Hicklin found that shipments from a rare-bird farm were spreading diseased parakeets throughout the United States. Psittacosis (*Chlamydia psittaci*) is a bacterium whose reservoir is in parakeets, parrots, and lovebirds, and less frequently in poultry, pigeons, canaries, and seabirds. If humans inhale dust from dry droppings, they can come down with fever, headache, rash, and chills. In the elderly or immunocompromised, the disease can be life-threatening. Fortunately, it does not spread person to person.

In 1954 the disease jumped to turkeys in Texas, then Oregon. Nearly two hundred Texas turkey handlers came down with psittacosis, and one died. In response, turkey growers began to give massive doses of antibiotics to their flocks, a policy that would create problems in the postwar era.

The psittacosis outbreak proved what James Steele, the head CDC veterinarian, already knew. Zoonoses — diseases of humans that derive from animals — were a major problem. With Steele's urging, in 1953 the first veterinarians were accepted as EIS officers.

3

KILLER VACCINE, GOAT-HAIR ANTHRAX, RABID BATS, AND STAPH ATTACKS

POLIO IS CONQUERED, declared the April 12, 1955, banner headline of the *Pittsburgh Press*. Variants of the jubilant message appeared in newspapers across the country. On the tenth anniversary of the death of Franklin Delano Roosevelt, polio's most famous victim, the results of the largest medical study in history were announced. The Salk vaccine, made from inactivated poliovirus, clearly prevented polio in most cases.

Edward R. Murrow announced on national television that the news had "lifted a sense of fear from the homes of millions of Americans." In the 1950s, at a time when most infectious diseases could apparently be controlled by antibiotics, sanitation, and clean water, polio was a mysterious, seemingly unstoppable disease that paralyzed and sometimes killed. It struck particularly hard in the antiseptic suburbs. Despite closing swimming pools and movie theaters, and massive spraying with DDT to kill flies then thought to transmit the virus, polio claimed new victims every summer.* In 1952, the worst polio epidemic year on record, there were more than fifty-seven thousand cases nationwide. In one Milwaukee family, four out of six children developed bulbar polio, which attacks the cranial nerves that control

---

*Polio is spread by the fecal-oral route.

breathing. Those who survived bulbar polio ended up in iron lungs for life, but many, including all four Milwaukee siblings, died.

Since 1951 Epidemic Intelligence Service officers had been studying and attempting to combat polio. Then Jonas Salk perfected his killed-virus vaccine. EIS officers helped supervise a massive field trial that proved the vaccine was a success.

That same day, April 12, 1955, the government authorized the vaccine's use, and six manufacturers released it for the inoculation of the country's first and second graders. Ten million doses were distributed, most of them free, thanks to the National Foundation for Infantile Paralysis. For the first two weeks of the campaign, the major problem was an insufficient amount of available vaccine.*

The Cutter Incident

On Sunday morning, April 24, an Idaho pediatrician notified the local public health officer that a first grader who had received the Salk shot had developed paralysis in her inoculated left arm. The shot had come from vaccine made by California-based Cutter Laboratories. The state health officer, assuming that the first grader had been exposed before she was vaccinated, did not notify the CDC.

The next day Chicago-based EIS officer Bob Mellins got a call from a doctor who had used the Cutter vaccine on several patients. One of them had developed paralysis in both legs after an injection in the buttocks. Mellins called Langmuir, who notified William Workman, head of the NIH Laboratory of Biologics Control, the agency charged with authorizing and auditing the vaccine. Workman, like the Idaho public health officer, assumed that the child had been previously infected.

On April 26 calls from California announced five more Cutter cases. "I became as convinced as anyone could be at this stage that the cases were attributable to a common source, the Cutter vaccine," Alexander Langmuir recalled. At an emergency meeting of public health

---

*The polio vaccine helped to set a precedent in which drug companies, not the government, produced vaccines. Since vaccines are not used repeatedly by an individual, they are not big moneymakers, and this fact would lead to vaccine shortfalls in the years to come.

experts that day in Washington, D.C., Langmuir urged that the Cutter vaccine be recalled immediately, but others disagreed, not wanting to scuttle the vaccine program. They could not reach consensus and so left it up to Surgeon General Leonard Scheele, known in public health circles as "Shilly-Shally Scheele" for his indecision. After much consultation, on April 27 he ordered the cancellation of that day's scheduled Cutter inoculations and urged Cutter Laboratories to withdraw its product. The company complied.

The next day Scheele asked Langmuir to set up a system to track all polio cases. Until then, EIS officers had performed routine surveillance only on diseases rare in the United States, such as diphtheria or malaria. This was of another magnitude altogether, and Langmuir jumped at it, eager to prove the importance of the EIS and CDC. He assigned a new EIS officer, Neal Nathanson, to head the new Polio Surveillance Unit (PSU).

"When the first Cutter cases happened, I was the only one with nothing to do, so I was drafted to start the PSU," Nathanson remembered. He and EIS statistician Jack Hall compiled a daily report and sent it to the surgeon general, state epidemiologists, and others with a need to know. Nathanson and Hall issued their first report on May 1, 1955, featuring twenty-two vaccine-associated cases.

In each state, a polio reporting officer (usually a state health official) was designated. EIS officers were dispatched to investigate each reported case. In all, twenty-two EIS officers were assigned to investigate polio cases, but as Langmuir wrote, "All of our Epidemic Intelligence Service Officers now are alerted for first priority duty to investigate cases of poliomyelitis anywhere in the country."

By May 4, thirty-six Cutter cases had been reported, but there were also cases apparently associated with vaccine from another manufacturer, Eli Lilly and Company. Three days later, Hall estimated the "expected" rate of polio, based on previous years, and found that "among the 2,250,000 children who received Lilly vaccine a total of seven cases was expected by chance alone and a total of six has been reported to date."

Most of the cases continued to be associated with the Cutter vaccine, and these occurred at a rate much higher than that expected by chance. On May 7 the first Cutter death was reported — a two-year-old boy in New Orleans.

At an emergency meeting, all six vaccine makers admitted having trouble with inactivating the virus. "We found a lot of virus in some of [our safety tests]," the Lilly scientists revealed. The Wyeth Laboratories representative also acknowledged that many lots had failed.

In an interview published in the May 6 *U.S. News & World Report*, Surgeon General Scheele expressed "complete faith" in the Salk vaccine, saying that "among the millions receiving the inoculations, some are likely to develop the disease. That does not mean, however, that the polio results from the vaccine."

The very next day Scheele ordered the suspension of the entire vaccination program, and on May 8, in a televised address, he announced the temporary withdrawal of polio vaccine from the market until a team of inspectors could visit every manufacturing plant.

Most people infected with the poliovirus never develop symptoms. Only one in two hundred becomes paralyzed. Others develop milder symptoms such as fever and temporary muscle weakness. Yet even those carrying inapparent infections can shed the live virus in their stool, and the virus can then spread to family members or other contacts. On May 8 a twenty-eight-year-old Tennessee mother contracted bulbar polio. She had not been vaccinated, but her two children had been injected with the Cutter vaccine a month earlier. The next day a young Atlanta mother, whose baby had received the Cutter product, died of polio.

EIS officers around the country soon reported that seventy-four unvaccinated family members had been paralyzed after children in the family had received the Cutter vaccine. In addition, a number of community contact cases were identified. Paul Offit, a professor of immunology and author of the book *The Cutter Incident,* wrote, "At least 220,000 people were infected with live polio virus contained in Cutter's vaccine; 70,000 developed muscle weakness, 164 were severely paralyzed, and 10 were killed."

The future of the polio vaccine program — and other vaccine ini-

tiatives — was at risk. Fortunately, the polio surveillance figures implicated just two bad lots of Cutter vaccine as the prime culprits, and following the epidemiological evidence, research laboratories were able
to isolate live virus from these lots. The Laboratory of Biologics issued revised requirements for vaccine manufacture to ensure that the
virus was thoroughly inactivated.

Gradually, most of the lots from the five companies aside from
Cutter were recleared, and the Salk vaccination campaign officially
resumed in June. But during the rest of 1955, only the bravest parents
allowed their children to be injected. Then a polio epidemic in Massachusetts provided chilling evidence that those who were unvaccinated had a much higher risk of contracting polio.

The work of EIS officers and the Polio Surveillance Unit proved
that national surveillance was essential to provide accurate, timely information on important diseases.

The Wyeth Problem

But this version of history, in which the EIS and Langmuir saved the
day by implicating only the Cutter vaccine, is not the entire story.
Langmuir attempted to minimize publicity about other problems, in
an understandable attempt to save the polio vaccine, which he knew
could prevent much suffering and death in the United States and the
rest of the world.

There were also alarming cases associated with the Wyeth vaccine,
distributed in Pennsylvania, Delaware, Maryland, the District of Columbia, and part of Ohio. The vaccination program in these areas had
begun a bit later than in the rest of the country. In the PSU bulletin issued on May 9, 1955, Neal Nathanson reported the first paralytic
Wyeth case in a seven-year-old Pennsylvania boy, followed by a girl in
the same state two days later.

On May 14 a Delaware Wyeth case appeared in the PSU report,
and three days later two more cases set off alarm bells. "Of five Wyeth
associated cases now accepted, three have shown a correlation between site of inoculation and site of first paralysis," wrote Nathanson.

One of the paralytic cases was associated with lot 235, and two with lot 236.

The cases continued to come in. On May 23 three more were reported from Pennsylvania, where EIS officers Philip Brachman and Peter Isacson worked frantically, finding three more Wyeth-associated suspects.* On May 27 they reported four new Maryland cases, all of which had a history of family contact with a child vaccinated with Wyeth lot 236. Wyeth was asked to withdraw the unused portion of that lot.

A confidential report in the CDC files entitled "The Wyeth Problem," dated August 31, 1955, and written by Langmuir, Nathanson, and Hall, with input from EIS investigators Brachman and Isacson, concluded that "Lot 236 was related in a causative way with at least some of the vaccine associated cases." In Pennsylvania, there were the incriminating paralyses in inoculated arms, but otherwise, the picture was confused, because an unusual amount of natural polio was simultaneously occurring in the same area. In Maryland, however, there was little polio other than fifteen contact cases associated with Wyeth lot 236.

The matter might have rested there had it not been for seven-year-old Pamela Erlichman, who was first paralyzed in her left arm, then the other three limbs. She subsequently died. In December 1955 her tortured father, Pennsylvania pediatrician Fulton Erlichman, demanded an investigation. At a three-hour meeting with Pennsylvania health officials, Langmuir, and EIS officers Brachman, Hall, and Edgar Pattison, Erlichman spoke emotionally of his "sense of moral guilt" for allowing his daughter to receive a vaccine that was not "wholly safe."

In 1963 Langmuir and Nathanson published a comprehensive set of papers on the "Cutter Incident," but Langmuir chose not to publicize the "Wyeth Problem." He never authorized the publication of the

---

*Even as the Wyeth cases flowed in, Langmuir wrote in a May 24, 1955, letter, "It seems to me, however, there is equally abundant evidence that no live virus in an infectious form is present in any of the other vaccines [aside from Cutter]."

detailed papers on the suspect Wyeth lots. By not making the Wyeth Problem public, Langmuir undoubtedly thought that he was protecting the polio vaccine program.*

The Goat-Hair Hazard

In July 1954 Langmuir sent Philip Brachman to New Orleans to investigate a man ill with suspected anthrax. "I knew nothing about anthrax. I ran to the CDC library and checked out a medical textbook to read on the airplane. When I got to the hospital, here was this farmer with a rather large, dark black lesion on his back. It didn't look like the anthrax picture in the textbook. Everyone was looking to me as the anthrax expert." Brachman faked it. "It could be anthrax," he said. "We'll have to wait for the cultures to see."

Caused by the spore-forming *Bacillus anthracis,* anthrax most commonly infects animals. Its spores can lie inert in soil for years and then reactivate to cause disease and death in humans, usually through infected skin lesions. Such cutaneous anthrax is usually not lethal if treated promptly with antibiotics. Inhalational anthrax is the most deadly form of the disease, occurring when the minuscule spores are breathed deep into the lungs.

Brachman's experience in New Orleans was typical of that of many new EIS officers. They frequently had to become instant experts while reading frantically on an airplane or train, and they often ended up knowing more than local public health officers by the time they reached the epidemic location. Brachman would go on to become one of the world's leading authorities on anthrax in all its forms.

As an EIS officer, Brachman was stationed in Philadelphia, assigned for half his time to the Wistar Institute, associated with the University of Pennsylvania. There he conducted a longitudinal study

---

*Initial paralysis in the inoculated limb within two weeks of a polio vaccination was a strong indication that the vaccine contained live virus. By this criterion four of the six original vaccine manufacturers allowed some live virus to slip through the inactivation process, though Cutter was the worst offender. After more stringent safeguards were installed, there were no more such paralyses.

of respiratory disease in fifty local families. The remainder was spent working for the secret biological warfare specialists at Fort Detrick, Maryland. The Fort Detrick scientists had developed an experimental anthrax vaccine, and they wanted Brachman to test it on humans. Although anthrax occurred sporadically on U.S. cattle ranches, it was primarily an occupational disease afflicting people who worked with goat hair imported from Iran, Iraq, Pakistan, and India. The hair was used to make inner linings for suits and ties, as well as carpet pads. The raw material arrived in bales liberally studded with dried skin, blood, and excrement. The underpaid employees who ripped them apart sometimes contracted cutaneous anthrax when spores found a skin abrasion.

Brachman first established baseline data, defining the extent of the anthrax problem in mills, most of which were located in Philadelphia. Then he inoculated volunteer goat-hair workers in three Pennsylvania factories; half received the experimental vaccine, and half a placebo. The vaccine worked, with few side effects.

At the time, it didn't bother Brachman that he was working for Fort Detrick, where army scientists were also brewing vats of anthrax spores for possible biological warfare applications. "I had nothing to do with the offensive end of it," he said, "but I think it's absolutely horrible now."

Brachman so enjoyed his anthrax research work and the preventive nature of public health that he asked if he could stay on at the end of his two-year EIS stint. "It's never been done, but let's do it," Langmuir said. Brachman then supervised a succession of his own EIS officers. In May 1957 he added a fourth goat-hair mill in Manchester, New Hampshire, to his vaccine study. Then he flew to study anthrax in the Middle East and southern Europe, leaving EIS officer Stan Plotkin in charge.

Although nearly half of the employees in the Manchester mill had been vaccinated, none of the vaccinated group worked in the carding or combing departments. On the morning of August 27, 1957, a worker in the combing department felt hot and achy. His doctor diagnosed the illness as flu. Two days later the worker's neck was swollen. Hospitalized at 4:45 A.M., he died at 6:00 A.M. of what turned out to be inhalational anthrax.

Two more fatal inhalational cases from the carding room followed on September 1 and 2. A week later a fourth victim came down with the disease, but he survived. A New Hampshire pathologist called the CDC and was routed to Langmuir, who sent Plotkin to the scene. Langmuir then contacted Brachman, who flew back from Rome.

Perhaps, Brachman and Plotkin surmised, other inhalational cases had occurred in the past and had gone undiagnosed. They examined the autopsy protocols of sixty-eight mill employees who had died since 1947 and found none that could be reasonably attributed to inhalational anthrax.

They also looked at the records for all lots of hair used during the epidemic period. It was believed that the incubation period for inhalational anthrax was from two to six days, with cutaneous anthrax taking a bit longer. Only one lot was used within the ten days previous to the onset of each case — lot 321-B, black goat hair from India. The hair probably "contained organisms possessing unusually high virulence," the EIS officers concluded. From then on, all plant employees were given the experimental anthrax vaccine.

In 1958 Brachman had to complete his two-year medical residency. In order to retain him, Langmuir created the Career Development Program. The CDC would pay for Brachman's two-year residency at a much better salary than the hospital rate if he promised to return and serve at least three more years at the federal disease agency. He set a precedent for many future EIS officers who would make a career at the CDC.

Zombies in Hidalgo County

Doon Yuen was born in a village in southern China in 1922. Renamed Tom Chin on Angel Island in San Francisco Bay by immigration officials, he was twelve when he arrived in Hamilton, Montana, the home of the Rocky Mountain Laboratory, a branch of the National Institutes of Health. The young Chinese boy, an amateur entomologist, was befriended by scientists there. He earned a medical degree and a master's in public health, and served during the Korean War as a public health officer.

When he joined the Epidemic Intelligence Service in 1954, Tom Chin was assigned to the CDC Kansas City field station. On August 24, 1954, a call for help came from Hidalgo County, Texas, where there was a huge polio outbreak with an unusual number of adult victims.

When Chin and fellow EIS officer Calvin Kunin arrived, an elderly woman had just died. Chin joined the pathologist for the autopsy and insisted on getting a piece of brain, which he sent to a CDC lab. The lab isolated the St. Louis encephalitis (SLE) virus, so named because of a 1933 epidemic in St. Louis. The virus was also found in local *C. quinquefasciatus* mosquitoes.

This was not polio, but one of the largest SLE outbreaks ever described. The disease primarily affected the elderly. There were 373 reported cases, with 10 deaths, but Chin estimated that more than 1,000 cases had probably occurred. In Hidalgo County there were many Mexicans who had entered Texas illegally. They probably suffered in silence, unlikely to seek medical services for fear of deportation.

Kunin concentrated on clinical descriptions of the encephalitis cases. He wrote that "the onset was relatively abrupt." Some went into convulsions. Others proceeded to "disorientation, stupor, and coma." Within a few days their faces lost expression. Or, as Kunin put it in an interview, "they were like zombies." Fortunately, when the encephalitic brain swelling subsided, most recovered and returned to normal.

Rabid Bats

In 1951 a Dallas woman died after being bitten by a rabid insectivorous bat, and several more such cases occurred in the next few years. U.S. public health officials were alarmed, since dogs, cats, foxes, and skunks had until then been the primary rabies carriers.

In 1955 Kenneth Quist, a veterinary EIS officer, was assigned to help entomologist George Menzies study the situation. The two ventured into Frio and Bracken caves in central Texas to capture and band some of the millions of Mexican free-tailed bats, trying to track where they migrated in the winter. The noise was eerie, as the bats' chattering echoed from the walls. The animals salivated as they chattered. "It was like walking into a mist," Quist remembered. The men were also concerned with the dermestid beetles that seethed in undulating waves, eating the dead bats that fell to the cave floor. Natural history museums used the beetles to reduce specimens quickly to skeletons. A visitor who tripped and hit his head on a rock could quickly become skeletal, which is why bat cave investigators always worked in pairs.

Quist and Menzies collected dead or dying bats, bringing them back to the lab for tests. They were able to isolate the rabies virus in about 10 percent of them. They were extremely careful as they handled the bats. Without prompt treatment, rabies is always fatal and is a particularly gruesome way to die. After initial symptoms of fever, headache, and a scratchy throat, the muscles stiffen, and painful spasms of the pharyngeal muscles occur whenever swallowing is attempted. A flow of thick saliva pours from the mouth. The victim develops severe hydrophobia, so that even with intense thirst, he refuses to drink. He becomes terrified, enraged, and may attempt to bite others.

The men worked over the Christmas holidays, rushing to band more bats before they migrated for the winter. On January 1, 1956, Menzies returned to his Austin home feeling feverish. He began to salivate the following morning. Two days later he died, leaving a wife and two young children. No one knew how he had contracted rabies, since he had not been bitten. If Quist waited to see whether he developed symptoms, treatment would be too late. He took repeated painful shots of immune horse serum, which made him extremely sick, as well as an experimental rabies vaccine. He did not contract the disease.

In subsequent years, other EIS officers put sentinel animals such as foxes inside double cages in the Texas bat caves to ensure that the bats could not bite them. Many of the animals died of rabies. Apparently breathing the mist of the rabid bats' saliva was enough to catch the disease.

The Hospital Staph

Near the end of June 1955 EIS graduate Rei Ravenholt, epidemiologist at the Seattle-King County Department of Health, got a call about an unusual number of breast abscesses among new mothers who had delivered their babies at Fort Lawton Army Hospital in Seattle.

Ravenholt and Jerry LaVeck, another recent EIS grad doing his residency in Seattle, called mothers who had delivered babies in the hospital that year. A disturbing story emerged. Many infants had developed an oozing sore within two weeks of birth. Then, in another week or two, breast-feeding mothers got breast abscesses. Cultures of the pus revealed *Staphylococcus aureus.*

Staph bacteria are ubiquitous in nature. Virulent strains can form toxins and cause skin abscesses, pneumonia, septicemia, and a wide array of other human ailments. "The baby boom was creating a deluge of births, and hospitals were improvising," Ravenholt said. "There were mobile carts with eight babies like peas in a pod. With harried nurses who forgot to wash their hands, the opportunities for cross-infection were innumerable."

Ravenholt and LaVeck discovered the same pattern in several private hospitals in the area. Some of the babies contracted severe pneumonia and ended up in different hospitals, further spreading the bacterial infection. Twenty-three of them died, and Ravenholt suspected that the actual death toll was higher. This strain of staph had developed resistance to penicillin, though it was still sensitive to newer antibiotics.

Ravenholt called Langmuir and told him that staph was the leading infectious cause of death in Seattle and a major national health issue. "You're full of crap," Langmuir responded. But he subsequently told EIS officer Russ Alexander, "Hit the library and find out about staph." Alexander found a few references to hospital staph outbreaks in other countries, but nothing in the United States.

Alexander and lab scientist Elaine Updyke flew to Seattle, where they confirmed Ravenholt's assessment. Langmuir sent EIS officer Don Wysham to Seattle to continue the studies. In a two-week period in November, Wysham found fifty-two staph infections leading to five deaths.

Over the next few years staph epidemics swept through hospitals in most of the world, leading to a CDC focus on hospital infections in general, and to the founding of infection control units in hospitals throughout the country.

Near the end of October 1958, Saint Joseph's Children's Hospital in Atlanta notified Langmuir of an alarming number of postoperative staphylococcal wound infections. EIS officer André Nahmias, assigned to the case, discovered that there had been twelve infections attributed to one thoracic surgery team since July 17. After eliminating problems with the particular operating room and the possibility of a contaminated piece of machinery, Nahmias focused on a human source. He determined that "Surgeon C" was the only one of the operating room personnel who had attended all twelve of the operations in question.

Cultures from patients were typed as strain 80/81, which was resistant to penicillin, erythromycin, and Aureomycin. This increase in drug resistance was a disturbing development in the three years since Ravenholt had found resistance only to penicillin.* Surgeon C carried the same strain in his nostrils. After a round of antibiotics still effective against the staph, he was clear of the infection and was able to rejoin the thoracic team.

André Nahmias went on to become the self-described "czar of staph" at the CDC, writing extensively about hospital epidemics and drug-resistant strains.

---

*"Many of the major achievements in public health in recent years have been realized through the use of new drugs and chemicals," observed a 1957 CDC report. "Despite their great merit . . . their widespread employment has created a paradoxical situation . . . The growing resistance of certain organisms to antibiotics and drugs . . . constitutes one of the most pressing problems confronting health workers today. Antibiotic resistant strains of *Staphylococcus* are producing infections . . . among hospital patients all over the world."

4

PANDEMIC FLU, PURPLE ENTERITIS ON MARS, POLIO PROBLEMS

IN 1957 A NEW STRAIN of influenza, first identified in late February in China and dubbed "Asian flu," spread rapidly around the world. By mid-June, outbreaks occurred in California, among other places at a conference for high school girls in Davis.

At the end of June a California delegation of 100 people, including a Davis conference attendee, traveled by train to Grinnell, Iowa, for a religious convocation that would be attended by 1,688 participants from forty-three states and nine foreign countries. When most members of the California group arrived in Grinnell with the flu, a state health officer sent a telegram to the CDC. Recent EIS grads Tom Chin and Grace Donovan arrived to monitor the situation.

The airborne disease raced through the overcrowded conference dormitories. The convocation was canceled, but the flu virus was seeded across the country when it went home with the attendees.

Influenza did not spread readily during the summer, but the disease was likely to reach epidemic proportions in the fall when school commenced. Donald A. (called D.A.) Henderson, Langmuir's chief EIS officer* — an ambitious young man destined for great things — asked

---

*The chief EIS officer was basically Langmuir's administrative assistant.

fellow EIS officer Yates Trotter to set up a flu surveillance system, is-suing twice-weekly reports.

School started early, in July, in Tangipahoa Parish, Louisiana, in order to free children to help pick spring strawberries. Students were sneezing by July 31. Within a few days a thousand children were absent from twelve schools. EIS officers Fred Dunn and Don Carey arrived on August 7, by which time ten of the parish's schools had closed.

The Louisiana epidemic peaked around the time of their arrival, with a 65 percent attack rate. By the end of September over 100,000 American cases of Asian flu were reported in thirty-seven states.

This new flu strain was causing the second major influenza pan-demic (a worldwide epidemic) of the twentieth century. The first pandemic of 1918, in combination with pneumonia, killed more than 20 million people worldwide, and half a million in the United States. The 1957 flu was far less lethal. "Clinically, the disease was relatively mild and complications were few," Dunn wrote in his report. But it could be fatal to the elderly or those already ill. CDC statisticians measured "excess mortality" compared to normal flu years. "Mortal-ity rates have been affected strikingly, although they do not approach those of the 1918–1919 pandemic," wrote Dunn.

The type A influenza virus comes in multiple varieties, with two types of protein—hemagglutinin (H) and neuraminidase (N)—wrapped around the RNA that takes over the host cell interior. The H protein locks onto matching receptors on the outside of respira-tory-system cells, allowing the invasion. Then the N ruptures the cell to allow the replicated viruses to spread. The types of influenza virus are named for the particular type of protein they carry: H_1N_1, H_1N_2, H_2N_2, and so on. The flu virus is particularly prone to mutation and adaptation, so that each year's variety represents a slight change, called genetic drift. Every year biologists must guess which flu vac-cine is likely to work. Occasionally, however, there is a shift, a major change of one or both protein types, which can cause a pandemic. Such a shift occurred in 1957 with the Asian flu, H_2N_2.

Drug companies rushed to produce an effective vaccine, which EIS officer Bruce Dull tested on inmates in the Atlanta Penitentiary.

"We rewarded volunteer inmates with cake and ice cream," he recalled. They were also rewarded with fairly effective immunity. Because of its time-consuming manufacture, vaccine was in short supply, so most was reserved for essential occupations.

Appearing on NBC, Langmuir predicted that the epidemic would subside by Christmas. "Santa Claus won't catch Asian flu," he quipped. Indeed, the epidemic reached a peak in early November, affecting one in four Americans, and by December seemed to be ending.

An unexpected second wave began in January 1958, peaking in late February and finally subsiding in April.* Future Epidemic Intelligence Service officers would never let the chief forget his mistaken forecast. Subsequent EIS diplomas featured a line drawing of Langmuir in a little rowboat, with the second wave towering overhead, about to engulf him.

Fighting Smallpox in East Pakistan

In the spring of 1958 Langmuir learned of severe smallpox and cholera epidemics raging in East Pakistan (now Bangladesh). The State Department was lukewarm about his offer to help until it heard that the Soviets were sending in a team of scientists. Then Langmuir got an urgent go-ahead.

Cholera was endemic (always present) in East Pakistan, rather than epidemic. The older Russian scientists chose to deal primarily with this bacterial diarrheal disease, while staying comfortably in Dacca. "The Soviets were heavy old lab people," recalled Jake Brody, one of seven EIS officers on the team. "We were lithe and all under thirty, and we ran all over the country, looking for smallpox, the more urgent problem."

Despite the existence of an effective vaccine, smallpox ravaged poverty-stricken countries. The ancient viral disease, *Variola major* (there is also a less lethal version, *Variola minor*), first causes fever, headache, backache, and vomiting — similar to influenza — followed

---

*Epidemiologists are not sure why flu epidemics generally occur during cooler months. Perhaps it is because people are inside and closer together. No one knows why there is sometimes a second wave of flu.

by a severe rash, beginning on the face and extremities. Smallpox virus also attacks the throat, lungs, heart, liver, and other internal organs. The virus escapes through the broken pustules to infect others. The fatality rate in East Pakistan was 40 percent.

The EIS team found that the smallpox epidemic had begun in 1957, with eleven thousand reported deaths for the year. In the first few months of 1958 fourteen thousand people had died of the disease. The government of Pakistan had issued an urgent international appeal for vaccine in April, resulting in a plentiful supply, primarily from the Soviet Union and the United States.

There were already Pakistani vaccination teams in each of the seventeen states of the country, but no one knew how many people were actually being immunized or what the pattern of smallpox spread was. The local health officers needed surveillance and assessment help in order to deploy their forces intelligently. Each EIS officer, teamed with a Pakistani medical student or doctor who would serve as interpreter and assistant, went into the field, where they conducted surveys, collected data, and helped with vaccinations.

One of the EIS officers deployed to East Pakistan, Malcolm Page, wrote to his future wife: "It is so difficult to travel through the villages and find the people. They are always out in the fields or somewhere. Whenever we come in sight, the women run into hiding and just won't come out—maybe if we're lucky they will stick their arms out the door but many won't even do that without their husband's permission, and of course you can't find their husbands. The children run into the jungle, climb trees etc. . . . In addition they have absolutely no refrigeration and much of the vaccine being used is dead and of no value. Smallpox seems to be on the decline in most areas but there remains about an overall 35 percent of the people completely unvaccinated."

A coup on June 20 toppled the East Pakistan government, and the new regime decided to use Pakistani natives rather than American epidemiologists to fight smallpox. In their final report, the EIS officers noted, "Our findings must be regarded as tentative because . . . our period of observation has been brief, [and] because the data we have collected is derived from very small samples." Nonetheless, their

seventeen-page report noted that people vaccinated long ago sometimes got milder cases of smallpox, which made them "even more effective spreader[s] of infection." The officers traced smallpox along
railroad lines, transmitted by rail workers and their families. There
was an excess of deaths in unvaccinated children younger than nine.
The report recommended continued surveillance, weekly reporting,
and refrigerated wet vaccine.

The EIS had uncovered much important information on the
spread of the disease in a relatively short period. Yet their recommendation to keep the wet vaccine cold didn't help much, since, as Page
had noted, East Pakistan had almost no refrigeration.

At the end of the training course in July 1958, EIS officers put
on a satirical skit they called "Purple Enteritis on Mars," a send-up
of the East Pakistan venture. Full of in-jokes, innuendo, and self-
mockery, the skit would become a tradition during the annual April
conference.

Polio in the Ghettos

After the Cutter Incident of 1955, the inactivated Salk polio vaccine
(IPV) had been safely made, and it steadily reduced the polio level in
the United States and elsewhere with an estimated 90 percent effec-
tiveness. But where polio did strike, the types of victims changed substantially. Before the vaccine, epidemic polio had afflicted everyone,
but particularly the white middle and upper classes. In contrast, the
1956 epidemic in Chicago was concentrated in the black ghetto, where
the children were not getting vaccinated. The American Medical Association had fought free immunization as "socialized medicine."

Nonetheless, the total number of polio cases in the United States
fell steadily in the first few years in which the Salk vaccine was used.
There were 38,476 cases in 1954, before the vaccine, then 28,985 in
1955, 15,140 in 1956, and only 5,485 in 1957.

But in 1958 there was a slight rise to 5,787 cases. The most severe
epidemic occurred in the poor sections of Detroit, with more than
half of the cases among unvaccinated children under five. Another severe polio epidemic occurred on the Blackfoot Indian reservation in

Montana among unvaccinated young children. The year 1959 turned out to be significantly worse than the previous year, with a total of 8,425 polio cases nationally.

Trials in Léopoldville

Criticism of the Salk vaccine mounted, particularly when a few children who *were* properly inoculated still got polio. Some of these cases were in fact not polio but aseptic meningitis or newly discovered echoviruses, the so-called orphans that gradually were identified with diseases.* Nonetheless, interest mounted in the oral polio vaccine (OPV), with live attenuated (weakened) virus, which caused the immune system to react by creating antibodies.

OPV had several advantages over the Salk vaccine. It could be taken by mouth rather than injection. It was cheaper to make. It reproduced quickly in the intestines, giving gut immunity. When excreted, it sometimes spread by the fecal-oral route and thereby could immunize other family members and contacts.

Three competitors vied with one another in the creation of a vaccine, developing slightly different strains and processes: Herald Cox of Lederle Labs, Hilary Koprowski of the Wistar Institute, and Albert Sabin of the University of Cincinnati. EIS officers Stan Plotkin and Joe Pagano, based at the Wistar Institute, worked with Koprowski on his oral polio vaccine studies.

Langmuir and Koprowski clashed both personally and professionally. The EIS chief refused to allow Plotkin, who went on to become one of the giants in the vaccine field, to present a paper on his polio vaccine work, saying that he was too young and inexperienced.

Langmuir, meanwhile, had become increasingly disturbed by evidence that some of the live polio vaccine — particularly Type 3 — apparently reverted to virulence in monkeys and in people, thus causing rather than preventing polio. He visited the Wistar Institute, meeting with Koprowski, Plotkin, Pagano, and others in March 1959. "The issues were discussed with considerable heat," Langmuir reported. He

---

*Echo stands for enteric cytopathogenic human orphan.

refused to allow Plotkin to conduct research as an official EIS officer in a large field trial of seventy-five thousand children in the Belgian Congo, but he did permit him to take sixty days' leave with the understanding that he was working only for Koprowski.

Plotkin ended up going to the Congo, where he supervised ill-planned trials in Léopoldville (now Kinshasa) in April and May of 1959. "There was a problem with controls. It was a mess," he recalled. "At least I was thorough and systematic, which enabled us to extract some useful data. I discovered that the efficacy of vaccine in a tropical setting is not very high. Oral polio vaccine doesn't work very well there because there are so many other competing intestinal infections in developing countries."

Plotkin was nearly killed by angry villagers who thought that the scientist's taking of blood from femoral veins in the children's thighs (for antibody testing) was actually a neutering operation. "The Belgians had arranged the trials and were only using African natives, not white children, so this caused suspicion. I had to be rescued by the army."*

Nightmare in Nebraska

Albert Sabin eventually prevailed over Koprowski and Cox. In 1959 he gave his vaccine to Soviet scientists, who inoculated 10 million Russian children and claimed complete success with it. As pressure mounted in the United States to authorize use of the Sabin vaccine, Surgeon General Leroy Burney approved it for trial manufacture in August 1960.

Ironically, after the frightening 1959 rise in polio, Salk vaccinations kept whittling away at the national statistics. By 1961, when its reputation was at its lowest, the Salk vaccine had nearly succeeded in eliminating polio from the United States, with under a thousand paralytic cases.

---

*Many years later, in his book *The River,* Edward Hooper charged that Plotkin had inadvertently started the AIDS epidemic through the Congo polio injections — a charge that Plotkin and others have convincingly rebutted.

But the political winds all blew toward the new Sabin vaccine. Late in 1961 the government authorized the use of Sabin's Type 1 strain, followed in 1962 by Types 2 and 3. Congress allocated $1 million to purchase Sabin vaccine for a free stockpile to be administered by the CDC, then passed the Vaccination Assistance Act of 1962, authorizing continued support.

The Type 3 vaccine was licensed on March 27, 1962, and in April mass vaccination programs commenced in several states. On May 22 an Oregon Type 3 case was reported in which a vaccinee was paralyzed within thirty days of taking the oral dose. There were four more such Oregon cases as well as suspicious reports from Arizona and Ohio in the next few months. On July 25 EIS officer Jim Bryan flew to Oregon to investigate.

On September 8 Surgeon General Luther Terry was asked to speak in Omaha, Nebraska, where he learned from local health officials that several paralytic cases had occurred after a statewide Type 3 Sabin campaign. The Nebraska Department of Health had not reported any of them to the CDC. Three EIS officers and a recent EIS grad investigated. They found and visited ten Nebraska cases that were clearly vaccine associated, occurring within thirty days of ingestion of Type 3. There was no wild polio in the state during this period, and the virus from the victims' stools proved to be "tame," similar to that in the vaccine. Six of the ten cases were adults. The association rate was determined to be 10.7 cases per million doses — about twenty times higher than the average rate of OPV-related polio in the rest of the country.

Why did the vaccine cause so many cases in Oregon and Nebraska? They were relatively rural, isolated states in which many people, including adults, were susceptible to polio, having never encountered the virus as infants. Adults who contract polio are prone to even worse paralysis than children.

On October 2 the Ad Hoc Committee on Oral Vaccine met in a contentious session, with Sabin vigorously defending the vaccine. "Embarrassed to be on Committee," Langmuir scribbled in his notes. In the end, the committee issued a wishy-washy recommendation that Type 3 be used cautiously in adults over thirty.

The following month Langmuir wrote to a British colleague: "The present situation with us is hopelessly snarled in violent views on both sides." Sabin refused to admit that his vaccine had caused polio anywhere, at any time. "We have just completed a very intensive search for cases in Nebraska," Langmuir continued. "There are eight pretty convincing cases* with residual paralysis that fell in a logical incubation period after Type 3 vaccine. Half of these are in children, which casts doubt on the validity of our present position, excluding only adults from use of Type 3."

Despite his severe misgivings, in public Langmuir continued to support the mass oral polio vaccine program and the official statement that in certain cases there was a "very small risk" associated with the vaccine. He never allowed the detailed EIS paper on the Nebraska cases to be published, afraid it might harm the vaccine program and lead to lawsuits. Instead, the Nebraska data were buried in a 1964 paper covering all vaccine-associated polio cases, which indicated a national average of 0.40 paralytic cases per million doses of Type 3 vaccine.

Polio in Paradise

In spite of the lingering questions about Type 3, OPV quickly became the standard vaccine in the United States and most of the world. Oral vaccine is the most suitable for use in severe epidemic conditions, because of its ease of administration, rapid efficacy, and fecal-oral spread to contacts. It is also inexpensive.

Jim Bryan demonstrated the benefits of OPV in a 1963 outbreak in the Marshall Islands, at that time part of the remote U.S. Trust Territory in the Pacific Ocean. The major island of Kwajalein Atoll was reserved for three thousand Americans and their families. Of the twenty-five hundred natives crowded onto the tiny nearby island of Ebeye, some four hundred Marshallese commuted by water taxi each

---

*At Sabin's urging, the committee eliminated two of the ten cases. During his presentation at the April 1963 EIS conference, EIS officer Bob Eelkema commented, "Well, those two didn't pick up their mats and walk because of that decision."

day to work on Kwajalein as laborers and domestics for American families. The domestics frequently brought their children with them.

On January 7, 1963, a nine-year-old American girl on Kwajalein was diagnosed with bulbar polio and was evacuated to Hawaii for an iron lung. Type 1 poliovirus was isolated from her stool. A three-year-old Marshallese boy developed leg paralysis on January 12. Over the next few days, six more children on Ebeye came down with paralytic polio. Travel was quarantined between the two islands on January 16. The native children were in particular danger, never having been exposed to polio.

A naval medical team arrived from Hawaii with Type 1 oral vaccine on January 19, by which time there were twenty-five paralytic cases on Ebeye and a second American case on Kwajalein. The entire population of both islands was fed vaccine, and the navy team flew back to Pearl Harbor.

On January 29 a radio message from a distant atoll, Rongelap, reported that 16 of the 208 people on the island were paralyzed. Trading ships were spreading polio. The CDC in Atlanta got an urgent summons to vaccinate the entire island chain. EIS officers Jim Bryan and Ron Roberto, along with another CDC veteran, arrived with the vaccine on February 14.

Bryan flew with a navy epidemiologist to Majuro, the capital of the Marshalls, where the epidemic was still raging. "We took six weeks to immunize the islands, working in concentric circles around the epidemic. These guys would fly me in to an atoll on an amphibious plane. They couldn't get too close because of the coral reefs, so they would blow up a one-man raft for my interpreter, who carried a briefcase and the vaccine, and I would swim in," Bryan said. "We could hit two or three atolls a day that way."

Less than half of the Marshall Island population was exposed, and polio never reached the other island groups. Despite the severity of the epidemic, with an attack rate of twenty per thousand persons exposed (many times higher than any U.S. experience, and not equaled since anywhere in the world), the oral vaccine prevented a tragedy of far greater magnitude.

5

NEW DISCOVERIES AND MYSTERIES
IN THE EARLY SIXTIES

ON FEBRUARY 3, 1961, a naval commander called the CDC about infectious hepatitis in the civilian population of Pascagoula, Mississippi, where nuclear submarines were being built. A sub was about to take a long cruise, and the commander was concerned about a possible hepatitis outbreak onboard.

Arriving at Pascagoula, EIS officer Jim Mason discovered an unusual pattern. "Normally, hepatitis A cases involved children and often their parents as secondary victims. In this case, there were almost no childhood cases. And most of the adult cases were men."

Mason found that the only connection between the victims was that all had eaten raw oysters within six weeks of contracting the disease. From a random phone survey in Pascagoula, Mason learned that about 30 percent of those he called — the "controls" — had eaten raw oysters versus 100 percent of the victims.*

It's clear that raw oysters are involved, thought Mason, *but how did the controls who ate them avoid hepatitis?*

The answer lay at the mouth of the river, where a sign warned that

---

*This is an early example of a case-control approach rather than a cohort study of an entire population, as in a church supper. In a widespread epidemic, it is easier to choose random controls from the community.

it was illegal to harvest oysters in that area. Because of the shipyard, the Pascagoula community had grown too quickly and had overtaxed its sewage system. "Most of the sewage flowed directly into the Pascagoula River," Mason recalled.

As rich organic material flowed by the river mouth, filter-feeding oysters grew exceptionally fat and juicy, accumulating a supply of hepatitis virus from the fecal matter. Three brothers couldn't resist the illegal oysters. They tonged them at night and sold them in Pascagoula and to an oyster bar in Mobile, Alabama.

A flurry of hepatitis cases in Mobile led Mason to the oyster bar. Often, in an epidemic, such outliers — cases remote from the primarily affected community — can serve to point to the cause. "I found that the bar bought gunnysacks of oysters from the brothers," he said. The controls had eaten raw oysters caught in cleaner waters. For the first time in the United States, seafood was recognized as a source of hepatitis. Ultimately, Mason found eighty cases in five states due to the Pascagoula brothers, who were prevented from tonging more contaminated oysters.

Upon his return to Atlanta, Mason joined EIS officer Bill Elsea as a member of the Hepatitis Surveillance Unit. Within two months, their unit learned of dozens of adult hepatitis cases in Newark, New Jersey, where businessmen seemed to be the primary victims. Elsea, sent to investigate, asked them, among other questions, whether they had eaten raw oysters, but they had not. "So I decided to ask if they had ingested clams recently. I found that 60 percent of them had." The cherrystone clams came from polluted Raritan Bay, New Jersey. The outbreak grew to more than five hundred cases in New Jersey and New York City.

The CDC had no regulatory power, however, and industry lobbyists kept the clams on the market. D.A. Henderson, head of the Surveillance Unit, told a reporter that "eating raw shellfish from Raritan Bay is playing Russian Roulette on the half shell." Thus EIS officers and their supervisors sometimes had to rely on publicity to protect the public's health.

Salad Whiz

In December 1961 Don Millar, Langmuir's chief EIS officer, went to Jacksonville, Florida, to Cecil Field Naval Air Station, which supported aircraft carrier pilots. An epidemic of infectious hepatitis, affecting only officers, was under way. "They were very concerned that someone in the prodromal [early] phase would be a bit fatigued and fly into the rear end of a carrier," Millar recalled.

He and fellow EIS officer Paul Joseph spent two weeks investigating the outbreak. The twenty-two victims had all eaten at the bachelor officers quarters (BOQ) mess hall, also frequented by married officers visiting from aircraft carrier units. The navy kept detailed records of menus and who ate at the BOQ on particular dates. All of the victims had been there on October 26 or 27. But because more than a month had elapsed since then, the victims couldn't remember precisely what they ate.

Millar and Joseph came up with a food-preference questionnaire focused on foods they didn't eat. None of the twenty-one cases who responded said they never ate potato salad or ice cream — meaning that *all* of the cases sometimes ate those two items. Of the 116 control respondents who ate at the BOQ but didn't get sick, 29 percent said they never ate potato salad, but only 5 percent never ate ice cream. "So we figured potato salad was the likely culprit," Millar said.

When the EIS officers tested the food handlers, only JL, an enlisted man, carried the hepatitis virus. "He had been arrested in Alabama for pissing on a police officer's boots when stopped for drunk driving," Millar said. "His wife told us that on occasion, he deliberately peed on his bed. So we decided that he had probably urinated into the dressing used on the potato salad."*

Contaminated Blood

In the fall of 1962 EIS officer George Grady interviewed hepatitis patients in a dozen Boston-area hospitals. He spoke to those with

---

*The hepatitis virus is usually carried in excrement, but it can also travel in urine.

infectious hepatitis (now called hepatitis A, with a shorter incubation period) and serum hepatitis (hepatitis B, with a longer incubation). One-fifth of the patients had recently eaten raw clams or poorly
cooked shellfish, but the majority had been infected with hepatitis B
in the hospital by transfusion with contaminated blood.

The year before, a record seventy-two thousand cases of hepatitis
were reported throughout the United States. Most deaths were probably due to hepatitis B. "The seriousness of serum hepatitis resulting
from faulty sterilization techniques was vividly shown [in 1960] in
an outbreak involving over forty cases and fifteen deaths in one physician's practice," observed Langmuir. A New Jersey osteopath-psy-
chiatrist had treated 250 depressed outpatients with drugs, including
tranquilizers, vitamins, and "energizers." The doctor used the same
tubing for all intravenous barbiturates, allowing cross-contamination.
He was inadvertently injecting patients with toxic doses of hepatitis B
virus, as EIS officers Ted Eickhoff and Ron Altman documented.

EIS officers thus confirmed that in addition to raw shellfish and
disgruntled kitchen staff, intravenous injections could be the source
of hepatitis epidemics. Ironically, hospitals posed the biggest threat.

Salmonella Odyssey

In the fall of 1961, eleven of the eighty-five people in tiny Come By
Chance, Newfoundland, were afflicted by one of the most common
of all food-poisoning bacteria, one of the two thousand or so species of *Salmonella*. This one, however, was unusual in North America — *Salmonella thompson*. The victims had all eaten angel food cake
made from a Betty Crocker mix prepared in the United States.

As Canadian epidemiologists had already traced the cases to the
cake mix, EIS officer Eli Friedman was dispatched to Come By Chance
to find out what had contaminated the mix. "When I read the box, it
said, 'Do not overcook,' so that the cake would remain moist. Among
the ingredients were powdered eggs, a natural for *Salmonella*."

Friedman then flew to Hammond, Indiana, to visit the H & M
Hatchery, which had supplied the eggs. Chicken feces there tested
positive for *Salmonella thompson*. Friedman found out that the chick-

ens were fed fishmeal. This led him to Wildwood, New Jersey, where a huge fish plant processed menhaden. "At the plant, I found that the fish were contaminated with S. thompson," he said. Along with EIS alum Kenneth Quist,* Friedman went out on one of the fishing boats. He inserted cotton swabs into the newly caught fishes' cloacae (anuses), put the swabs in sealed culture tubes, and shipped them back to the CDC labs. They reported no trace of Salmonella, so the source must have been in the fishmeal plant.

Friedman and Quist diagnosed that no matter the source of the contamination, the fishmeal was not being heated sufficiently to kill the bacteria. They suggested changes in the production system.

Friedman ultimately concluded that sewer rats in the plant may have been a source of the Salmonella. "Happily, Dr. Brachman [the head of the Salmonella Surveillance Unit] did not ask me to go and find out how the rats had been contaminated," he quipped.

In April 1963 Philip Brachman got phone calls from New York City and Philadelphia about Salmonella derby cases, all from large general hospitals in each city. By July, forty hospitals in ten states had reported a total of 775 cases. Sixteen people with salmonellosis died, most of them elderly patients.

While other EIS officers investigated a cluster of cases in New York City, Friedman and Jim Bryan went to Philadelphia. They were interested primarily in the initial cases. No patients had been interchanged between all the hospitals. Many had initially entered the hospital for other gastrointestinal diseases, so perhaps some common procedure or piece of equipment was the culprit. But nothing came of that hypothesis.

Because of their surgery, most of the patients had been placed on highly restricted diets, and the only food item consumed by all the S. derby victims was raw or undercooked eggs as part of their liquid nutrients. Friedman and Bryan discovered that about half of the hospitals' patients received raw eggs on any given day, but that 90 percent of the victims had consumed them within forty-eight hours of becoming ill.

---

*See pages 29–30, where Quist survived the bat caves and rabies scare.

The epidemiologists traced the eggs back through large distributors, to wholesalers, then regional processors, and eventually to twelve thousand individual poultry farms. A handful of Pennsylvania farms supplied all of the affected hospitals. *Salmonella derby* was recovered from slurries of cracked eggs from the farms.

Salmonella cases kept piling up, mostly from chickens or their eggs — sometimes in eggnog, or frozen eggs used to make lemon meringue pies, or dried egg products, or undercooked chicken. DEATH LURKS IN THE KITCHEN, a *Time* magazine headline warned in September 1964. The following month Brachman sent recommendations to state health departments, and the FDA subsequently passed regulations requiring that eggs be inspected (and diverted for pasteurization if cracked), then graded and sanitized on the outside.

Searching for the Most Lethal Plague

In July 1964 EIS officers Jim Gale and Palmer Beasley, along with a CDC plague specialist, flew to La Paz, Bolivia. Fort Detrick biological warfare specialists wanted a live sample from a lethal bubonic plague outbreak to add to their bank of virulent organisms. From La Paz, the three Americans flew to eastern Bolivia, then took a truck to the eastern slope of the Andes, where they mounted pack animals for the two-day trip up to the remote village of Descargadero.

Where thirty-two Quechua Indians had once lived, there had been thirteen cases of plague with eight deaths. All but three of the surviving inhabitants had fled. Plague was relatively rare by 1964 and, if diagnosed promptly, could be countered with antibiotics. In Descargadero, somehow a rat flea carrying *Yersinia pestis,* the plague bacillus, had arrived and infected an eighteen-year-old boy. It appeared that the bacteria then were spread by fleas on humans, an unusual transmission route.

One of the remaining villagers showed the American researchers the grave of the fifth victim, who had died twenty-one days before. "We dug her up," Gale recalled. The body was buried without coffin or shroud. Wearing a pair of gloves, Gale cut off the little finger of the right hand. "The plague organism survives in bone marrow better than anywhere else," he explained. "I wasn't that worried. In the remote possibility I caught anything, tetracycline would knock it out. Also, young EIS officers have a certain immortality complex."

Two days later, back in civilization, they mixed the bone marrow material with saline solution, then injected a live guinea pig, which contracted plague. The Americans sacrificed the animal, then removed the spleen where the plague bacilli were concentrated, iced it, and brought it back to Fort Detrick. The EIS officers had arrived too late to help prevent more deaths, harvested the bacterium for military purposes, and showed little respect for the dead. "I think back and am surprised I went along with it," Gale said. "But supposedly the bacterium was meant for defensive purposes, to create a vaccine against it."

The following year Gale investigated an apparent outbreak of encephalitis among Mayans in Quetzaltenango, Guatemala. There he found patients in a comalike state. Many had died a slow, agonizing death. "I learned that none of the victims had fever, and there were no mosquitoes at that high altitude. So I began to think about a toxic product." He found out that the previous winter, there had been a poor harvest, so rather than starve, they had eaten wheat seed that had been treated with pink methylmercury fungicide. His discovery prevented further deaths.

The First Chronic Disease Investigation

Late in 1960 and early in 1961 three students at St. John Brebeuf, a parochial elementary school in Niles, Illinois, died from acute leukemia. Two other students, still alive, were also suffering from leukemia. The school's principal called a cancer research hospital in Chicago, which contacted the CDC. EIS officer Clark Heath, twenty-eight, arrived on March 27, 1961, to investigate.

Heath discovered three more Niles cases. A three-year-old boy, whose two older siblings attended St. John Brebeuf, had died of leukemia in 1957. A six-year-old girl, whose older brother also attended the school, had recently died of the disease. So had a ten-year-old

Lutheran girl whose best friend was one of the deceased Catholic school students.

Heath determined that the incidence of leukemia in Niles (21.3 cases per 100,000) was nearly five times the rate in the rest of Cook County (4.6 cases per 100,000) over the same time period. The only known etiology for the disease was radiation, but a Geiger counter failed to show unusual levels of radiation in the elementary school or the homes of deceased students, and Heath didn't find any carcinogenic household chemicals or pesticides.

There had also been an unusual number of cases of rheumatic fever (caused by streptococcus bacteria) among students in recent years, and when Heath plotted the cases, they fell roughly at the same time as leukemia onsets. Did strep somehow trigger leukemia in susceptible children? In addition, during the same period, seven Niles babies died soon after birth of congenital heart defects. Did the same thing that caused leukemia also contribute to birth defects?

Niles was a new postwar suburb. The population, over twenty thousand when the EIS officer arrived, had grown tenfold since 1950. In his comprehensive article, published in 1963, Heath called it a "microepidemic" and hypothesized that children thrown together in new communities might develop leukemia because of exposure to an infectious agent to which they had no immunity.

Despite extensive surveys and blood tests, there was never any proof that the cluster was more than a chance event — a conclusion that would become all too familiar to EIS officers in the next decade of leukemia sleuthing. Heath would train and supervise most of those officers.

Cholera in the Philippines

In 1961 a deadly El Tor strain of cholera began to afflict people in Indonesia. Untreated cholera can kill through dehydration in less than twenty-four hours. The bacterium spread quickly throughout Southeast Asia, into the Philippines and Thailand, to Taiwan, then west into Iran, Turkey, and Africa. It was the beginning of the seventh cholera pandemic of modern times.

In 1962 a CDC team, including EIS officers Paul Joseph, Wiley Henry Mosley, and a CDC lab scientist, went to Negros Occidental, the western side of an island in the central Philippines, where they established headquarters in an empty school building converted to an emergency hospital in Bacolod City. The cholera victims were hooked to IV lines with salt water and electrolytes to replace the diarrheal stream that poured out of them through holes in the cots into buckets below.

The first distinct outbreak of cholera had occurred from November 1961 through January 1962. Mosley and Joseph knew that cholera bacteria were usually spread in polluted water. The public water supply in Bacolod City did not contain the cholera *Vibrio,* however.

Through retrospective interviews with victims and surviving family members, they found that the epidemic pattern indicated a common-source outbreak that began suddenly in November 1961, built to a peak in December, and then gradually declined. The victims were concentrated primarily on the coast, but cases also appeared simultaneously and apparently at random in the island's interior. The EIS officers learned that a popular Filipino delicacy, tiny shrimp called *hipon,* was often eaten raw. The *hipon* season began in late September and extended through January, matching the epidemic's timing. "Everyone we could locate from the first epidemic wave had direct contact with raw shrimp," Mosley recalled.

The EIS officers located the probable index case,* a thirty-four-year-old photographer who lived on the seacoast in a house on stilts, where his toilet emptied directly into the ocean. On November 4, at 11 P.M., he suffered the onset of severe diarrhea. By 1 A.M., unable to walk, he was taken to the hospital. No one knew how he contracted cholera, but as the final report noted, "because of the pattern of *hipon* fishing, the *hipon* distributed in the Bacolod area would be caught literally in his backyard." Once again, raw shellfish from polluted water had led to a devastating epidemic.

---

*An index case is the first recognized victim in an epidemic.

A Parent's Worst Nightmare

For a week an eight-year-old girl in North Carolina suffered from intermittent upper respiratory symptoms. Just as she seemed to be getting better, she became lethargic, then vomited. She later became restless, irritable, and confused. Rushed to an emergency room, she drowsed, went into convulsions, fell into a coma, and died the following day.

This pattern recurred in sixteen North Carolina children between January 2 and April 16, 1962. All but one were white children. Ten were girls. Most were elementary school age. The cases were scattered in rural areas around the state. Autopsies revealed severely swollen brains and fatty livers. George Johnson, an EIS officer based in North Carolina, noted that the peak of the cases coincided with the top of the 1962 influenza B epidemic curve. Had the flu somehow precipitated this awful syndrome?

The following year three Australian physicians published an article describing the same phenomenon. The lead author, R. Douglas Reye, provided the name by which it is now known, Reye's syndrome.* Though it had acquired a name, however, it remained an unsolved mystery for years to come, even as subsequent EIS officers struggled to identify its cause.

Big Chief Langmuir

During the 1960s Alexander Langmuir was in his prime as the chief of the Epidemiology Branch of the CDC. Among his EIS officers, whom he called his "boys," he inspired awe, fear, admiration, respect, and sometimes loathing. Langmuir valued loyalty, and that meant personal fealty to him and the CDC. In 1961, when Russ Alexander told him he was taking a job at the University of Washington, Langmuir nastily responded, "You'll never make it in academia."

"Working closely with Alex was a treat and a challenge," Alexander recalled. "He didn't really care about how much work something took, he just wanted it done. And he relished an argument. He just said

---

*Later called just Reye syndrome or Reye-Johnson syndrome.

what he thought and didn't care about the consequences." As another EIS veteran observed, "Alex was often wrong but never in doubt."

Langmuir could also be incredibly supportive of his EIS officers, whom he always backed in public. He gave savvy advice on how to work with state and local health departments. "When you go on an outbreak, always look for the mid-level person who has worked in a department a long time and knows how everything works, how to get things done in a hurry," he would tell EIS officers.

Upon his arrival at the CDC, one of the first things he did was to call a meeting of the state public health officers, who were often hostile to the feds, and ask them to come up with a list of diseases that should be regularly reported, along with the name of one person to contact for information about that state's cases. That person became known as the state epidemiologist. The resulting organization, the Conference of State and Territorial Epidemiologists (CSTE), has worked closely with the CDC ever since.*

During the July training course for new officers, Langmuir would have EIS officers call in from the field during an outbreak so that he and the trainees could ask them questions on a speakerphone. It was exciting, in the moment, and dramatic, with Langmuir always at center stage.

He insisted on multiple drafts of EIS officers' reports and papers. As a result of this painful exercise, EIS officers learned to write clear, concise, comprehensible reports, many of which appeared in the *Morbidity and Mortality Weekly Report* (*MMWR*), originally a dry statistical publication about reportable U.S. illnesses and deaths. Langmuir managed to appropriate the weekly from the National Office of Vital Statistics on January 1, 1961. Under his eagle eye, the *MMWR* became a readable source of current information on breaking epidemics.

Langmuir's demanding approach didn't suit everyone, but it inspired many. "Alex made me feel like I could do anything, that given a problem, somehow I could solve it," recalled EIS alum John Boring. "I think *confidence* was one of Alex's great gifts to us," added EIS veteran

---

*CSTE is now called the Council of State and Territorial Epidemiologists.

Andy Vernon. "He assured us that these were soluble problems, if we just approached them in the right way."

For Langmuir, the right way was the pragmatic way—get out there, get the basic facts, and act on them. "Alex detested complicated statistical arguments," said Boring. "If you did it right, we would all see it, it would be glaringly obvious."

"He was never frightening to me," EIS alum Stan Foster recalled. "He had a real interest in people and their families. He really cared about people." Still, the EIS usually came first. "I was out in the field so often," recalled Russ Alexander, "that my wife had to complain to Alex that I seemed to be gone whenever she was ovulating, and it was blocking our attempts to start a family. He let me stay home until she conceived, and then I was off again."

Langmuir's own family life was troubled. In 1940 he married Sally Harper, who bore five children in thirteen years: Anne, Paul, Susan, Lynn, and Jane. Langmuir was a workaholic who traveled frequently. When he was home, he preferred rapid-fire questions to more relaxed dinner-table conversation.[*]

In 1960 six-year-old Jane fell from the balcony of their home, surviving a blow to her head. She died three years later of hydrocephalus from scar tissue buildup. "When Jane died, I went to the Langmuirs' home after the funeral," recalled former secretary Martha Waits Brocato. "It was the only time I saw Alex Langmuir totally broken. But when he came back to work, he didn't talk about it." Indeed, many EIS officers didn't even know that Langmuir had offspring.

His surviving children sometimes spoke bitterly about their father.[†] "It took a real toll on his family for him to be so incredibly attuned to his officers," Susan Langmuir observed. "All my life, I've met EIS graduates who say, 'Oh, wow, your father changed my life, he was the most powerful influence on me, the reason I'm in public health. And he was the best teacher I ever had, staying up with me until 2 A.M.

---

[*] During one dinner, Langmuir offered a dollar to anyone who could tell him where the islets of Langerhans were. Paul rushed to the atlas but couldn't find it. His father eventually told him that they were part of the pancreas.

[†] Anne Langmuir died in 2004.

to hammer out an article.' And I felt like saying to them, 'Yeah, but he was lousy at helping me with long division.'"

She recalled a few tender, special moments. "Once a month, he'd make us pancakes that spelled our names, and sometimes we'd sing 'McNamara's Band' while Mom played the piano." On some weekends he took them on rural back-road explorations. "We'd get to an intersection, and Dad would ask us kids, 'Right, left, straight, or backwards?'"

Lynn Langmuir, whose birth concided with the EIS's founding in July 1951, said, "He was a pompous ass, and really difficult. I was totally not important to him; it was really painful. He loved me, but I don't think he liked me that much." Paul Langmuir, who talked to his father more about his career and the EIS, wasn't so negative. "I didn't see Dad that much, but I would say he was a great father." Still, Paul never felt that he measured up to expectations. "I was bright but dyslexic. I didn't qualify."

Susan Langmuir felt that her father was a sexist. "We [the daughters] were supposed to be magnolia blossoms. Girls were just not on Dad's radar screen." At the same time, Langmuir was a political and social liberal. He believed strongly in a woman's right to appropriate birth control or an abortion. He was an advocate for all forms of public health. It was largely due to Alexander Langmuir's curiosity and encouragement that the EIS and CDC moved into many new areas, such as cancer clusters research and family planning.

"Although he is controversial at times, I think there are few who would question the tremendous contributions he has made," wrote D.A. Henderson of Langmuir in 1963.

6

THE DIASPORA

URGENT. GET SMALLPOX SPECIMENS FOR LAB. EIS officer Don Millar got the cable from D.A. Henderson the day before he was to fly home from Indonesia in late November 1962. He had joined a World Health Organization (WHO) mission to assess that country's Malaria Eradication Program, leaving his wife and two children back in Atlanta. The WHO program to rid the world of malaria by spraying DDT on indoor walls was an ambitious undertaking, but Millar had found that anopheles mosquitoes remained untouched in the seventeen thousand smaller Indonesian islands. Henderson considered smallpox a more likely target for eradication since its virus afflicted only humans, with no other reservoir or vector such as mosquitoes to worry about. Hence his special interest in specimens.

Millar quickly found a hospital with two dozen smallpox patients in different stages of the disease. "I made slides of the fluid and put some scabs in test tubes, then carefully packed them," he said. Somehow he got through U.S. Customs. "I was concerned because I had worn my tie in the smallpox hospital and might have draped it over the patients while I was getting specimens. I had an unvaccinated infant daughter." Taking no chances, he flushed the tie down a toilet at New York's Idlewild Airport.

When he reported to work, Millar learned that he would be Henderson's deputy, specializing in viral diseases such as smallpox and measles. He stayed in that CDC position when he graduated from the EIS.

In July 1963 the Jamaican minister of health had asked the CDC for help in vaccinating the children of Kingston against diphtheria, a growing problem in the crowded urban setting. Langmuir grabbed the opportunity to send his "boys" to test vaccines and technologies, so Millar led a team of EIS officers and other CDC personnel to conduct a mass vaccination campaign that tested a combined diphtheria-pertussis-tetanus shot and the new measles vaccine.

The EIS officers brought fourteen electrically powered jet injector guns — invented by the U.S. military — to administer the shots by pressure without needles, along with a technician to maintain the guns and a generator for rural areas where electricity was not available. With the help of local health personnel and university students, the team immunized nearly 100,000 children, attracting their parents through radio, newspaper, and sound trucks, and offering entertainment, pep rallies, and raffle prizes. Midcampaign, a popular Jamaican folk singer recorded the "Immunization Calypso."

The mass immunization clearly reduced diphtheria transmission, with only eleven new Jamaican cases diagnosed by the following May. It was less effective in halting tetanus, which killed half of its victims on the tropical island. Most of those deaths occurred in newborns delivered by local midwives, who applied contaminated mixtures of herbs and secret ingredients to the umbilical stump.

After the main immunization effort, EIS officer Ron Roberto tested a new slanted nozzle for the jet guns, intended to deliver small-pox vaccine intradermally, just under the skin. The U.S. Army, which had commissioned the modified injector, paid the CDC to test it in various venues.* The gun worked. It offered a fast, efficient alternative to the multiple needlestick method into a drop of vaccine on the arm.

---

*The army was interested in a quick, easy way to vaccinate new recruits. The jet injector gun was also used on volunteer prisoners.

The EIS Wives Club

To cope with the loneliness she experienced while her husband traveled to exotic climes, Joan Millar founded the EIS Wives Club. "We tried to support one another, to feel unity in a group," she recalled. "It was very difficult to be left all the time. We could be at a dinner party, and in an hour, he had to rush home and pack and be off. The wives had no say in this. You just had to accept it."

When mail from an EIS husband arrived two weeks after it was written, the EIS Wives Club would meet. "We would call all the other girls, get together for dinner, and read the letter aloud — all but the very personal parts. There was a special feeling at CDC, that you were part of a wonderful thing that was happening in health. Our job was to maintain the home and children." Although a few women (mostly nurses) had been admitted to the EIS program, Langmuir preferred male doctors, and it would be another fifteen years before that pattern began to change.

Dengue Fever

In August 1963 EIS officer John Neff flew to Puerto Rico, where a dengue fever epidemic was raging. It had been twenty years since the dengue virus, spread by the *Aedes aegypti* mosquito that breeds in stagnant freshwater puddles, had appeared in the Western Hemisphere.

In Puerto Rico, Neff was joined by two other EIS officers, a sanitary engineer, two CDC entomologists, and a statistician. Since they had arrived early in the epidemic, they had a rare opportunity to do a prospective study, tracking the disease as it spread. Neff chose the village of Guaynabo on the north coast, where no dengue cases had yet been reported.

The team stayed in a San Juan hotel but drove daily to Guaynabo, where they tracked every household in two neighborhoods, on the north and south sides of town.

Dengue fever did indeed spread throughout Guaynabo in the fall of 1963, infecting over a third of the residents, causing fever, headache, chills, eye pain, muscle aches, and rashes. Neff and his colleagues discovered that even those over twenty-five, who had previously contracted dengue and consequently had antibodies in their bloodstream, were not immune to this new strain. They also found that the mosquitoes stayed remarkably local, so that they could trace the slow spread of the disease first among household members, then to neighbors.

Neff's study was purely descriptive epidemiology, with no attempt to intervene to stop the disease. "Alex and I worried over this," he recalled, "but it rained every other day, so it was impossible to remove the breeding pools in the garbage people threw out their windows." None of the homes had screens, and they would not have kept the mosquitoes out anyway, since there were gaps in the shack walls.

Even though Neff and his colleagues did nothing to prevent the current dengue outbreak, their findings added to the body of knowledge that would make prevention more effective in the future by documenting how and at what rate it spread. Sometimes EIS officers did rush in and save the day, but more frequently they sought evidence that might incrementally lead to solutions.

Larry Altman, Literary EIS Officer

When Alexander Langmuir asked the EIS class of 1963 for a volunteer to edit the *Morbidity and Mortality Weekly Report,* Larry Altman's hand shot up, much to the relief of his classmates, who wanted exciting assignments, not a boring editorial position.

As a teenager, Altman had worked summers in Massachusetts for the *Quincy Patriot Ledger,* continuing his job there when he attended Harvard. He loved journalism, but because his father was a radiologist and his uncles physicians, it was a given that he would go to medical school. Now the freshman EIS officer saw a way to put journalism and medicine together.

"I thought the health field should be covered no differently from defense or diplomacy," Altman said. "The public needed to be informed." At the same time, he made it clear he wanted to be sent on outbreaks, not just sit in his Atlanta CDC office. In September 1963 Altman went to Maysville, Kentucky, a hamlet where a family eating home-canned pickled corn contracted type B botulism. "The local physician had prescribed chewing tobacco as therapy. One child died.

I wrote this up for the *MMWR* and Alex Langmuir had a stroke. He thought we were making fun of local physicians, who were important sources of information."

Botulism is caused by *Clostridium botulinum,* a bacterium that can only reproduce in the absence of oxygen. The spores of various varieties of botulism are hardy and live in soil. Types A and B are most common. Type E, which survives in lake beds, is usually found in fish. It isn't the bacteria that hurt people, but the toxin they produce. Adequate heat kills the poison, so most commercial products are safe. Products incorrectly canned are usually the source of botulism poisoning in the United States. Botulinum toxin paralyzes and suffocates about 10 percent of those who don't receive antitoxin, and it can leave others with disabilities such as blurred or double vision.

On October 7, 1963, Altman got a call from the Tennessee state epidemiologist. In Knoxville, a thirty-two-year-old father and his ten-year-old daughter had died, and three people in other families were sick with suspected botulism. That afternoon Altman joined Danny Jones, an EIS officer assigned to Tennessee. They visited the three hospitalized patients.

All three had eaten smoked whitefish chubs. "Vacuum-packed. Ready to eat. Keep under refrigeration," the label stated. Contacting other hospitals and doctors, Altman and Jones learned of six more Tennessee cases, all of whom had eaten the whitefish. Their trace-back investigation determined that the fish had been left unrefrigerated for hours on a loading dock, allowing the bacteria to produce toxin in the airless packages. The CDC lab identified type E toxin in unsold packages and the victims' leftover fish.

Altman dictated his *MMWR* story over the phone. Because of prompt press coverage and an FDA recall of the product, the cases stopped. The final tally was seventeen cases in Tennessee, Alabama, and Kentucky, including six deaths. "The abrupt end of the outbreak documented the crucial need to inform the public immediately about health threats because a delay of even a few hours could be life-threatening," Altman observed.

While visiting friends in New York City late in 1963, Altman heard women talking about rubella going around. This virus, popularly called German measles (though unrelated to measles), produces only mild fever and rash, but it can cause pregnant women to give birth to children with congenital defects.

"I came back and told D.A. Henderson and Don Millar about it," Altman recalled, "and Don said, 'My god, look into it.'" At the time, rubella was not a nationally reportable disease. Altman examined the meager existing records and found a seven-year recurring pattern in which epidemics began on the East Coast and then spread across the country. He called state-based EIS officers to alert them. An Atlanta obstetrician told Altman that first-trimester abortions were on the increase because of rubella, as women with German measles were choosing to end their pregnancies. The EIS officer included that tidbit in the *MMWR* article on the possible onset of a rubella outbreak.

When Alexander Langmuir read it, he was outraged. "He said that I had put the U.S. surgeon general in the position of defending abortions," Altman said. Yet he had indeed sounded an early alarm for a major 1964 rubella epidemic that resulted in some twenty thousand babies born with congenital rubella syndrome.

"I saw the *MMWR* as a newspaper. Alex believed that critical information should go to those with a need to know, but that did not always include the general public." After Altman's first EIS year, Langmuir relieved him of his editorial duties.

The Flip Side of Smallpox Vaccination

Beginning in 1964 Don Millar headed a tiny Smallpox Unit with EIS officers John Neff and Ron Roberto. Even as the CDC crew was gearing up to immunize more people against smallpox with jet injector guns, Colorado physician Henry Kempe was agitating for the cessation of all smallpox vaccinations in the United States. He claimed that the potential adverse effects were not worth the risk.

Life-threatening complications could follow smallpox vaccination in some cases. Postvaccinal encephalitis (swelling of the brain) could lead to convulsions, coma, and death. Preexisting eczema became much worse. Those with compromised immune systems could contract *vaccinia necrosum,* a horrendous ailment that killed and blackened the skin around the smallpox vaccination site, then inexorably ate away the rest of the body. "It was terrible to see," Neff recalled. "You could cut off someone's arm, and it would still keep growing throughout the rest of the body. The fatality rate was nearly 100 percent."

There were also less lethal but more prevalent adverse reactions, such as rashes and secondary infections. Neff decided to focus on adverse reactions that occurred in 1963. There was no official channel to report reactions to the vaccine, but Millar suggested an interesting approach. Vaccinia immune globulin (VIG), made from blood contributed by servicemen who had been recently vaccinated against smallpox, helped counteract severe adverse reactions. VIG was distributed by the American Red Cross to seven U.S. medical consultants who specialized in reactions. Any physician with a patient suffering from a severe smallpox vaccine reaction obtained the VIG from one of these consultants.

Neff met with each of the seven, including Henry Kempe, and collected their records. He also asked the American Red Cross for records of VIG distribution, looked at national death certificates that listed postvaccinal encephalitis as the main cause of death, and contacted state epidemiologists. At the same time, Kempe conducted a national survey of U.S. pediatricians, asking them to report all smallpox vaccine complications they had ever observed, and Neff picked up relevant data from Kempe's findings.

Only partial data were available for each case. "I tried to match records from these various sources and found about 450 cases with enough information to contact the doctors directly," Neff said. That gave him the numerator for the number of adverse reactions per vaccination, but he still had no idea how many smallpox shots had been administered in the United States during 1963. Then he discovered that the National Bureau of the Census had conducted an immunization survey, sampling 35,000 random households. Interpolating from the results of that survey, he estimated 6 million-plus primary vaccinations in 1963.

There were 433 people hospitalized as a result of smallpox vaccinations in 1963, about 70 cases per million shots. A total of 7 had died, yielding a rate of just over one death per million from primary smallpox vaccinations. One infant with postvaccinal encephalitis was left alive with severe brain damage. Two of the children died from contact with a vaccinated sibling.

Neff wasn't satisfied with his obviously incomplete data from a hodgepodge of patched-together sources. With the help of EIS officer Mike Lane, Neff conducted a more thorough survey in four states where he called upon EIS colleagues to send detailed questionnaires to physicians. There were no deaths reported, but the number of complications was much higher than the national study—more than 450 cases per million vaccinations. In other words, these were milder but more prevalent reactions to the vaccine than the more serious cases that required VIG treatment.

Through his research, Neff came to admire Henry Kempe for his passionate willingness to question the status quo. Yet Neff was distressed that Kempe was preparing to offer flawed, inflated figures at a May 1965 annual meeting of the American Pediatric Society. "I told Alex Langmuir that I intended to challenge Kempe with my own data," Neff said. Langmuir suggested that such a confrontational approach from a young EIS officer would amount to professional suicide. "Don't challenge him directly," Langmuir advised. "Just present your data and let it speak for itself." Neff took the advice.

The May meeting sparked an intense debate among public health practitioners. Many were appalled at Kempe's suggested elimination of routine smallpox vaccination in the United States. Neff and his CDC colleagues called only for halting smallpox shots for infants younger than one, who accounted for a disproportionate number of adverse reactions and deaths. That modification was implemented soon afterward, but the debate over domestic smallpox vaccinations continued until routine vaccination in the United States was finally stopped in 1971.

In the wake of Neff's findings, Don Millar realized that the threat of smallpox importation into the United States had not been studied sufficiently. He assigned EIS officer Tom Mack to assess this element. Studying the European importation outbreaks, Mack concluded that there was much less risk for Americans, because "we demanded a record of recent smallpox vaccination for anyone coming into the USA." As long as Americans traveling to countries with endemic smallpox were appropriately vaccinated, Mack saw no great danger of imported cases. But the country's doctors were not yet ready to take the next logical step and cease routine smallpox vaccination.

Tropical Jet Gun Ventures

The Smallpox Unit continued to test new delivery technology. The electricity needed to power the intradermal jet injector guns made them difficult to use in remote areas of developing countries. A foot-powered version, dubbed the Ped-o-Jet, was developed by the army, and in March 1964, four EIS officers brought the new device to the islands of Tonga, where they could vaccinate a "virgin" population to test various dilutions of the vaccine and the resultant take rates (i.e., the vaccine "took" when a smallpox scab developed).

Bill Foege, the son of a Lutheran minister, was one of the EIS officers sent to Tonga and was destined to become a towering figure in public health. Stationed in Colorado, he also spent three months in India in 1963 as a replacement for a Peace Corps physician and saw smallpox cases there.

In less than two months, the small EIS group vaccinated fifty-six thousand Tongans. The jet guns sometimes jammed and needed frequent cleaning, but they worked, and dilutions up to fifty parts water to one part vaccine were effective.

In late September 1964 John Neff and Don Millar flew to Brazil at the invitation of the Pan American Health Organization (PAHO), which had mounted a smallpox campaign starting in 1950. PAHO wanted help in Brazil, where smallpox (*Variola minor,* the less virulent strain) remained endemic, and in Peru, where an epidemic had just begun near the Brazilian border.

Millar and Neff flew to a number of Brazilian cities and villages, including Moju, which required a seven-hour trip up the Amazon.

The mayor summoned the six hundred villagers with a loudspeaker system. "We lined them up and finished over half within an hour," Neff wrote to his wife. They then took the Ped-o-Jet house to house. "Home again by moonlight. We sat on the roof of the boat quietly, sang songs, and listened to the jungle noise." Neff complained that he was "sick of traveling so much," especially since his wife was pregnant. "How are you feeling? Is the baby growing rapidly now?"

In response, Lee Neff wrote an unprecedented letter for an EIS wife. "Come home," she wrote. "Come home now. Do not go to Peru with Don." She wanted him there when their child was born. During her pregnancy, John had contracted rubella while testing the jet gun on prisoners. Lee had taken gamma globulin, but both parents knew that the baby might be born with congenital rubella syndrome. Neff obeyed his wife's summons, leaving Millar to go to Peru alone.

Neff arrived home in time for the birth of a healthy daughter, but he had to leave two weeks later. By the time his two-year EIS commitment ended, Neff had set an EIS record for time away from home. To preserve his marriage, he left the CDC in favor of an academic career in public health, though he continued to track adverse reactions to smallpox vaccines.

In late January 1965 Don Millar led another CDC team back to vaccinate residents of Amapá Territory, the poorest, most remote region of Brazil. The goal was to train local public health teams and to vaccinate as many people as possible in villages of three hundred people or more during a three-week period. The EIS officers traveled by jeep, boat, dugout canoe, monoplane, and a bus body set on railroad wheels.

In the capital city of Macapá, the CDC team advertised their "war on smallpox" using a sound truck with samba dancers and musicians. As the truck rolled along, the EIS officers fired saline solution from their jet injectors into the air. The campaign was a resounding success. Except for nine hundred multiple pinprick vaccinations done as part of a comparative study, all forty-eight thousand shots were given by jet injection.

The Ped-o-Jets were speedy, reduced manpower needs, used less vaccine, and cost one-third as much as traditional methods. They also required less skill and training and produced very high take rates among primary vaccinees.

Opportunistic Evolution

The creation of the Smallpox Unit exemplified the way the EIS organization grew and changed. With the Career Development Program retaining more EIS officers within the CDC after further education, Langmuir concluded that the amorphous duties of D.A. Henderson's Surveillance Section and Philip Brachman's Investigations Section had to be subdivided into units, and even that approach could not contain the growing cadre of administrative officers. "I was beginning to realize that it would be wrong and actually impossible for me to retain such a large group of epidemiologists [entirely] within Epidemiology Branch," Langmuir later recalled. "I quietly encouraged what I call the EIS Diaspora." Some EIS alums remained under Langmuir's wing, while others served the CDC elsewhere.

Based in Kansas City, Tom Chin headed the CDC field stations, which specialized in histoplasmosis, plague, Rocky Mountain spotted fever, and other esoteric ailments. Bob Kaiser supervised the Parasitic Diseases Unit, including malaria. Jim Mason had gone to the Laboratory Branch, and John Boring left to supervise the special epidemiology lab. Clark Heath returned to CDC to head the Leukemia Surveillance Program, while Bob Warren directed the Childhood Virus Disease Unit. D.A. Henderson and Don Millar headed the smallpox program within the Epidemiology Branch. All were EIS alums, and all but Chin were based in Atlanta.

While smallpox took center stage, EIS officers continued to work on other diseases. In 1964 Gene Gangarosa entered the Epidemic Intelligence Service at the age of thirty-eight, already a world-renowned cholera expert with experience in Indonesia, Thailand, and Pakistan. After serving a year as Langmuir's chief EIS officer, Gangarosa joined Brachman's section, where he initiated surveillance on an entire category of diseases for the first time, investigating food- and waterborne diseases in general in the Enterics Unit.

Around the same time, the Pakistan-SEATO Cholera Research Lab, run out of Dacca (now Dhaka), East Pakistan, asked Langmuir and the CDC to take over its epidemiological programs. Langmuir rehired EIS alum Wiley Henry Mosley and sent him to East Pakistan in the summer of 1965, also assigning Bill McCormack as the first in a series of EIS officers who would study cholera in Dacca and at the Matlab field station, located in a canal-laced, densely populated area. Mostly, they tested a series of cholera vaccines, none of which worked very well.

A Shady Request

Near the close of 1964 Larry Altman was sent to Africa to help the U.S. Agency for International Development (USAID) set up a measles immunization program. One in ten African children died of measles, in combination with malnutrition and other afflictions. USAID had agreed to pay for the campaign but needed someone from the CDC to supervise the measles program.

USAID proposed to eliminate measles by immunizing a quarter of the children annually for four years. "Only an idiot could have designed these trials," said Altman. No one had thought about the susceptible babies born in the interim period.

USAID spent several months organizing Altman's trip, and once he arrived in Africa, it took another two months before the trucks, generators, and other equipment finally arrived from the United States in late November.

Writing back to EIS colleagues on December 17, Altman recounted what had happened during a village immunization effort. "About 1:30 P.M., both [jet] guns failed to operate. I looked around for some help and discovered that I was jammed in by hundreds and hundreds of Africans. . . . I pushed my way out and saw chaos in the street. About 100 yards away, an AID vaccination truck was in flames. . . . As I raced up the street, I saw them drag away a chauffeur, who was clutching his face."

The native driver nearly died from his burns. The refrigerator on the vehicles required butane gas, and the trucks had been designed so that the gas flame was back-to-back with jerry cans storing extra fuel. The cans had exploded. It turned out the trucks wouldn't work in temperatures over 90 degrees Fahrenheit. When he explained this to USAID headquarters in Washington, D.C., bureaucrats cabled back that he should park the trucks under trees. "I looked out of my Quonset hut," Altman recalled, "and the tallest tree was a tiny shrub." He sent a telegram in reply: "SEND EMERGENCY SHIPMENT 10,000 DUTCH ELM TREES. IF UNAVAILABLE, WILL TAKE 10,000 AMERICAN CHESTNUT TREES."

Because Altman was vaccinating during measles season, the Chinese communists spread rumors that the American vaccine *caused* measles. During his nine months in West Africa, Altman did manage to vaccinate many children against measles, but mostly he served as a foot in the door for the CDC.

Salmonella Strikes Again

In May 1965 *Salmonella typhimurium* caused a huge diarrhea epidemic in Riverside, California, afflicting an estimated 20 percent of the 100,000 residents. The illness killed an infant, an anemic sixteen-year-old girl, and a fifty-five-year-old woman with cancer.

Langmuir sent a team of EIS officers and CDC personnel to Riverside. Food histories among cases and controls failed to single out milk, eggs, poultry, or any other food product. Most patients lived within the city limits. What common source within the city could it be?

Everyone on the team hazarded his best guess. On a scrap of paper, EIS officer Palmer Beasley scribbled "water" — an unusual medium for the *Salmonella* bacterium. He was right. The city of Riverside prided itself on its pure water from deep wells. It was not chlorinated, and somehow *Salmonella* had contaminated the system. No one ever figured out how the organism had gotten into the water. Until then, no American municipal water system had produced a major epidemic in modern times. This outbreak hastened the trend toward chlorinated water supplies, especially in Riverside.

An Unsolved Outbreak

On August 6, 1965, administrators at St. Elizabeths Hospital, a large psychiatric facility in Washington, D.C., called the CDC to report that some kind of pneumonia was afflicting patients, several of whom had died. EIS officers John Bennett and Bill Stuart were sent out. Supervisory EIS alums came later as reinforcements.

They took blood samples and pathology slides of lung tissue, but every test came out negative. The ailment caused fevers that spiked to 102 degrees Fahrenheit, chills, confusion, weakness, lethargy, and a dry cough. In severe cases, it led to congestive heart failure and coma. Sixteen patients died. Some of the psychiatric patients were impossible to interview, complicating the investigation.

The epidemiological evidence suggested an airborne ailment. Most of the first wave of cases occurred on the west side of the 350-acre campus. Of the eighty-one cases, seventy-four had either slept by windows (open all summer, since there was no air-conditioning) or had ground privileges, allowing them to walk around freely.

In July 1965 construction crews had installed a new water-sprinkling system on the west-side grounds, and on July 18 a thunderstorm with high winds uprooted several trees, throwing up more dust. The disease peaked five days after the closure of the excavation site. Whatever caused it didn't seem to spread. There were no cases among medical caregivers, for instance.

"We looked at a host of possibilities," John Bennett recalled. "I was there for a month on and off, but we came up with zilch." It would take many years for the mystery to be solved.*

Prelude to Smallpox Eradication

On May 21, 1965, John Neff, Don Millar, and Tom Mack flew to Washington, D.C., to look into a suspect smallpox case, a hospitalized woman who had just flown in from Africa. When the CDC lab confirmed her rash as smallpox, the EIS officers and reinforcements vir-

*See page 178.

tually shut down the nation's capital while they traced and vaccinated every possible contact. Mack even flew to the woman's hometown in Ghana before the CDC lab realized that it had made a mistake: it was a chicken pox case after all. The false alarm led to a much-improved smallpox lab and reinforced the importance of eliminating smallpox elsewhere in the world.

In the meantime, USAID officials planned to continue their measles eradication program in West Africa, and following Larry Altman's return to the United States, they wanted D.A. Henderson to send nine more EIS officers for six months each.

Where would I find nine officers willing to leave their families for six months? thought Henderson. He came back with a counterproposal that he knew would be turned down. "We proposed a five-year combined smallpox-measles program in all of West Africa, in one contiguous block," Henderson said. The inexpensive freeze-dried smallpox vaccine didn't require a cold chain to keep it refrigerated all along the route. With the jet gun, eradication might be feasible. Instead of the $7 million measles-only program in six countries, Henderson suggested a $35 million program in eighteen countries.

As he predicted, USAID turned down his proposal, and he thought he was off the hook. "But LBJ was casting around for a program he could announce as the U.S. participation in International Cooperation Year [1965]." In September 1965 Bill Stewart, an EIS alum, was appointed U.S. surgeon general. He backed the CDC proposal, and LBJ liked it. USAID was told to fund the smallpox-measles program. Suddenly the CDC had to ramp up for a major international program that would employ around forty-five people.

Alexander Langmuir exploded. He doubted the CDC's ability to administer such an ambitious undertaking. He certainly did not want many of his EIS officers involved, which would keep them from other important projects. Although Langmuir approved of brief overseas ventures, he didn't like the idea of extended stays without his close supervision. "Take what you want," he told Henderson, "and get out." Henderson's new Smallpox Eradication Program set up shop outside

Langmuir's purview. The rift was traumatic for both men. Henderson had been Langmuir's golden boy, a contender with Brachman to succeed him as the chief of the Epidemiology Branch.

With the initiation of the Smallpox Eradication Program in West Africa, the diaspora of EIS alums was complete, and the CDC's biggest challenge lay ahead.

7

FIGHTING POX, PANDEMICS, AND SPECIAL PATHOGENS

IN MAY 1966, after a bitter debate, the World Health Assembly passed by two votes a resolution to fund a campaign for worldwide small-pox eradication. Marcolino Candau, the Brazilian director general of the World Health Organization, was opposed to the smallpox pro-gram because, after more than a decade in operation, the WHO ma-laria eradication program was foundering. Why add another expen-sive program?

Irritated at the United States for joining the Soviet Union in press-ing for smallpox eradication, Candau insisted that an American take charge so that when the program failed, the United States would be viewed as the responsible party. He chose D.A. Henderson, who had been spearheading the West African measles-smallpox program funded by USAID.

With smallpox eradication added to the measles program in Janu-ary 1966, EIS officer Ralph "Rafe" Henderson (no relation to D.A.) and others had rushed from country to country to facilitate the sign-ing of project agreements in West Africa. Each nation differed in its ap-proach, politics, and demands, and some refused to sign for months.

For each of the eighteen countries in the West African smallpox-measles project, D.A. Henderson had recruited a medical officer and operations officer. The medical officers joined the regular incoming

EIS officers for their July 1966 training course. Meanwhile, the non-medical operations officers learned to repair Dodge pickup trucks. They would administer the smallpox program, keep the trucks running, and free up the physicians to be epidemiologists.*

After the EIS course, the two groups trained together, with the medical officers also getting a quick lesson in auto mechanics. Don Millar, D.A. Henderson, and John Neff lectured on smallpox, while Bernie Challenor, the first African American EIS officer,† and Rafe Henderson (back from Africa) taught classes on measles. In the evenings, the new recruits took a crash course in French.

In November 1966 D.A. Henderson and his family departed for Geneva to work at the World Health Organization (though CDC continued to pay his salary), where he would supervise the worldwide smallpox eradication effort, including the fledgling CDC program in West Africa. He left Millar in charge of the CDC Smallpox Eradication Program. Meanwhile, the medical and operations officers flew to find new homes and roles in West Africa. Rafe Henderson and his new bride, Ilze, lived in Lagos, Nigeria, where he would be the second in command at regional headquarters. Bernie Challenor took charge of Togo, Dahomey, and Ghana. Official smallpox eradication was scheduled to begin in January 1967.

Serendipity in Ogoja Province

The CDC eradication program faced incredible challenges: poor or nonexistent roads; political unrest; hundreds of different tribal languages, religions, and cultures; sometimes uninterested governments; and frustration with USAID interference.

For a disease that had been the scourge of humanity since the time

---

*Several operations officers were CDC Public Health Advisors (PHAs), typically humanities graduates hired after World War II to track syphilis contacts. They had excellent interviewing and communication skills and, when the syphilis program merged with the CDC in 1957, some PHAs rose to become important CDC administrators and problem solvers.
†As a new EIS officer in 1965, Challenor could not find housing near the CDC headquarters in northeast Atlanta. "Let him live with others of his kind," a CDC administrator told a concerned fellow EIS officer. Challenor settled in southwest Atlanta and sought overseas assignments.

of the pharaohs, little was known about how smallpox spread or how it could best be stopped. It was believed that the only way to eradicate it was through vaccination of at least 80 percent of the population, supplemented by mop-up operations. Authorities assumed that transmission would take place primarily in crowded urban slums.

EIS alum Bill Foege soon learned that those assumptions were incorrect. After his time as an EIS officer, Foege had earned a master's degree in public health from Harvard, then moved to eastern Nigeria with his wife, Paula, and their three sons to serve as a Lutheran medical missionary. In 1966 he joined the CDC smallpox-measles program, on loan from the Lutherans. Nigeria, the largest country in the region, would be the linchpin of the eradication effort.

On December 4, 1966, a missionary notified Foege by radio of a smallpox outbreak in Yahe, a remote village in Ogoja Province. Negotiating their motorbikes over bush trails, Foege and several colleagues arrived in Yahe with a Ped-o-Jet and a limited supply of smallpox vaccine. After immunizing the villagers, they pieced together the story of the epidemic.

In August 1966 a man from a nearby village had come down with smallpox after returning from a trip to the north. The disease spread slowly throughout that village until October, when, through contact, it arrived in Yahe, seven miles away. On November 4 the first Yahe victim died. At least fifteen cases developed over the next month, prompting the call for help.

With limited resources and vaccine, Foege could not use a mass vaccination strategy for the entire area, so he pursued a delaying action. He radioed missionaries to look for smallpox in as many villages as possible. Foege and his colleagues decided to use the jet guns in Ukelle and Yala, market centers where smallpox was most likely to appear.

Foege's surveillance-containment method would eventually revolutionize smallpox eradication methods. The notion of searching for cases (surveillance) and vaccinating all possible contacts (containment) was not new — D.A. Henderson had included it from the outset in his game plan—but no one had thought it could replace mass vaccination. "We weren't looking for a new strategy, just using vaccine effectively," Foege said. "We tried to map smallpox outbreaks in eastern Nigeria, and they seemed to travel seasonally, from north to south. So beginning in January 1967, we focused on stopping its advance from the north."

To deal with another outbreak in Abakaliki, a market town to the north, and nearby Effrium, Foege's team mounted a mass jet-gun campaign in the area in May 1967. In a week, sixty-two thousand people were vaccinated, in part because the chief told villagers to come see Foege, who at six foot seven was advertised as "the tallest man in the world." To allay fears of vaccination, Foege immunized himself repeatedly. Nearly 90 percent of the population was reached, and the outbreak, which had killed 180 people, was apparently halted.

In July 1967 civil war erupted, with the eastern enclave, where Foege worked, calling itself Biafra. Foege, arrested briefly in Biafra as a possible spy, fled to northern Nigeria, where he was arrested again because he had worked in Biafra. (By that time, his family had returned to the United States.) As a persona non grata, he moved back to Atlanta to help administer the eradication program. Amazingly, smallpox had been eliminated from the Biafran region just before the war began.

Harmful Fetishes

When the Biafran War began, U.S. policy allowed no American dependents into Nigeria. So in July 1967, just as Rafe Henderson's EIS service was ending as second in command in the Lagos regional office, he and his wife, Ilze, returned to French-speaking West Africa. In Dahomey, Rafe helped form Les Douze (the dozen), a team that quickly responded to smallpox outbreaks, arriving on motorbikes.

Les Douze carried vaccine and newly introduced bifurcated needles, which would revolutionize smallpox vaccination. These simple, efficient needles, with tiny forked ends, held a drop of vaccine. While the jet guns worked well in northern Nigeria, where the Muslim emirs could assemble whole village populations, the bifurcated needles were ideal for house-to-house treatments.

In November 1967 Bernie Challenor investigated a rumor of smallpox in Toglekope, a village in Togo that had been mass-vaccinated twice. He was dismayed to discover eight cases, seven of whom had been hidden in the bush during the vaccinations, apparently out of superstition or fear.* Fetish priests had attempted to stop the outbreak by forbidding people to whistle or eat certain foods. The next month, in the village of Hon in Dahomey, Challenor found that one hundred of the six hundred inhabitants had contracted smallpox over the last nine months. Forty had died. Because of the local worship of Vodu-Sakpata, a smallpox god, the villagers strongly resisted vaccination. However, the chief had lost faith in the fetish priest, and he organized teams that "chased and rounded up people in the bush, and when necessary searched individual homes," wrote Challenor. They were forcibly vaccinated.

The first year of the smallpox eradication program was frustrating, chaotic, and enlightening. Smallpox did not spread as readily or rapidly as health officials had assumed. With sufficient surveillance and vaccination, disease transmission could be contained. But it could continue to smolder in slow transmission in rural populations.

New Funding for State Officers

In 1966, with new federal funding, Langmuir got twenty-four additional EIS officers who would be state-based, spending half their time on measles immunization and the other half chasing down other disease outbreaks. With the Vietnam War heating up, it was easy to recruit young physicians eager to avoid the draft. In self-mocking mode, they called themselves Yellow Berets.

Pediatrician John Witte was appointed to head the measles program with one foot in Langmuir's Epidemiology Branch and the

---

*In some areas in Nigeria, EIS alum Stan Foster reported, "The people believe that we are using human brains as vaccine."

other in the Immunization Branch. EIS officer Lyle Conrad served as his assistant. While Witte dealt primarily with measles administration, Conrad served as the support system for the state-based officers, a role he would grow into over the next three decades.

The graduates of the overflowing 1966 EIS course fanned out to the states, initiating intensified measles immunization campaigns, along with DTP (diphtheria, tetanus, pertussis) and oral polio vaccines. Langmuir added urgency to the campaigns by declaring that measles could be eradicated from the United States within six months. New CDC director David Sencer modified that goal somewhat, saying that measles in the United States should be eliminated by the end of 1967.

The measles vaccine, licensed in 1963, was expensive, and few inner-city or poor rural children had been immunized. Maternal antibodies protected newborns, so that the vaccine didn't work well until the babies were a year old, and it was hard to get all parents to bring their children in at that time for the shot. In addition, measles was perceived as a relatively harmless disease. Yet it affected 4 million U.S. children annually, four thousand of whom developed encephalitis that could leave them mentally impaired. Some five hundred children died every year of measles complications.

EIS officers assigned to the states helped to coordinate free mass vaccinations. After measles became an officially reportable disease, surveillance was stepped up. When a measles epidemic was reported in Snohomish County in Washington State in late November 1966, three EIS officers flew out to mount a vaccination campaign. In Texas, EIS officer Vic Zalma decorated his white van with red spots and the message MEASLES MUST GO.

Even before the allocation of federal money, EIS officer Beryl Rosenstein had helped mount a mass measles vaccination campaign that virtually eliminated the disease from Rhode Island. When twenty-nine-year-old Bill Schaffner reported for EIS duty in that small state in August 1966, his job of measles vaccination had already been done, so he set up a surveillance system that investigated 106 suspect cases. Only 49 were measles, most of them imported by military families.

Schaffner crisscrossed the state, investigating a report of cutaneous anthrax, a typhoid carrier, mumps and influenza epidemics, and cases of swimmer's itch, and joined other EIS officers in his native New Jersey for an epidemic of hepatitis B among needle-sharing heroin addicts.

He also gave lectures on epidemiology and appeared on a local television show, discussing, among other things, "The Common Cold and the Hazards Associated with Miniskirts." He was typical of many state-based EIS officers, who were delighted to find themselves free to roam their territory, set up new programs, and respond to emergency calls. They made a decent living, took a broad view of public health, and could have a huge impact. They were also aware, of course, that had they not been EIS officers, they might well be serving as physicians in Vietnam.

Measles Refuses to Go Away

The 1967 measles eradication campaign did not succeed. Although measles incidence was cut by nearly 90 percent, the CDC estimated that approximately 7 million children remained unvaccinated. Out of the 276 measles cases that were reported in Chicago in January 1968, over half of the victims were preschoolers. The epidemic began in the slums. Working mothers who left their infants with neighbors in informal day-care situations facilitated the spread. Armed with forty-five jet guns and forty thousand doses of vaccine, twenty-two EIS officers and ten Public Health Advisors descended on Chicago for a mass immunization campaign in elementary schools and neighborhood clinics. Others went door-to-door in housing development high-rises in an effort to get vaccine to preschool-age children, though many occupants wouldn't open their doors. In the middle of the campaign, on April 4, 1968, Martin Luther King Jr. was assassinated. Rioting broke out, and the CDC had to withdraw the EIS officers. It would take another thirty-one years before a comprehensive, revised immunization program would finally eliminate indigenous measles from the United States.

Malarial Woes

The CDC took on another difficult eradication program in 1966: malaria. The ancient disease, which probably had killed Alexander the Great, affected 100 million people annually, and approximately a million of them died. The disease in humans is caused by four types of *Plasmodium* protozoa, but the two most common are *vivax* and *falciparum*. Their complex life cycle requires time inside a female anopheles mosquito and then inside a human being, where the protozoa feed on the liver and red blood cells. *P. falciparum* is the most lethal variety, especially if it gets into the brain, where it causes hemorrhagic cerebral malaria.

With USAID providing the funds, EIS officers traveled around the world to assess WHO-sponsored Malaria Eradication Programs. Alan Hinman, who joined the Epidemic Intelligence Service in 1965, knew Spanish and moved to El Salvador, where he evaluated malaria eradication programs for the remainder of his EIS time and then as a regular CDC employee. "Malaria eradication was not working," he recalled. Not only were mosquitoes developing resistance to the DDT sprayed on interior walls, but the one-size-fits-all program did not take into account cultural or economic differences. "In Haiti, the huts were so small that in the evening people sat outside and got bitten," Hinman said.

In 1967 EIS officer Tom Vernon was assigned full-time to the Nepal Malaria Eradication Program. Over the next two years, whenever a remote malaria outbreak was reported, a helicopter dropped him as near to the affected village as possible, though he sometimes had to walk for days to reach it. "The Nepalese were the most incredibly hospitable people I've ever known," Vernon said. "Wherever I went, I was welcomed with big smiles, children gathering around."

The program was going relatively well in the eastern two-thirds of Nepal by 1968, reaching a low level of twenty-five hundred cases. But in Ceylon (now Sri Lanka) and India, in areas where DDT spraying had been discontinued because the disease had nearly disappeared, malaria exploded, causing a worldwide reevaluation of the program.*

In 1969 Vernon wrote a controversial report in which he cautioned against extending the expensive eradication program to remote, sparsely populated western Nepal. Instead, he suggested routine surveillance and control. In his final January 1970 report, he called the Nepal program "one of the most successful," but concluded that "malaria eradication will not be achieved by 1973," USAID's target date. Some householders were refusing to allow more DDT into their homes, "fed up with as many as nine years of spraying." Vernon bluntly stated: "USAID/Nepal should . . . abandon the myth of time-limited eradication." Given all the obstacles and setbacks that malaria eradication efforts faced, many were growing skeptical about the program in other countries as well.

Hong Kong Flu

When an influenza epidemic hit Hong Kong in July 1968, no one at the CDC was alarmed until specimens revealed that this flu was a new strain, H3N2, which presaged the third worldwide flu pandemic of the twentieth century, following 1918 and 1957. The disease hit Singapore in mid-August, then Taiwan, Malaysia, Vietnam, and the Philippines. In September 1968 a Marine colonel, just back from Vietnam, came down with the flu, becoming the first American case of what came to be called Hong Kong flu. Drug companies began to prepare vaccine against the new virus. By the middle of November there were outbreaks in nine states as well as Puerto Rico, and in December Hong Kong flu swept the country. EIS officers documented that flu vaccination against the previous years' strains was useless.

EIS officer Steve Schoenbaum in the CDC Influenza Section was

---

*In February 1968 EIS officer Bert DuPont joined a malaria eradication assessment team in West Pakistan. Although the program reported very low malaria rates, DuPont found that they were in fact quite high. Reports had been falsified, money misused. "The concept of malaria eradication for large geographic areas died a rapid death that day in Karachi," he recalled.

charged with tracking the pandemic and its impact. With Steve Mostow, his partner from the CDC lab, he had initiated a study of a new "ultracentrifuged" flu vaccine made by pharmaceutical company Eli Lilly that, it was hoped, would avoid adverse reactions caused by impurities in the egg embryos used to grow the virus. In 1967 and the spring of 1968, Schoenbaum and Mostow injected varying strengths of the new vaccine into volunteers at the Atlanta Federal Penitentiary.

"Our prison study didn't go through any kind of review," Schoenbaum recalled. It did, however, incorporate informed consent. "Prisoners who are minors or mentally incompetent will not be accepted as volunteers," the protocol stated.*

The study proved that the Lilly vaccine worked without undue adverse reactions, even at high concentrations. Then Hong Kong flu arrived. Schoenbaum conducted trials in late November 1968 with an ultracentrifuged vaccine produced from the new H3N2 strain, and several older vaccines, this time using prisoners at the Georgia State Prison in Reidsville. When Hong Kong flu hit the prison in late December, the new vaccine reduced illness by 70 percent among the immunized inmates.

But the unlicensed experimental Lilly vaccine couldn't reach most people. The pandemic, which affected one out of five U.S. citizens, killed thousands of elderly or already ill people, including actress Tallulah Bankhead and former CIA director Allen Dulles.

Doc, How about a Worse Bug?

While Schoenbaum tested flu vaccine on Georgia prisoners, EIS officer Bert DuPont induced diarrhea in Maryland inmates to test a *Shigella* vaccine. The volunteer prisoners signed informed consent forms and presumably understood what they would endure for their two-

---

*In 1965 Public Health Service doctor Herschell King conducted malaria drug studies at the Atlanta Federal Penitentiary in which volunteers were given malaria. King was uncomfortable with his assignment. "Many of the prisoners of marginal intelligence weren't capable of understanding what they were getting into," he recalled. He quit and joined the Epidemic Intelligence Service in 1966.

dollars-a-day pay, though some opted out of the program after a painful bout of bloody diarrhea. "Most of them were macho types," DuPont said, "who came back and said, 'Doc, that dysentery was bad, but I hear you have a worse bug than that. Let's have it!'"

In one study, DuPont fed 197 unvaccinated volunteers a virulent strain of *Shigella flexneri* in doses from 180 to 100,000 cells. The human experiments eventually demonstrated that the bacterium required an extremely low infective dose. "We showed that it takes just one or two *Shigella* bacteria to make people sick," DuPont said.

Once he determined the dose and natural history of the infection, DuPont tested different types of live attenuated *Shigella* oral vaccines to see if they would provide protection. He also fed virulent bacteria once again to those who had already had shigellosis, to see if a one-time bout provided immunity.

These "challenge" studies revealed that those who had already had the disease or received the vaccine were partially protected for a limited time. Unlike viruses, which usually provoke highly effective antibodies that last for years, bacteria do not stimulate long-term immunity. "We proved that our vaccine could prevent some cases of shigellosis," DuPont said, "but it was not effective enough to be licensed."

The EIS officer got much of his funding from the U.S. Army's Fort Detrick, which tested possible biological warfare agents such as Q fever, typhoid, and Rocky Mountain spotted fever on prisoners. "All of these organisms were susceptible to antibiotics, so the prisoners were never in any real danger," he explained.

DuPont also helped identify another mysterious cause of diarrhea and nausea that had traditionally been called winter vomiting disease. He got his samples from an epidemic in a Norwalk, Ohio, elementary school where 80 out of 232 children became ill on October 30 and 31, 1968, with abdominal cramps, diarrhea, and projectile vomiting. By the end of the next week, exactly half of the children had become sick, along with 120 secondary cases in their families.

Investigating EIS officers Jonathan Adler and Ray Zickl could find no agent or source for the epidemic, so they sent stool samples to Du-

Pont. He fine-filtered them to remove any bacteria, leaving only the possibility of viruses present, then fed the residue to prison volunteers, many of whom developed winter vomiting disease. "We established the infectivity of the disease with solid evidence that it was a virus," said DuPont. It remained only for Al Kapikian of the NIH to find the evidence under his electron microscope a few years later, when it was named Norwalk agent, subsequently shortened to norovirus, one of the most prevalent causes of food- or waterborne diarrhea.

Two Million Cases of Salmonellosis

During the late 1960s EIS officers investigated numerous *Salmonella* outbreaks. After five years of active surveillance, the Bacterial Diseases Branch estimated that 2 million cases occurred annually in the United States, with a fifth resistant to some form of antibiotics.

In January 1967 four EIS officers converged on Ward 39, the pediatric diarrhea unit of the Cook County Hospital in Chicago. There, over the previous few months, 110 infants had been diagnosed with multiple-drug-resistant salmonellosis. Ironically, they had come to the hospital suffering from another form of diarrhea, but this was a nosocomial outbreak — spread within the hospital itself. Nine of the vulnerable babies had died.

The EIS officers quickly assessed the situation. Ward 39 accepted babies from the Chicago slums. Handwashing facilities in the overcrowded and understaffed facility were inconveniently located, so the overworked paramedics rushed from infant to infant without washing. The EIS officers recommended closing Ward 39 and sending babies elsewhere, but for-profit hospitals refused to take the indigent cases — an example of how frustrating EIS investigations could be, since officers had no power to enforce their lifesaving recommendations.

In April 1967 EIS officer Robert Armstrong and two associates were called to New York City to investigate cramps, diarrhea, fever, and vomiting among guests at catered bar mitzvahs. They uncovered fourteen outbreaks in New York, New Jersey, and Connecticut, affecting as many as nine thousand people. The only food all victims had eaten was a nondairy kosher ice cream called Chiffonade made with raw eggs supplied by a Manhattan egg broker.

"We met Max, the egg broker," Armstrong remembered. Max bought cracked eggs, many of which leaked and were covered with bits of straw and chicken droppings. Yet a rabbi had candled the eggs in a strong light to make sure they weren't fertilized — no meat, thus kosher. The eggs were full of *Salmonella*. The health department insisted that the Chiffonade maker stop using raw egg products, and the outbreak stopped.

On September 2, 1967, the town of Oxford, Nebraska, held its annual Turkey Days celebration. Huge pits were dug with backhoes, logs burned to embers, turkey meat wrapped in aluminum foil had been placed on the coals, and dirt piled back over the food. The low heat incubated *Salmonella* bacteria. Of the seven thousand who attended, about two thousand got ill after eating turkey sandwiches. The more sandwiches they ate, the sicker they got.

Two days after the barbecue a seventy-nine-year-old woman was hospitalized and misdiagnosed as having paratyphoid, a particularly nasty form of *Salmonella*. She subsequently died, and the Nebraska Department of Health sounded the alarm. Statewide media urged anyone who got sick after attending the barbecue to obtain antibiotic therapy. When EIS officers Bernie Aserkoff, Ken Maier, and Bill Woodward arrived a week later, they discovered that the epidemic involved not paratyphoid but *Salmonella typhimurium* and other common serotypes.

Everyday salmonellosis is a relatively brief, self-limiting illness of two to five days in otherwise healthy people. Aserkoff realized that here was an opportunity to study the effect of antibiotic use. "We found that most people who were treated didn't get better faster," he said. "In fact, the infection stayed in their systems longer." Not only that, but treatment fostered antibiotic resistance.

In the spring of 1968 *Salmonella* began to rage through a Baltimore nursing home. Because of Aserkoff's study, EIS officer Bert DuPont declared that antibiotics should be withheld in all but the most severe cases. The bacteria spread. "As I watched the infected old folks go into renal failure and develop pneumonia and sepsis, I changed my mind," said DuPont. He realized that in the elderly, even a mild form of *Salmonella* could be deadly, and antibiotics could save their lives, even if the infection lasted a little longer.

Profuse Diaphoresis in Infants

In a little St. Louis hospital run by the Salvation Army, some thirty babies a month were born to unwed mothers. The nurses and doctors ran an immaculate operation with complete prenatal care, delivery, and nurturing of newborns. On April 17, 1967, a week-old baby developed a mild fever, then became slick with sweat, his tiny heart beating rapidly. Transferred to a major hospital nearby, the child was treated with antibiotics but died within twenty-four hours.

Immediately after this death, three more babies began to sweat profusely. They survived following blood transfusions. Blood cultures of the babies were negative for any known infection. The hospital closed its nursery for ten days of thorough cleaning.

A month later another baby died suddenly with the same symptoms, and three more infants barely survived after transfusions. Second-year EIS officer Randy Eichner was called in and found that the babies had all been full-term pregnancies and appeared normal. They had been delivered by different doctors. The maternal vaginal canals had been cleaned with an iodine compound before delivery. All babies had been suctioned with a bulb and given the same eye ointment and vitamin injections.

Finally Eichner found a possible cause. Since July 1966 surfaces in the nursery had been cleaned with a disinfectant containing four phenol derivatives, including hexachlorophene, which had been shown to cause newborns to go into convulsions if used repeatedly without rinsing. The nursery was closed again and soaped down, new linens were purchased, and the disinfectant had been discontinued. Case closed.

Two months later, on August 29, another baby at the St. Louis hospital began to sweat profusely, and the hospital immediately called the

CDC. Eichner had graduated from the EIS, so officer Robert Armstrong prepared to investigate using Eichner's notes.

He noticed that chemical analysis of the babies' blood had found traces of phenolic hydrocarbons. After a quick literature search, he discovered that pentachlorophenol, used primarily as a wood preservative, had caused exactly the same symptoms in other outbreaks.

When he arrived at the small hospital in the morning, Armstrong began in the attic. "I found every box, bag, container, and took them apart." By the afternoon, he had worked his way down to the basement laundry room, where, in a storeroom, he turned a large cardboard barrel around and saw the label for Loxene, a whitening agent. Among its ingredients was pentachlorophenol, and the label warned, NOT TO BE USED IN HOSPITALS.

"The laundry ladies told me that they put it in the washer for the terminal rinse for diapers and all hospital linens," Armstrong recalled. He asked them to stop using it, called the health department, took samples, and locked up the barrel. The chemical was easily absorbed through the skin, especially a baby's wet skin covered by a diaper.

After a previous outbreak of infant illness in a North Dakota hospital had cast suspicion on Loxene, the company had added the cautionary label. Now Wyandotte, the manufacturer, denied any negligence — the label had said it shouldn't be used in hospitals. Armstrong was not persuaded, especially after his own blood, submitted as a control, was found to have a relatively high level of penthachlorophenol. The St. Louis hotel where he had stayed during the investigation also used Loxene for its sheets and towels.

While the U.S. Department of Agriculture had regulatory power over the laundry product, "their officials didn't see the necessity to recall the product," Armstrong remembered. "The USDA was just a front for industry."

Armstrong went to CDC director David Sencer. After reviewing the data, Sencer called the president of Wyandotte and told him to recall the product and never sell it again in the United States. Although the CDC had no regulatory power, Sencer promised that he would make a very public stink about it if the executive did not agree. That was the end of Loxene.

Hospital Infections

In 1966 Philip Brachman and John Bennett started the Hospital Infections Section and began to prepare a CDC manual to help hospitals reduce the spread of communicable diseases. Two years later, twenty-nine-year-old EIS officer Bill Scheckler initiated a surveillance program of eight U.S. hospitals called CHIP (Community Hospital Infection Program), logging fifty-four thousand air miles in two years. His studies showed that about 5 percent of infected patients acquired the microbes while in the hospital, a figure still regarded as typical.

In September 1968 Scheckler and two other EIS officers went to the Johns Hopkins Hospital in Baltimore, Maryland, where drug-resistant *Klebsiella* was causing life-threatening septicemia by getting into patients' bloodstreams. Scheckler and his colleagues found that many of the victims had indwelling intravenous plastic catheters, so they cautioned against their overuse and emphasized the proper procedure for their insertion and daily care.

In November of the same year, Scheckler investigated a staph outbreak among newborns at Morrisania City Hospital in the Bronx, tracing it to "Mrs. X," a practical nurse who had worked in the nursery for thirty years but who carried staph 80/81 in her nose.

And so it went. In mid-1969 Brachman asked Scheckler to expand the eight reporting hospitals to over thirty in a voluntary confidential program they named the National Nosocomial Infections Study (NNIS).

EIS officer Julie Garner, a nurse, joined the Hospital Infections Section in 1969 and refined the definition of hospital-acquired infections so that infection-control nurses could defend identification of them. "It was a hot issue," she recalled. "Doctors and hospital administrators often preferred to say that a disease had originated in the community."

Handling hospital outbreaks was always a delicate matter. "We usually tried to keep things away from the press. We didn't name hospitals in our Epi-Aid reports.* We learned a lot and recommended changes, but a lot of things were never made known to the public."

In December 1969 the chief of pediatrics at Atlanta's Piedmont Hospital called the CDC for help. Over the past three months, eight babies born at the hospital had developed Group A streptococcal infections, mostly on their umbilical stumps. In addition, he had learned that ten mothers had developed strep infections after they left the hospital.

Garner and fellow EIS officer Steve Zellner investigated the outbreak. Suspecting there were more cases, they conducted a telephone survey of randomly selected families, discovering that a quarter of the Piedmont newborns had contracted strep infections, along with many mothers and other family members. A student nurse had probably introduced the strep infection to the neonatal ward, where nurses spread the bacteria from baby to baby over a three-month period, but no one had known the extent of the problem because most babies developed the infection after they had been discharged.

The infants then on the ward received a ten-day course of penicillin, a cohort system of baby care was instituted, and nurses and doctors were reminded to wash their hands thoroughly between caring for each infant. The outbreak was halted.

The following year Garner spoke at a CDC-sponsored conference on hospital infections, where she found a distinct male physician bias against female nurses. A doctor commented from the audience that it was a waste of time training nurses to do disease surveillance, since the only surveillance they would be conducting within five years would be on their children's behavior at the supermarket. Langmuir defended Garner, who would remain at the CDC as a leader in the hospital-infections field for three decades.

---

*Each time an EIS officer was sent on an official CDC investigation, it was called an Epi-Aid. An Epi-1 documented the initial problem and response. EIS officers wrote detailed Epi-2 reports upon completion of the investigation.

Special Pathogens

Another new CDC division, the bacterial Special Pathogens Unit, was created in 1967. Headed by EIS officer Marc LaForce, it was a catch-all division for unusual bacterial diseases that didn't fit elsewhere, and in time it became one of the most cutting-edge, sought-after EIS assignments.

In November 1967 the CDC got a request from the government of Nepal to investigate an epidemic in a remote Hindu village. A large cattle die-off was reported, and human victims suffered with large black sores. It sounded like anthrax. Philip Brachman, the anthrax expert, went to Nepal along with LaForce, veterinarian EIS alum Arnold Kaufmann, and a CDC statistician. The outbreak turned out to be the plague, not anthrax. "It was the same type that had attacked Europe in the black death," LaForce recalled.

The index case was a sixteen-year-old girl who tended cattle. When she died, her body was thrown in the river. Two weeks later her replacement, a twenty-four-year-old man, fell ill with a bloody cough, diarrhea, and vomiting. After his death, the plague spread throughout his family and four other nearby households. LaForce concluded that it had been transmitted through fleas in humans as well as airborne droplets.

In the United States, meningococcal meningitis (*Neisseria meningitidis*) killed two women on Sunday night, January 14, 1968, on the same ward of a Mississippi mental institution. Meningitis, the inflammation of the covering of the brain, can be caused by many invaders of the bloodstream and cerebrospinal fluid, including bacteria, viruses, fungi, or protozoa. Bacterial causes, such as those in the Mississippi State Hospital, are the most frightening. The bacteria can remain latent in the nasal passages, but once symptoms of fever, headache, and stiff neck develop, the disease can kill in a matter of hours.

By the time EIS officers LaForce, Lowell Young, and Jacques Caldwell arrived on Tuesday, another of the fifty-six women on the floor had died, and a fourth was hospitalized. The sulfonamide meant to stop the bacteria had no effect. The EIS officers recommended massive doses of penicillin for all patients. They also took nasopharyngeal swabs of everyone on the floor. Five were asymptomatic carriers, but within the next few days, two of them came down with active meningitis. Eventually, eleven of the women contracted the disease.

Bacterial meningitis usually attacks children, yet these victims were around sixty. What had caused this outbreak of a sulfonamide-resistant strain? The EIS officers hypothesized that a flu virus that had hit the Mississippi hospital may have made older meningococcal carriers more likely to become active cases.

8

ERADICATION ESCALATION

IN THE LATE 1960S some EIS officers began to move into the realm of chronic disease epidemiology. In North Carolina, Peter Schrag investigated byssinosis, a lung disease that afflicted many longtime employees in the cotton mills. "Doctors were not reporting it, but 30 percent of those who worked in the carding rooms of the textile mills were quite ill after twenty years of exposure to cotton dust," Schrag recalled. "It was as if they had asthma — shortness of breath, wheezing."

The EIS officer investigated a mill in Eden, North Carolina, but company executives were unhappy with the findings. The owners justified the oppressive work conditions by reminding the poor white employees that they were lucky to have jobs, and that they were superior to even poorer blacks.

Schrag was frustrated that nothing had been done to regulate the industry by the time he left the EIS in 1968. The following year he called Ralph Nader and prompted him to write an exposé in *The Nation*. "But we can't call it byssinosis," Nader said.

"How about white lung, for cotton?" Schrag suggested.

"That's too clean-sounding," Nader answered. "Let's call it brown lung" — the name it has been called ever since.

EIS officers Jim Merchant and John Hamilton followed Schrag in North Carolina and continued to conduct brown lung studies, proving that the worst health problems occurred in the carding rooms, which produced the most cotton dust. Their published studies were seminal in changing the acceptable standards for dust in U.S. textile mills.

The Population Explosion, IUDs, and Abortions

"By preventing babies from dying," Alexander Langmuir told a reporter in the mid-1960s, "we have created the population explosion. I believe that, if necessary, 50 percent of the country's health effort should go to the solving of this problem." At that time, there were 3.5 billion people on earth, with growth to 6 billion projected by the year 2000. In 1963 economist Stuart Chase predicted that millions of people would starve unless drastic birth control efforts were promoted.

In 1964 Langmuir assigned EIS officer Nick Wright to work in a postpartum family-planning clinic at Grady Memorial Hospital in Atlanta. Wright implanted up to five hundred intrauterine devices (IUDs) per month in new mothers. "These were mostly young black women after their first or second child," he said. "I offered contraceptive advice and service if they wanted it." (Birth control pills were much more expensive at the time.) "The demand was overwhelming."

When he went to south Georgia to offer family-planning services, Wright found the same interest level. "I trained local doctors to insert IUDs and asked them to give free clinics twice a month." He successfully started 159 clinics in small rural Georgia counties and met some memorable clients. When he asked a recently widowed woman whether she still wanted an IUD, she said yes, adding, "My husband may be dead, but I'm not."

Wright's EIS experience influenced his career path; he left the CDC to work in family-planning programs overseas. To replace him, Langmuir recruited three new EIS officers in family planning for the class of 1966. Bob Hatcher, who had served as a pediatric resident in Wright's clinic, worked at a health facility in Columbus, Georgia. Charles McGee, an obstetrician, worked in Louisiana. Langmuir

chose thirty-two-year-old Carl Tyler as the primary officer who would
work at Grady and build the program.

Tyler was married, had four children, and had already served for
two years as a Public Health Service obstetrician-gynecologist. "The
moment of birth excites me more than any other part of life," he said,
and as an EIS officer he saw an opportunity to assure safer, planned
births. He did not, however, approve of abortions, other than in extreme cases.

Langmuir sent him on an educational round-the-world trip in January 1967. Tyler stopped in Geneva to visit the World Health Organization, then flew to Karachi, West Pakistan, going into urban neighborhoods, where he spoke with midwives promoting contraceptive
services. Then he went to Dacca, East Pakistan, and to the rural Matlab outpost.* The visit there had a major effect on Tyler. "Nothing
prepared me for the profound poverty surrounding Matlab."

After further stops in Calcutta, New Delhi, and Bangkok, Tyler returned to Atlanta a changed man. "I yearned to save all the women in
the world who had pregnancies they didn't want." Gradually, his opposition to abortion eroded.

Under Tyler, the Family Planning Evaluation Unit expanded. In
July 1967 five EIS officers came aboard, including Ron O'Connor, who
spent a year continuing to develop programs in rural Georgia. During
his second year, O'Connor collected data on patients in Georgia, then
other states. "We wanted to know how successful different interventions were," he recalled. Did women stay on the pill? Did their IUDs
remain in place?

EIS alum Rei Ravenholt had meanwhile become the new population chief at the U.S. Agency for International Development, where
he jump-started birth control programs around the world. Ravenholt
turned to O'Connor as a consultant.

In November 1968 EIS officer John Asher initiated abortion surveillance at Atlanta's Grady Memorial Hospital. Of the ninety intentional abortions during the following year at Grady, thirty were medi-

*See page 67.

cally approved, while the other sixty came to the hospital because of complications from illegal abortions. Asher concluded that a "rational approach . . . will require a combination of improved contraceptive services and wider availability of safe hospital abortion." Nearly 20 percent of Atlanta's babies were born out of wedlock, and half of the mothers were teenagers.

In 1969 EIS officer Roger Rochat joined the Atlanta family-planning group. He evaluated the impact of Georgia's liberalized abortion law, passed in April 1968, that required three physicians to agree to each abortion. "I looked at the first year's data and found that the women getting abortions were mostly young, unmarried, urban white women. In contrast, those who had been dying of illegal abortions over the last twenty years had been mostly older, rural black women." He concluded that legalizing abortion while simultaneously making it difficult to access was unlikely to stop deaths from illegal or self-induced abortions.

Rochat also studied the impact of Georgia family-planning programs on fertility. At a national meeting, he presented his data, which showed that African American women with access to contraceptives were having fewer children. "A white female obstetrician accused me of being a racist," Rochat said. Langmuir defended him, commenting, "We must have an objective evaluation of our programs, without regard to politics or ideology." But keeping politics and ideology out of abortion issues would prove impossible.

Tracking Leukemia Clusters

As an EIS officer, Clark Heath had investigated a cluster of childhood leukemia in Niles, Illinois.* In 1965 Langmuir lured him back to the CDC to head a new Leukemia Section with funding from the National Cancer Institute.

Over the next two and a half years, EIS officer Peter McPhedran crisscrossed the country in pursuit of leukemia clusters, but despite

---

*See pages 49–50.

tantalizing circumstantial evidence, he could not nail down an etiology. Here are two summaries of two typical investigations:

In March 1966 a possible cluster in Sussex County, New Jersey, was reported. Since January 1965 there had been six cases of acute leukemia in the county. Two victims were first cousins, so perhaps there was a genetic component. One had been subjected to annual bone X-rays—might the radiation have led to the disease? Another had painted fence posts with a wood preservative containing pentachlorophenol—an environmental toxin? McPhedran brought blood specimens back to the CDC chromosome laboratory, but they found no answers.

In Douglas, Georgia, children in three successive families who lived in a modest cinder-block home had contracted leukemia. McPhedran interviewed all the families and visited the house, taking water samples and checking radiation levels. Nothing.

After his EIS service, McPhedran went on to a career in blood disorder research, while Heath continued to send out EIS officers in a vain search for that one leukemia cluster that would lead to an answer. Though human leukemia remained a mystery, such diligent shoe-leather investigations exemplified the EIS approach—thorough, logical, probing, always looking for the key to the mystery but not always finding it.

Birth Defects Surveillance

Clark Heath was also interested in birth defects, since congenital heart problems appeared to be linked with leukemia incidence. In addition, children with Down's syndrome frequently had leukemia, prompting Heath to set up a cytogenetics lab to study chromosomes.

In 1967 EIS officer Allan Ebbin, matched with Heath's new Birth Defects Unit, initiated the Metropolitan Atlanta Congenital Defects Program. He and nurse Suzanne Schimpeler persuaded twenty hospitals in the greater metropolitan Atlanta area to cooperate.

"Each week we rounded at the hospitals and got reports of congenital anomalies," Ebbin recalled. This was the first birth defects sur-

veillance ever conducted in the United States. Once baseline information for "normal" defects was established, it would be easier to spot
problems such as the deformed babies caused by thalidomide consumption, which no one had recognized until 1961, four years after the
drug went on the market.

In his hospital rounds, Ebbin saw a wide array of abnormalities.
Whenever an apparent increase in a condition occurred, he would
contact the families to ask about drug usage, exposure to illness during pregnancy, family history, and any other possible common asso-
ciations between the cases. As with the leukemia investigations, there
were no obvious answers at first, but in time the study of birth defects
would yield dramatic results.

In 1968 pediatrician Godfrey Oakley joined the birth defects team
as a freshman EIS officer. His first paper observed that the older a
woman was, especially after thirty-five, the greater her chances of
having a Down's syndrome child. Oakley remained with the CDC
for the rest of his career. "It is a major life-altering event when there
is a birth defect in a family," he said. "People think God made them
happen. Bullshit. Eventually, we will figure out what causes all birth
defects."

Skull Valley Sheep Deaths

On March 14, 1968, six thousand sheep in Utah died. Chemical warfare specialists at the remote Dugway Proving Ground had been testing VX, a deadly nerve gas, the day before as they had done for years.
Pilots would release the gas near the ground, then pull up and jettison
the empty tanks. But this day, around 5:30 P.M., the gas kept discharg-
ing from the new high-pressure test dispensers after the pilot pulled
up. Wind blew the nerve agent west over the mountains where shepherds tended their flocks.

When the news hit the major media, the military called in a CDC
team of veterinarians. The two EIS officers who did the frontline
work were Dan Hudson and Dennis Stubblefield. The investigation
was top secret. One of the army officers asked Hudson what his clear-

ance was. "I told him I was about five-eleven. He didn't think that was funny." Later, Hudson watched from a helicopter as men in protective suits led sheep into an area where VX gas had been directly sprayed. "The sheep died within a second. They had given us ten atropine antidote capsules that you could automatically pop into yourself. I asked the sergeant how many I would need to be safe. 'Son, I wouldn't worry about it,' he said. 'Those are just for looks. You'll be dead before you get the first one out of your pocket.'"

The next year President Richard Nixon unilaterally ordered all offensive U.S. biological warfare research to be stopped. That had a major impact at Fort Detrick, but it inexplicably allowed the chemical warfare tests to continue at Dugway Proving Ground.

Pontiac Fever

On Friday afternoon, July 5, 1968, the director of the Oakland County Health Department, based in Pontiac, Michigan, reported to the CDC that most of his employees were sick with headaches, chest pains, aching muscles, chills, and fevers. He himself was ill.

That night Tom Glick, an EIS officer in the Viral Diseases Branch, and EIS colleague Ira Kassanoff departed for Pontiac along with a CDC lab scientist. The three investigators worked alone over the weekend in the sweltering health building, which housed the administrative staff, medical and dental clinics, and a diagnostic laboratory in the basement. They didn't turn on the air-conditioning for fear of spreading the disease.

The epidemic had begun on Tuesday, July 2, affecting over half those who worked there. More got ill the following day. By the time the EIS officers arrived, 90 of the 104 employees were sick. Inspired by an auto advertising slogan popular at the time, "Dodge Fever, Catch It!" Glick named the mysterious ailment Pontiac fever.

Four employees who had gone on vacation at the end of June were fine, so it appeared that whatever afflicted people had begun on Monday, July 1. Although the epidemic clearly stemmed from a common source, it couldn't be the water fountain, which twenty-four

employees denied using. Many clinic patients and visitors also contracted Pontiac fever. The severity of the disease was the same, regardless of exposure time.

The epidemiologists concluded that the disease must be carried in
the air. By Monday morning, most employees were feeling better and
returned to work. With the outside temperature over 90 degrees Fahrenheit, they turned on the air-conditioning. The EIS officers continued to track down leads.

What recent changes had taken place? Workmen had installed
lightning rods on the roof. In June the nearby sanitarium's parking
lot had been torn up and extended toward the health building, raising clouds of dust. Some pipes had been repainted in the basement.
There had been torrential rains near the end of June, followed by a
heat wave.

By Tuesday night Glick and his colleagues had severe headaches.
They felt terrible and could only lie miserably in bed. They had Pontiac fever. Using their own cases, it was easy to calculate a two-day
incubation period. The air-conditioning system must be spreading
whatever it was.

Over the next few weeks, the CDC sent two waves of reinforcements, including veterinarians, toxicologists, zoologists, sanitary engineers, mycologists, and bacteriologists. Many of them got sick, too.

The building was shut down on July 15. Blood and stool samples
were checked, but lab experts could find nothing. Recent EIS grad
Mike Gregg, the head of the CDC Viral Diseases Branch, arrived in
late July. He turned his attention to the air-conditioning, which con-
sisted of two separate systems. In one, air circulated over cooling coils
sprayed with recycled water from the tank at the base of the unit. The
second took in fresh air that was cooled as it passed near the cooling
coils and led into the building. Gregg stood inside the huge intake
duct on the roof for fifteen minutes, just looking. He found a dead
bird. "I thought that the good Lord would give me an answer. Two
days later I got it," he said.

What he got was Pontiac fever. So did veterinarian Arnie Kaufmann, an EIS alum summoned to look at the dead bird. After they

recovered, Gregg suggested cutting into the air-conditioning ducts. The investigators found that the recycled water for the cooling coils looked foul, and the algicide intended to clean it was not getting in. On the other side, where the fresh air was being cooled, there was a puddle of wet dirt. There were cracks in both ducts so that cross-contamination was occurring. In addition, the exhaust for one system was too close to the intake for the other on the roof.

The source of the epidemic was identified. After the air-conditioning system was thoroughly disinfected and rebuilt, the building was opened again, and no further cases occurred. Gregg, Glick, and the rest of the team returned to Atlanta with a liter of the dirty water. For the next few months Kaufmann subjected guinea pigs to an aerosolized spray of the water, and they got sick, with nodules on their lungs. But the lab could not identify any disease agent.

In their paper on the outbreak, the EIS officers concluded that Pontiac fever was "an example of the hazards that may in obscure ways be associated with man's manipulation of his environment."*

Oral Rehydration Therapy and Rice-Water Stools

At the Matlab outpost of the Cholera Research Lab in East Pakistan, EIS officers were conducting field trials of a revolutionary oral treatment for cholera. In fall 1968 Roger Rochat and Barth Reller arrived at Matlab, where they slept in hammocks on an old prison barge and cared for cholera patients, who lay in a hospital on blue cholera cots with holes cut in the bottom, evacuating nearly continuously into the yellow buckets underneath.

Rochat and Reller fed victims a life-giving elixir made with sodium chloride, sodium bicarbonate, glucose, and potassium citrate — salt, baking soda, sugar, and a source of potassium. Dubbed oral rehydration therapy (ORT), the treatment, developed the year before by David Nalin and Richard Cash, proved to be simple and effective, as long as the patients were not already in shock and near death.

ORT revolutionized the treatment of cholera, a disease that could

---

*For the solution of the Pontiac fever mystery, see page 178.

otherwise kill from dehydration within twenty-four hours. Only the most severe cases now required IV drips. Mortality rates dropped to 1 percent or less. It was one of the most important medical advances of the twentieth century.

"For each patient, we would dump their vomitus into their stool bucket, then make up an ORT solution in the same amount, to replace the lost fluid," Reller said. "One man set a record by expelling and replenishing fifteen gallons over a forty-eight-hour period."

In mid-December 1968 EIS officers Eli Abrutyn and John Forrest arrived at Matlab to replace Rochat and Reller and to continue the ORT study. "We had the idea that we could make up plasticine packets that could be mixed in a jug with water, like Kool-Aid," Abrutyn recalled. They made a Super 8 movie of their purchases of ingredients in the local bazaar to show how simple it was, even in such a remote place. It was a good idea but proved too complex an educational process, and mass-produced ORT became the inexpensive remedy in time.

On January 7, 1969, Abrutyn woke to an acute onset of watery diarrhea and painful cramps. "Everyone figured I probably had shigellosis," he said. "Our lab was only good for diagnosing cholera. They thought they had better get me back to Dacca."

In a speedboat with an IV pole taped to the gunwales for the four-hour trip to Dacca, he began to issue rice-water stools — clear diarrhea containing white flakes of the intestinal lining — a sure sign of cholera. It had never occurred to anyone, despite all of their contact with the bacteria, that an American might catch cholera. Because they were generally healthy and careful about washing their hands, they were thought to be immune. Besides, Abrutyn had been vaccinated against cholera a few months before.

The cholera vaccine was ineffective, however, and by the time he reached the Dacca hospital, his eyeballs were sunken in their sockets and he had lost nine pounds. Ironically, he needed quick intravenous rehydration rather than the oral solution he had been promoting. He felt well enough within a day to leave the hospital and switch to ORT.

Once he recovered, Abrutyn turned his experience into a third-person paper in *The Annals of Internal Medicine.* He wrote: "The patient was a 28-year-old American physician. . . ."

West African Smallpox Endgame

The CDC smallpox eradication program in West Africa had turned a corner, due in part to Bill Foege's use of selective rather than mass vaccination to stop an epidemic. Foege had joined Don Millar in the Smallpox Eradication Program offices at the Atlanta headquarters, where he helped to prepare new EIS and medical officers for Africa.

Foege was convinced that the surveillance-containment method — finding an outbreak and containing it by vaccinating only in that area — could interrupt smallpox transmission, especially with redoubled efforts at the end of the rainy season in October, when incidence was lowest. "We can break the back of smallpox in 1968," Foege told Millar.* They called the program "eradication escalation," a sly reference to the concurrent escalation of the Vietnam War.

The new approach worked, but it was not easy. In October 1968, for instance, a large outbreak in Upper Volta was finally contained, but it was traced to an index case from the remote village of Kouna, Mali. With CDC colleagues, EIS officer David Vastine walked six miles over a rocky, steep path to get to Kouna, where they discovered that less than a fifth of the villagers had smallpox scars. They vaccinated the village, and that was the last smallpox outbreak in Mali.

Biafra in Crisis

Even as eradication-escalation efforts were helping to wipe out smallpox, people were dying of starvation and disease in rebel Biafra (eastern Nigeria). Bill Foege flew back for the last three months of 1968 to work with the Lutherans and the Red Cross to coordinate relief efforts.

---

*While Foege is widely credited with the shift to surveillance containment, D.A. Henderson, who directed the worldwide smallpox eradication effort, asserted that in Africa "the mass vaccination component using potent, stable vaccine was the key for most of the countries."

When Don Millar ordered Foege back to Atlanta, EIS alum Lyle Conrad took his place until February 1969. Because of the Vietnam War, the new Nixon administration didn't want public health doctors working overseas too long, so international service outside Vietnam was irrationally limited to sixty days.

Conrad found a chaotic situation in Nigeria. "There was not enough food coming into the area to feed a half million refugees," he said. So they had to allocate food to the neediest. Severely malnourished children were easy to spot with their distended bellies and reddish blond hair. But how to judge otherwise? Height and weight ratios were the most reliable measures, but functioning scales were hard to come by. A Quaker relief agency had invented a simple method, substituting arm circumference (AC) for weight, and measuring height with a stick — the QUAC-stick method, which EIS officers adopted. They carried out surveillance as best they could and set up immunization clinics, particularly for measles, which killed more than half of the malnourished children. This was the first CDC involvement with nutrition.

Three EIS officers — Godfrey Oakley, Karl Western, and Jonathan Berall — arrived just after Christmas 1968 to conduct surveillance on malnutrition in the camps. "Who ever heard of three young Americans eager to run out to a battlefield and begin working?" Conrad wrote on January 26, 1969. "These three are chasing measles and smallpox to within two miles of the front routinely."

Oakley quickly learned to repair jet injector guns for smallpox vaccinations. He also served as a diversionary tactic by playing tennis with a notoriously brutal Nigerian general, giving famine relief teams time to get into the countryside. Stationed in Port Harcourt, Karl Western continued nutritional surveillance using the QUAC-stick method, but he encountered trouble on one mission. Dropped by a UNICEF helicopter in Calabar, he was crossing a river to do a nutritional survey on an island when he was picked up by a military motorboat. "They had heard that a white man was roaming around and concluded I must be a spy." Fortunately, he was able to convince the colonel to release him.

A Terrifying New Disease

On February 28, 1969, just before Lyle Conrad was due to leave Nigeria, he got a call from EIS alum Stan Foster, who ran the Nigerian smallpox eradication program. Foster asked for a medical consult on Lily "Penny" Pinneo, an American missionary nurse near death with a mysterious illness. The next morning, along with Karl Western, Conrad met Foster and missionary Herman Gray, who had been in the first EIS class, to see the patient.

Whatever afflicted Pinneo had already killed two fellow nurses — Laura Wine, who contracted the mysterious illness in the remote northeastern village of Lassa, Nigeria; then Charlotte Shaw, who had cared for Wine. Pinneo had nursed Shaw and assisted at her autopsy two weeks previously. Now she could not eat. She complained of excruciating pain in her throat, which was covered with yellow ulcerated nodules. She could barely speak. Her head and back ached. Her pulse was weak and thready. Her skin was rashed with petechiae (tiny red dots), probably an indication of internal hemorrhaging. She had a fever of 101 degrees.

Thus, four EIS men together by coincidence identified one of the first deadly hemorrhagic fevers. *That's what happens when EIS officers go into the great wide world with their sensitivity to trouble,* Conrad thought. *They run into things.* Finding that the first victim had contracted the disease in the village of Lassa, Western suggested calling whatever she had Lassa fever. Conrad accompanied the severely ill patient on a Pan Am flight back to the United States, where she survived, although the virus she harbored subsequently killed a laboratory worker.

"Total Debacle"

Smallpox dwindled throughout 1969, until a September outbreak in Dahomey (now Benin) was contained. Then, nothing. It appeared that smallpox might indeed have been eliminated in West Africa.* EIS officers continued to cycle into Nigeria for the relief effort, which was

---

*In the meantime, EIS alum Leo Morris was leading the effort to eliminate smallpox in Brazil. It was the last country in the Western Hemisphere with the disease (*Variola minor*). The last case of smallpox in Brazil was diagnosed in April 1971.

feeding 500,000 people a week and providing medical care for an additional 30,000.

It was clear that the Biafran enclave would soon fall, and the U.S. Department of State wanted someone from the CDC to conduct a nutritional survey. On October 14 Karl Western flew into Biafra with a State Department diplomatic team. The Biafrans, focused on negotiating a peace settlement, did not want a nutritional survey done. "I anticipated this," Western recalled. "I had brought two jerry cans of petrol, a letter of introduction from Bill Foege, and some whiskey for the missionaries." He slipped away from the negotiations and hitched a ride by holding up a jerry can. Since gas was rare, the driver stopped.

Western conducted a random population survey in thirty-six widely distributed sites in eight provinces of Biafra. Of the 2,676 villagers he examined, 31.4 percent were severely malnourished. There were few very young or elderly villagers, since most had died. "The most important question was how many people were in the enclave," he recalled. "Some said one million. Some said ten million." Western found that 67.2 percent of his sample had smallpox scars. Knowing that over a million doses of smallpox vaccine had been administered in the area during the campaign, he extrapolated to estimate a total Biafran population of 3.23 million. Of those, roughly a million suffered from advanced protein malnutrition. Amazingly, Western accomplished all of this in less than two weeks.

A few weeks after he returned to Atlanta, he sent two new EIS volunteers to Nigeria. One was Ohio native Paul Schnitker, twenty-eight, a Harvard Med School graduate. "We told officers to fly on Pan Am, but Paul wanted to go to London first," Western remembered, "and Nigeria Airways flew from there." On November 20, 1969, as Schnitker's plane approached Lagos, it exploded, probably because of a terrorist bomb hidden in luggage. He was the first and thus far only EIS officer to die in the line of duty.

On January 4, 1970, EIS officer Matt Loewenstein arrived in Port Harcourt. WELCOME TO NIGERIA, WHERE BABIES ARE HAPPY AND HEALTHY, read a sign near the airport. By the time the war officially ended on January 15, Loewenstein had set up in Owerri, inside the former Biafra, along with the Austrian Red Cross, Lutherans, and other agencies, trying to conduct surveillance and emergency feeding in the midst of utter chaos. Regardless of their condition, refugees streamed back to their home villages. "It was extraordinary, this desire to get home at all costs," Loewenstein remembered.

Attempts to feed refugees on the Port Harcourt–Owerri Road were disastrous. "Total debacle," Loewenstein wrote in his diary on January 15. "Dumped food . . . was never distributed. 200 bags already brought to Owerri are missing." He also discovered that many fearful, starving Ibos were fleeing into the bush. "Situation is very grave," he reported on January 18. "Only the healthy are on the roads. Sick in bush and small villages . . . One village had closed sick bay with 150 patients day before because of no food."

Loewenstein wrote on January 23: "People in Owerri are in danger of panicking. Supposedly help is on the way. . . . We will have to stop feeding in Owerri to prevent the thousands from storming the town each day."

By January 31 some order had been established. "I'm getting more optimistic," he continued. "We're now up to 85 sick bays and orphanages." Yet on the same day, he got a letter from the Egbu sick bay: "The little food which you brought us on the 27th Jan. 1970 is finished. The children are starving terribly."

Even when sufficient food arrived, getting it to the sick bays and feeding stations quickly was difficult. It took time to redistribute from warehouses, so Loewenstein did away with them entirely. Ten-ton Leyland trucks from Port Harcourt were met by smaller local trucks for distribution to sick bays.

Because of the extraordinary circumstances, Loewenstein got permission to stay beyond the sixty-day limit. By the time he left on March 28, 1970, the relief effort was functioning relatively smoothly, but the six-foot-plus EIS officer weighed 140 pounds, having lost 40 while in Nigeria. "I worked 120 hours a week," Loewenstein said. "You felt you would never again do anything this important in your life."

On May 21, 1970, the last case of smallpox in West Africa was diagnosed. Smallpox had truly been eliminated from the region, though it was still a problem elsewhere, especially in India.

The End of an Era

Alexander Langmuir opened the annual spring EIS conference on April 13, 1970, then turned the microphone over to CDC director David Sencer, who made a startling announcement. Langmuir was retiring. Philip Brachman would take over as director of the Epidemiology Program and the EIS. It was the end of the Langmuir era.

Sally Langmuir had died of lung cancer in February 1969. Langmuir's reaction had been to throw himself into work, including nights and weekends. Then he had quietly begun to court longtime friend Leona Baumgartner, the former New York City health commissioner now teaching at Harvard. They were married in June 1970, and Langmuir moved to Cambridge, Massachusetts, to be with her and to teach at Harvard Medical School.

Langmuir probably sensed that the Epidemic Intelligence Service had evolved to the point that it no longer needed him. The EIS thrived for its first two decades under his dominant micromanagement. But it was clearly getting beyond the point where one man could control the burgeoning program. Langmuir would remain an important influence on the EIS for the rest of his life, but the child had outgrown its founding father.

II

THE GOLDEN AGE OF EPI
(1970–1982)

9

NOT JUST INFECTIONS ANYMORE

IN APRIL 1970 the CDC's name was changed from the National Communicable Disease Center to Center for Disease Control. The organization had expanded beyond its original mandate and now dealt with international health issues, infectious or otherwise.

A few weeks later an outbreak rang in the new decade of disease investigation. On Monday, May 4, 1970, a few students at the Willis School — a junior high in Delaware, Ohio — felt hot and headachy, with sore throats and discomfort in their chests. Over the course of the week, the mysterious ailment hit 40 percent of the school's 960 students. On Friday the principal closed the school.

The Ohio Department of Health investigated, finding no water contamination and no viruses or bacteria in eighteen throat swabs, and called the CDC. EIS officer Alan Brodsky arrived on May 25. When interviews of the forty sickest students didn't yield a hypothesis, Brodsky developed a questionnaire for all who used the building. He also sent blood samples from two hundred randomly selected students back to the CDC labs for antibody testing.

The questionnaire revealed that students became ill whether they ate the cafeteria food or brought their own lunches, rode the bus or walked to school. The high school and nearby Ohio Wesleyan University had no epidemic. The illness rates in the classrooms were relatively uniform.

Brodsky reasoned that the disease was probably airborne. The CDC sent EIS officer Matt Loewenstein to help. He asked whether there had been any special activities. No. Well, wait a minute, there was Earth Day. On that day, the children were assigned different cleanup tasks, including raking and sweeping up debris around the school building.

Maybe it's histoplasmosis, thought Loewenstein.* Perhaps the students had stirred up histo spores, which grew best in bird droppings. He questioned veteran teachers. Why, yes, there had been flocks of starlings perched in the trees that once shaded the school's courtyard. Bird droppings were so thick that the trees had looked like they were covered in snow. The damaged trees were long gone, but the rotted bird droppings remained.

The students had raked the courtyard adjacent to the kitchen and cafeteria around lunchtime. On that hot day, the kitchen staff had reversed the exhaust fans to blow fresh air in, along with the invisible spores, so that anyone eating in the cafeteria ended up breathing them. Then the air circulated through both buildings. The results from the CDC lab revealed that histoplasmosis antibodies were in the blood samples.

It was ironic, wrote the EIS officers, that "as a result of a well-meant attempt at cleaning up the environment, the largest number of clinical cases of histoplasmosis ever reported in a single epidemic occurred."

Cute Connecticut Pets

When pediatrician Steve Lamm reported for work as a Connecticut-based EIS officer in August 1970, he came across a stack of laboratory reports on his desk. Noting that many were bacterial *Salmonella* isolates from children, he conducted a phone survey of affected families. Among other things, he asked about pets, and found that about a third of them had pet turtles. He then used children diagnosed with

---

*See Tom Grayston's investigations, pages 13–14.

viral diseases as a formal control group and learned that only one out of fifty such patients owned a pet turtle.

Lamm visited case families. "Johnny always washes his hands after playing with the turtle," one mother insisted. But when Lamm went to collect a water sample from the dish, the turtle wasn't there. Johnny was keeping the turtle snuggly under the roof of his mouth.

Lamm traced the pets back to the Louisiana ponds from which the eggs came.* He learned that the owners fed any cheap meat they could find to their turtles, including dead horses and offal from rendering plants. Eventually, he could name the specific pond where a turtle originated, simply from identifying the *Salmonella* serotype it carried.

Lamm found thirty-six salmonellosis patients from twenty-five Connecticut families with pet turtles. Eight of the victims were hospitalized for a total of ninety days, costing over $10,000. Extrapolating the figures, Lamm and his colleagues estimated that 280,000 cases of turtle-associated salmonellosis occurred annually nationwide.

In 1972 the FDA required that pet turtles be certified as *Salmonella*-free before sale, and in 1975, it banned all interstate shipment of pet turtles in the United States. But turtle exports continued. "Undaunted and without conscience," EIS alum Gene Gangarosa later complained, "the industry continues to export its lethal product . . . to distant lands."

Hurricanes, Cyclones, and Tidal Waves

On August 3, 1970, Hurricane Celia slammed through the heart of Corpus Christi, Texas. In response to fears of epidemics in the wake of the storm, EIS officer John McGowan set up disease surveillance. Although 50 million gallons of untreated sewage had flowed into the floodwaters, the EIS officer found the survivors needed food, shelter, and the restoration of public services but there were no epidemics.

Hurricane Celia marked the beginning of routine EIS involvement in natural disasters. EIS officers would frequently conclude that un-

---

*Although Lamm did not know it at the time, the CDC had made the turtle-*Salmonella* connection back in 1963, and veterinary EIS alum Arnold Kaufmann had been researching and writing about the problem for years.

justified panic over possible epidemics led to inefficient, wasteful allocation of resources. A case in point was the November 1970 cyclone and tidal wave that damaged the southern coast of East Pakistan, where 1.5 million people lived. The tidal wave struck in the middle of the rice harvest, when up to 500,000 migrant workers were living in the fields.

EIS officer Al Sommer, stationed in Dacca, and a few colleagues from the Cholera Research Lab scrounged up five tons of rice and precooked food, took a public ferry, then hopped an army patrol boat. As darkness fell, they arrived at Mempura, a large island, home to twenty-five thousand people before the storm. "There were bodies everywhere," Sommer said.

The next day they deputized local men to dispense food to women and children first. Ripping up empty bags, Sommer made a large X in the center of a field, hoping relief planes would see it and drop more supplies. Later that morning a cargo plane dropped hundred-pound sacks of rice. With food distribution functioning smoothly, Sommer took a walking tour of the island, finding few alive, but the survivors had little need for medical attention.

Sommer reported what he had seen to EIS alum Wiley Henry Mosley, who was organizing a rapid four-day assessment by helicopter. Four two-man teams — an EIS officer paired with a Pakistani — conducted surveys of eighteen sites, concluding that a minimum of 240,000 people had died. The actual mortality figure was probably half a million or more. There was no evidence of excess disease. The water was salty but drinkable in most places.

When the world learned that food and clothing were urgently needed, charitable donations began to pour in. "It was amazing to me, the stupid stuff we got," Sommer recalled. Electric blankets and ski clothing were dropped in bundles. Drug companies, seeking tax write-offs, sent outdated weight-reducing pills and tranquilizers. Various countries and nongovernmental organizations (NGOs) sent fully equipped field hospitals and surgical teams, for which there was no need. Heeding the EIS survey, the U.S. government diverted over $2 million originally allocated for hospitals to clothing and shelter.

The Bloody Birth of Bangladesh

Soon after Al Sommer returned to Dacca, war broke out between East and West Pakistan. With the end of British rule of India in 1947, Muslim-majority areas in the east and west, a thousand miles apart, had been partitioned to create Pakistan. More people lived in Bengali East Pakistan, but the Punjabis in West Pakistan held most of the wealth and power. When Bengalis won the 1970 elections, the ruling government refused to sanction the results. The Easterners protested. On the night of March 25, 1971, the Pakistani army launched a violent attack on the Bengali opposition, targeting minority Hindus and University of Dacca students and faculty. The following day East Pakistan declared war and independence, renaming itself Bangladesh.

The ensuing war amounted to a near genocide. Ten million Bangladeshi refugees (mostly Hindus) fled into India, where they lived in crowded refugee camps. Shortly before the war broke out, smallpox had finally been eliminated from East Pakistan. In the camps, however, the disease once again spread rapidly. The Indian government, already sympathetic to the Bangladesh cause, was alarmed at the health threat within its borders, and in December 1971, Indira Gandhi declared war on Pakistan. Less than two weeks later, the war was over. Up to 3 million people had been killed.

By the end of 1971 only four countries — India, Pakistan, Ethiopia, and Sudan — still suffered from endemic smallpox, but they were a constant source of reimportation for their neighbors. Now the refugees streamed back to what was left of their homes, seeding smallpox everywhere they went. Bangladesh quickly became the fifth endemic country.

In 1972 Sommer headed back to Bangladesh to help control the raging smallpox epidemic. Stan Foster, who had directed the Nigerian eradication effort, came with him, conducting a smallpox tutorial on the airplane. They concentrated on Khulna, a city in southwest Bangladesh where there were two disease foci — in the slums (*bustees*) and in a nearby refugee camp. Equipped with bifurcated needles, native teams trained in surveillance-containment methods visited smallpox compounds three times, but some refugees resisted vaccination.

Sommer and Foster found that the only effective method was to make vaccination mandatory before receiving food relief.

Within three weeks the worst of the smallpox was contained in the Khulna region. With the genie out of the bottle, though, it would take years to rid Bangladesh of smallpox again. Foster remained to lead that fight.

Before he left Bangladesh, Sommer, who would later save millions of children's eyesight and lives through championing the administration of vitamin A, helped Matt Loewenstein set up an ambitious health survey under the auspices of the UN relief operation in Dacca. Loewenstein randomly chose 315 villages throughout the country. Upon reaching a village, EIS officers interviewed twenty families in every other compound. They also used the QUAC-stick method to assess the nutritional status of children, while looking for swollen limbs indicative of edema caused by protein deficiency.

The survey began on May 3, 1972, and was completed by June 6. In his preliminary report, Loewenstein estimated that forty-five thousand had died from introduced smallpox, despite an 81 percent vaccination coverage. He stressed that "the children of Bangladesh suffer from an extreme degree of chronic caloric malnutrition."

"Housing conditions are presently grossly inadequate," he wrote, "with 2,100,000 persons having no house at all." More than 25 million people lacked a water supply within a quarter mile of their homes. Over all of these disasters loomed the population explosion. Bangladesh held 75 million people, with a density of 1,300 persons per square mile, growing at a rate of 3 percent per year. Thanks to the EIS-led survey, the world might be reminded of the country's plight, but crowded, undernourished, waterlogged Bangladesh still faced an uncertain future.

Legal Abortions Can Still Kill Women

On July 1, 1970, New York State legalized abortions on demand performed by a licensed physician up to twenty-four weeks of gestation. Within three weeks three women died of complications following abortions, prompting the New York City Health Department to ask the CDC for help in setting up a surveillance system. Carl Tyler in the Family Planning Evaluation Unit assigned the job to EIS officer Jimmy Kahn.

Kahn found that there were no set standards for abortions being performed in doctors' offices, clinics, and hospitals. He suggested that for every legal abortion, a termination certificate be submitted with detailed information, along with a weekly summary report. In October a new state code forbade abortions in private offices and specified that all operations after the twelfth week of pregnancy (i.e., during the second trimester) had to be performed in a hospital.

On September 3, 1970, before the new system was implemented, a nineteen-year-old Indiana woman had an abortion in a New York City physician's office. Two days later, back home, she was admitted to the hospital with nausea, vomiting, and intense pain. Exploratory surgery revealed a perforated uterus, pooled blood, and a dead three-month-old fetus. She died on September 22.

EIS officer Beach Conger was called to investigate the case on January 18, 1971. Between July 1, 1970, and the time of the investigation a half year later, the New York doctor had performed 1,668 abortions, or an abortion approximately every forty minutes. Conger documented that the abortion specialist had perforated six uteruses, and several other procedures resulted in incomplete abortions.

Clearly, New York surveillance alone was insufficient, since half of the women seeking to end pregnancies came from other states. Kahn asked major ob-gyn hospitals around the United States to report abortion complications in what he named the Sentinel Hospitals program. For the first time, there would be a way to monitor rates of postabortion complications and fatalities.

At the end of the first year of surveillance, Kahn reported that approximately 168,000 legal abortions had been performed in New York City, resulting in nine maternal deaths. Although no maternal deaths were acceptable, the overall New York City rate of 5.4 per 100,000 abortions was much lower than for legal abortions in Denmark, Sweden, or England. The program was certainly preferable to notoriously dangerous illegal abortions. And while antiabortionists pointed out that the rate of fetal death was 100 percent, at least the process was now open to scientific scrutiny.

In the spring of 1972, after Pennsylvania had joined the growing ranks of states allowing legal abortions, the Philadelphia Department of Health called the CDC when a postabortion hemorrhage left a woman in critical condition. EIS officers Gary Berger and Judith Bourne found that twenty women, mostly from Chicago, had taken a bus to Philadelphia on May 13, 1972, for legal abortions. The abortion clinic was trying a new, untested "super coil" method invented by Californian Harvey Karman. Up to twelve coiled plastic strips (actually made to bind small packages) were inserted between the wall of the uterus and the fetal sack, left overnight, then pulled out by attached strings. Induced labor followed. Over half of the women experienced complications. Fortunately, none died, but Berger and Bourne recommended that new abortion methods only be permitted following a detailed research protocol. "Some who used super coils would never be able to have a child," Judith Bourne Rooks recalled.

In January 1973 the U.S. Supreme Court ruled in *Roe v. Wade* that abortion must be legal nationwide.

The Drip of Death

On December 1, 1970, the University of Virginia Hospital notified the CDC of a cluster of seven septicemia cases. Somehow, two types of uncommon *Enterobacter* bacteria — *E. cloacae* and *E. agglomerans* — were getting into patients' bloodstreams. EIS officer Dennis Maki found that all victims had been on IV drips made by Abbott Laboratories, a firm that supplied IV fluid to 40 percent of the country's hospitals. Observing how the infusion products were administered, Maki couldn't detect any breaks in sterile technique.

A community hospital that used Abbott products also reported a cluster of IV-related *Enterobacter* septicemias. The EIS officer who conducted a case-control study in both hospitals looked at diet, medications, doctors and nurses in contact with patients, length of time between IV set changes, and bottle additives. At the same time, CDC lab techs took samples.

Only two items significantly distinguished cases from controls. For cases, the mean length of time the IV fluid bottle had been hanging was thirty hours. For controls, it was fourteen hours. Also, more cases than controls received additives to their fluid, though no common medication was added. After Maki recommended that the hospitals replace IV administration sets every twenty-four hours, septicemia cases declined but did not disappear.

Searching computerized hospital infection data, Maki found other hospitals reporting septicemia patients, all with *Enterobacter,* all using Abbott IV fluids. He notified Abbott officials, but they stood by their quality-control procedures. By the beginning of March, twenty-five hospitals using Abbott products were reporting septicemia outbreaks. The most vulnerable patients were dying.

Maki felt the answer *had* to be right in front of him. Using a hot wire, he cut through the top of an unused Abbott bottle and sampled the liquid. Nothing. Then he picked up the severed top with its bottle cap. He unscrewed it. There was a plastic liner. He pulled it out with sterilized pliers, cultured it, and found *Enterobacter.* In April 1970 Abbott had replaced the red rubber liner it had used in its bottle caps for thirty-five years with elastomer, a soft plastic. It turned out that the rubber fortuitously diffused a substance that killed microorganisms, including *Enterobacter,* but the new plastic liner did not.

Of the 378 patients who had developed *Enterobacter* septicemia in the twenty-five hospitals, just over 10 percent died. Extrapolating, Maki estimated that some 20,000 people in the nation's hospitals may have become ill, contributing to perhaps 2,000 deaths.

The company agreed to a voluntary recall of its IV products on March 22 while refusing to admit culpability. The septicemia epidemic abruptly stopped. Maki and a CDC lab worker got permission to visit an Abbott factory. There, they observed that capped bottles came out of the oven in batches of thirty thousand. To hasten cooling for shipment, they were sprayed with tap water containing *Enterobacter.* As the bottles cooled, the steam condensed and was pulled up into the threads of the bottle caps.

When nurses unscrewed the cap to attach the bottle to the administration set, sometimes a few bacteria would get into the fluid. The longer the infusion fluid was allowed to hang, the more bacteria multiplied. When nurses added medicine to the fluid, they customarily screwed the cap back on and shook the bottle, thoroughly mixing the medicine and shaking loose more bacteria.

As a result of the Abbott outbreak, screw caps were no longer used for intravenous fluids, and the importance of hospital surveillance became obvious. Eight of the twenty-five study hospitals recognized only in retrospect that they had experienced an outbreak. In 1972 another nationwide epidemic was prevented by rapid identification of problems with contaminated infusion products.

The Pursuit of Reye's Syndrome

Reye's syndrome,* the childhood killer, had been investigated by several EIS officers who had established that most of the cases were preceded by influenza or chicken pox. EIS officer Tom Glick set up the first informal surveillance system for Reye's syndrome. Over a thirty-month period from 1967 to 1969, he found sixty-two cases of Reye's syndrome, with a median age of six. Only fifteen survived. Thirty-three children had been treated with aspirin. "Most, if not all, cases of Reye's syndrome," Glick concluded, "are etiologically unrelated to exogenous toxins or common medications."

On November 3, 1971, EIS officer Larry Schonberger got a call from Duke Hospital where three infants with Reye's syndrome had been admitted in the previous eleven days. Two had died, and the third was clinging to life on a respirator. Schonberger set up a surveillance system at Duke and three other North Carolina hospitals. He found ten patients with Reye's syndrome by Christmas. Surprisingly, none had predisposing influenza B or chicken pox, though eight had some kind of cough, cold, sore throat, or congestion. Six survived. Schonberger conducted a study, using children of similar ages admitted to the hospital for nonviral diseases as controls. The results were inconclusive.

*See page 52.

One of the surviving patients was a two-month-old girl. Schonberger gathered all of her medical records and questioned the mother intensely. "I left still puzzled," he remembered, "but I kept those records."

Polio Epidemics and Policy Questions

In October 1972 Schonberger got a call from a New York medical resident whose patient, a teenaged boy, had developed paralysis while attending a Christian Science school in Greenwich, Connecticut. Teachers and students did not believe in medical interventions.

Schonberger uncovered paralysis in eleven children, none of whom had been immunized against polio. Initially, the school refused to cooperate, but once the CDC labs isolated poliovirus from a stool sample, the administrators relented and allowed them to immunize the staff and students. One mother told the EIS officer that she was proud that God had selected her daughter to test her belief. "Of the original eleven cases, three recovered, and they felt they had corrected their relationship with God," said Schonberger. Yet he wondered whether that meant those who were paralyzed would blame themselves for their condition.

Though impressed with the efficacy of the oral polio vaccine (OPV), Schonberger became increasingly concerned about the wisdom of relying only on the Sabin product. In 1971 there were twenty identified cases of paralytic polio in the United States, the lowest number recorded since the EIS had begun surveillance in 1955. But twelve of those cases were caused by the vaccine itself.* Because of the OPV's rare but predictable propensity to revert to a more virulent virus, recommendations for the OPV immunization had been changed in 1964, suggesting that only children under eighteen should receive it. By 1971 most of the OPV-related cases of paralysis occurred in parents or other adults in intimate contact with infants who had been recently vaccinated.

---

*Florida-based EIS officer Stan Music identified the case of twenty-five-year-old Sherry Givens, who was paralyzed after catching polio from her vaccinated baby. She unsuccessfully sued the vaccine manufacturer.

Oral vaccine was cheaper, easier to administer, gave gut immunity, and vaccinated others through contact. The official 1972 recommendations didn't even mention the Salk inactivated polio vaccine (IPV). "I began to question whether this was the right policy. Why not use both vaccines?" Schonberger expressed these doubts to his superiors. "All the people I looked up to and learned from at CDC accepted the appropriateness of OPV over IPV," he recalled. The debate over the use of oral polio vaccine in the United States would remain unresolved for years to come.

The Dusty, Leaden Streets of El Paso

When an El Paso, Texas, health officer called to ask for help evaluating a possible lead contamination problem, Phil Landrigan and fellow EIS officer Stephen Gehlbach met in Texas on March 27, 1972.

The 828-foot tower of the American Smelting and Refining Company (ASARCO) had dominated the El Paso skyline since 1967. ASARCO transformed ore into lead, copper, and zinc, and in the process spewed 313 tons of tiny lead particles into the air in 1971 alone. A local study had revealed heavy metal pollution of the soil.

When Landrigan and Gehlbach analyzed blood from children in El Paso's nursery schools, they found that 12 of the 485 children had levels above 40 micrograms per 100 milliliters, at that time considered the health danger threshold.* Eleven of those children lived within three miles of ASARCO. Four Mexican American toddlers who lived in what was referred to as Smeltertown, in the shadow of the ASARCO tower, had levels above 80 micrograms, though none had symptoms of acute lead poisoning.

Over the next few months Landrigan directed randomized studies around the ASARCO plant. Household dust in Smeltertown was found to contain up to 22,000 lead particles per million. Air sampling revealed lead particles in the air near the plant, but they rapidly decreased to background levels three miles away. Most of the particles were smaller than 5 microns, so they could penetrate and remain in

---

*The safe level is now considered 10 micrograms or lower.

the lungs. The children of Smeltertown were swallowing and breathing excessive amounts of lead.

In June 1973 Landrigan returned to El Paso where he and Randy Whitworth, a University of Texas psychologist, studied a group of Smeltertown children with blood-lead concentrations over 40 micrograms per 100 milliliters, comparing them to other local children with lower lead levels. They gave them IQ tests (in Spanish when appropriate) and measured their wrist reflexes. The children with higher blood-lead levels had lower IQs and slower reflexes. Lead poisoning represented a continuum of health problems.*

Landrigan stayed at the CDC following his EIS experience and eventually headed a new environmental health section. As a result of his work, the newly created U.S. Environmental Protection Agency eventually tightened industry standards.

EIS officer Richard Levine, stationed in Alabama, had helped Landrigan with the initial El Paso smelter investigation. Fired up about the lead issue, Levine called Alabama's air pollution section in the summer of 1972. Employees there showed him letters from a farmer whose property was adjacent to a secondary lead smelter in Troy, Alabama, that reprocessed car batteries. The farmer wrote that his cows were sick, and some had died.

In September 1972 Levine discovered that nine employees of the Troy plant had been hospitalized over the previous two years with symptoms of lead poisoning. Roscoe Moore, a veterinary EIS officer, came to help with the investigation. However much Levine, an aggressive New Yorker, and Moore, an African American, annoyed conservative white Alabama officials, their findings irritated them even more. "The families living adjacent to the smelter reported that since 1971 at least 21 dogs and cats had died after several days of vomiting, ataxia, irritability, apparent blindness, and convulsions," Levine and Moore reported. Thirty out of thirty-seven plant employees had blood-lead levels over 80 micrograms per 100 milliliters.

---

*Industry and regulatory officials often assume no toxic effect below certain levels, leading to a "hockey stick" graph with a straight line showing no effects until the critical level is reached, then the "stick" part of the graph with a straight line rising above that level.

Levine wrote a damning report and distributed copies to his boss and other state health authorities. "When I came in the next day, my desk had been ransacked," he recalled. "All my notes and copies had been destroyed." Alabama state health officer Ira Myers, an EIS alum, tried to have Levine recalled to Atlanta. Levine was sued by the lead company for libel and slander but was cleared in court.

Levine and Moore were finally able to publish their lead smelter investigation in 1976. "A disturbing postscript to the present episode," they wrote, "was the discovery that between July 1973 and January 1975, 21 additional workers from the Troy smelter were diagnosed as having had lead poisoning and six were hospitalized."

Bad Blood Spills Over

On July 25, 1972, Associated Press reporter Jean Heller broke the story in the *Washington Evening Star* of the Tuskegee syphilis experiment. Since 1932 the Public Health Service had been studying a group of poor black Alabama men with untreated syphilis. The program continued even after penicillin was recognized as an effective syphilis cure. The subjects were never told that they had syphilis, only that they suffered from "bad blood."

Soon after the article appeared, the Tuskegee study was terminated amid a firestorm of negative publicity aimed at the CDC, which had inherited the program. (The EIS was not involved, though Alabama public health officials and EIS alum Ira Myers had advised against halting the program in 1969.)

The article transformed American medical experimentation and ethics. No longer could prisoners volunteer to be injected with infectious microbes. Institutional review boards (IRBs) would ensure that informed consent and other safeguards were in place for human subjects.*

The Tuskegee revelations provided an indirect benefit, however, to EIS officer Jerry Faich, who was studying the relationship between

---

*When Alexander Langmuir attempted to defend the Tuskegee study to his Harvard Medical School class, urging historical perspective, some students stormed out in protest.

malaria, malnutrition, and anemia in a poverty-stricken area on El Salvador's Pacific coast. Faich was the only local doctor, and people asked him to treat their ailments. In 1972 he persuaded the wealthy plantation owners — growers of cotton and coffee and raisers of cattle — to fund a cinder-block clinic in the town of Santa Lucia, where he would volunteer.

"My immediate CDC supervisor told me I was out of bounds doing clinical medicine, that I wasn't licensed in El Salvador," Faich said. After the revelations about the Tuskegee syphilis experiment, though, CDC policy shifted. The organization needed to refurbish its humanitarian credentials. Late in 1972, when CDC director David Sencer visited El Salvador, he was pleased to see the Santa Lucia Clinic operating and commended Faich for starting it.

The Return of Lassa Fever

In the summer of 1972 a Lassa fever epidemic broke out in Sierra Leone. With cases mounting, EIS officers David Fraser and Carlos "Kent" Campbell went to Panguma, the center of the Lassa fever epidemic, accompanied by a team of CDC virologists and zoologists.

Campbell helped with the autopsy of a deceased pregnant woman. When the researchers cut into her abdomen, blood spurted, drenching everyone. Campbell didn't mention this incident in letters to his wife, Liz, who was already disturbed by EIS alum Larry Altman's article in the *New York Times*: U.S. TEAM JOINING FIGHT TO STEM RARE FATAL FEVER IN AFRICA.

This was the fourth known Lassa fever outbreak. The previous three had been nosocomial, transmitted and amplified in hospitals. This Sierra Leone outbreak appeared to be primarily community-based. While Fraser and Campbell conducted epidemiological studies, the other scientists collected and bled a variety of animals to identify the reservoir of the virus. Lassa had been identified in the lab as an arenavirus, similar to others that were carried in rodents or bats, so those animals were a particular focus.

The EIS officers pawed through hospital records, identifying sixty-three cases that might have been undiagnosed Lassa fever in the

Panguma region over the previous two years. They visited each of the patients' compounds, as well as choosing control compounds for comparison. It was easy to see how Lassa fever might not be identified in the midst of so many other common health problems, including malaria, measles, and tuberculosis.

In the compounds, up to forty-five people crowded into ten rooms. Polygamy was practiced in most Muslim compounds. There was no water purification or sewage, and children urinated or defecated anywhere. "Rodents of several types inhabit all houses and shops," wrote Fraser and Campbell in their report. "Large rodents, monkeys, and bats are commonly eaten by most of the population."

Lassa fever seemed to be particularly lethal to pregnant women — six out of seven died — but the overall fatality rate of hospitalized cases was 38 percent. The EIS officers began to suspect that Lassa might be less deadly and far more common than previously thought. Many people may have had mild cases and recovered without hospitalization.

The case-control study indicated that Lassa occurred most frequently in crowded bedrooms. The study was less helpful in identifying a possible animal reservoir. All case compounds had rats, but so did 94 percent of the control compounds. Bats were found in 22 percent of the case compounds and 15 percent of controls. The incubation period varied from three to sixteen days.

On October 8, 1972, Kent Campbell wrote to Liz that he found it "most astounding" that 60 percent of the Panguma hospital employees had tested seropositive for Lassa, including carpenters and masons who had little patient contact. "That leads us to believe that the seropositivity in the area may be up to 40–50 percent," he told her.

The EIS officers wanted to test the blood of retired Irish nuns who had served in western Africa over the past few decades to see how many of them had antibodies to Lassa. They got permission to visit Ireland and the elderly Sisters of the Holy Rosary.

Campbell and Fraser arrived in London on Wednesday, October 18, then went to Dublin to test the nuns. Fraser departed, as Liz Campbell flew in to join Kent for a brief vacation. On Sunday, October 22,

Kent suddenly felt awful, with a high fever, chills, severe headache, nausea, and diarrhea. He had been in Panguma the previous week, well within the incubation period for Lassa fever. He was rushed to the London Hospital for Tropical Diseases and placed in strict isolation. "For a certain time," recalled Liz, "I thought Kent would die." On the fifth day, a CDC colleague arrived with hyperimmune plasma from Lassa survivor Dr. Jordi Casals-Ariet. Soon after the serum was administered, Campbell's fever broke.

He and his wife were flown to New York City in a portable isolation chamber. After another two weeks, Campbell felt fine. It is not clear whether he had Lassa fever. His blood tested positive, but that might have been from Casals's immune serum. None of the Irish sisters' or priests' blood contained Lassa antibodies.

The following year CDC laboratories isolated the Lassa virus from the blood of *Mastomys natalensis,* feral African rats. The animal reservoir of Lassa fever was finally identified.

10
SURVEILLANCE AND CONTAINMENT

IN APRIL 1973 EIS alum Alan Hinman, the New York state epidemiologist, called the CDC for help. In early March a second-year resident in radiation therapy at Strong Memorial Hospital in Rochester had come down with a high fever, chills, sore throat, nausea, muscle aches, and photophobia (aversion to light). In the next five weeks, seven similar illnesses occurred in radiation department staff and those who cared for experimental lab animals.

EIS officer David Fraser joined Hinman's investigation. They bled the victims and a selection of hamsters, mice, rats, guinea pigs, and rabbits. Awaiting the laboratory results, they interviewed staff and reviewed medical records, identifying twenty-three apparent cases. All but five victims worked in the radiation department. Three of the five were animal handlers. One was a plumber who worked all over the hospital, and the last was a Xerox machine repairman.

The repairman gave the disease detectives their best clue. He had serviced the photocopy machine in the animal-holding room on March 16, 1973, then fallen ill on April 4. To reach the machine, he had walked down a narrow passage flanked by cages of rabbits and hamsters, subjects of X-ray experiments on implanted tumors.

Fraser and Hinman asked radiation department staff how frequently each of them used the Xerox machine. Those who copied the largest quantity of documents were most likely to have become ill, probably because they had inhaled a virus as they walked past infected animals.

Subsequent laboratory results confirmed an outbreak of lymphocytic choriomeningitis (LCM) among Syrian golden hamsters and the medical staff. The LCM virus was found in frozen samples as far back as 1961 from the Southern Research Institute in Birmingham, Alabama, which provided hamster tumors to researchers across the country.

Nine months later a nationwide LCM epidemic occurred, transmitted by pet hamsters raised by a part-time breeder who worked for the Southern Research Institute. The researchers surmised he had probably started his colony with infected hamsters he had liberated from his workplace.

Visual Chain of Transmission

Friday afternoon, May 11, 1973, fhe Fayette County, Alabama, health officer reported an outbreak of violent itching and rash at an elementary school. About a quarter of the 366 students had become ill, and 48 students and three teachers had been taken to the hospital. Aside from the rashes, victims suffered a variety of ailments, including headaches, coughing, nausea, vomiting, weakness, sore throat, burning eyes, abdominal pain, numbness, shortness of breath, and diarrhea. Twenty-one students lost consciousness for a time. Most recovered quickly, but a few remained hospitalized overnight.

The following morning Alabama-based EIS officer Richard Levine drove to Fayette County Hospital in the town of Berry. He examined the patients, including a teacher who told him, "It was like there was Red Devil Lye splashed all over my skin." The victims had no fever, no abnormal white cell count. The fading rashes were mostly on the patients' extremities, in areas where they had scratched. Levine told the school principal that he saw no reason to cancel school on Monday.

The EIS officer went home, then returned on Tuesday to find

the school nearly empty. There had been another outbreak. This time eighteen students were afflicted. Most had also been in the first epidemic.

Levine called the CDC for help. EIS officer Fred Romm came from Atlanta with a sanitary engineer. EIS officer Dan Sexton arrived from Mississippi with John Kaiser, a fourth-year medical student taking an epidemiological elective. The CDC engineer set off smoke bombs to study air circulation. The investigators examined seating charts to see who sat next to an open window. No meaningful patterns emerged.

The outbreak appeared to be limited to the elementary school. Because of the rapid onset and lack of fever, it probably wasn't an infectious disease. Investigators collected information on chemicals used at the school but found no answers.

Levine and Sexton gradually pieced together the story. Shortly before the morning recess on May 11, two sixth-grade girls, both vigorously scratching themselves, were sent out of class to sit on a bench at the end of the main hallway. During recess, their concerned friends from the fifth and sixth grades gathered around them. They, too, began to itch and scratch. Some ran into the restroom to splash water on their burning skin. Students already in the bathroom became affected. "A few minutes later the 4th grade recessed and joined the commotion at the end of the hallway," Levine wrote in his Epi-Aid report. Soon fourth graders also began to scratch themselves.

Third graders waiting for lunch caught the itching plague as well. The first and second graders, already at lunch, were mostly kept free of the ailment, while the special education students in a distant classroom remained totally unaffected. Shortly after noon, the desperate principal evacuated the school. The skin of several teachers began to burn as well.

A week later Levine interviewed seven fifth- and sixth-grade girls who had suffered repeated attacks. "I've got an itch!" a fifth grader announced, scratching herself violently. The other girls followed suit, scratching so hard that they began to bleed. Two fifth-grade boys came into the room. One began to scratch. The other developed a sympathetic rash without touching himself.

Having witnessed this third epidemic himself, Levine was convinced that it was mass hysteria. Those who came down with the ailment simply had seen someone else suffering from it — a "visual chain of transmission," as he eventually wrote in a published article. As with most such episodes, the majority of the victims were female.* The only ones exempt were the special education students — perhaps because they were not "smart" enough to become ill. After the third outbreak, the local board closed the elementary school for the rest of the year, which was nearly over anyway.

The Cholera Center

After a little over a year in Alabama, having witnessed a hysterical epidemic and enraged state officials with his reports on lead, Richard Levine took a position at the Cholera Research Lab in Bangladesh conducting vaccine trials for the balance of his EIS service.

Day or night, speedboats brought patients from 234 nearby villages. From the upper deck of the old prison barge where he lived three days a week, Levine "saw the boats come in with cholera patients and their family members. People would be pooping in the boat on the way down." Employees flipped the boats over and washed the diarrhea, replete with cholera vibrio, into the adjacent canal. Family members, often asymptomatic cholera carriers, excreted directly into the canal. In addition, the hospital sewage system leaked into the waterway.

Examining hospital records, Levine found that during five epidemics occurring from November 1968 through February 1971, the cholera hospitalization rate in "area C" on the canal was 15.6 cases per 1,000 people a year, compared to a rate of 2 cases per 1,000 in all villages. The reinfection rate for area C was thirteen times as high as other villages. "Contamination of canal water can overcome any

---

*Why females appear to be more susceptible to psychosomatic disorders is a contentious issue. Explanations have included: 1) Women are more emotional and sensitive. 2) The imagined ailments stem from women's oppression. 3) It is a cultural phenomenon. 4) It is genetic.

immunity resulting from repeated exposure," Levine wrote in one of two papers reporting his results.

Once again, Levine was the bearer of controversial news. Even though he carefully concluded, "The benefit of the hospital to the community in terms of lives saved greatly outweighs the few extra cases in the hospital vicinity," CDC authorities would not approve the papers. So Levine and his coauthors submitted them to a British journal, *The Lancet,* which published them. Soon thereafter, new sanitary precautions were initiated.

Day-Care Diapers

At the April 1972 EIS conference, North Carolina–based EIS officer Steve Gehlbach told his colleagues, "The increasing number of facilities providing day care for groups of infants and toddlers may create new health problems in the control of fecal-oral spread of disease."

In Gaston County, North Carolina, during a six-week period, Gehlbach explained, a *Shigella* epidemic in one day-care facility had caused diarrhea, fever, and vomiting in eighty children and four nursery workers. In another day-care center, nonsymptomatic children spread hepatitis A, giving the infection to four parents and the center's cook.

In January 1973 EIS officer Jack Weissman investigated two urban shigellosis outbreaks that implicated day-care centers. In Cleveland, Ohio, 121 cases had occurred in a few weeks' time, primarily among blacks in the poorest area of the city. "Children ages 1–5 who left the home to mingle with other children in day care settings were significantly more likely to introduce shigellosis into their households," he wrote. Perhaps the disease spread easily because many of the younger children shared bedrooms with siblings or parents in the crowded Cleveland slums.

One week later Weissman was summoned to Lexington, Kentucky, where 112 cases of *Shigella* had been reported. Again, the initial cases were younger, and 22 of them had been in day care. "As increasing numbers of women continue to join the labor force," the EIS officer concluded, "more and more preschoolers will be brought in close contact with one another in day time care facilities." That meant more diarrheal diseases for the toddlers and their families.

Cruise Blues

With both husband and wife working, more couples had disposable income for luxury vacations, but pleasure seekers still got ill sometimes.

In October 1973 sixteen recently returned passengers from the SS *Statendam*, operated by Holland America Line, had experienced diarrheal illness due to *Salmonella bareilly* or *S. senftenberg*, both relatively rare serotypes. On December 19, 1973, the *Statendam* sailed on a nine-day Caribbean Christmas cruise, during which 55 of the 750 passengers complained of diarrhea. For the next five cruises, a CDC team, including EIS officers Mike Merson and Dale Lawrence, distributed a diarrhea questionnaire to all passengers. On each cruise, between 6 and 10 percent reported a diarrheal illness. Swabs from crew members revealed ten salmonella varieties. Many of the afflicted crew worked in the ship's galley.

Food preparation methods were alarming. Raw and cooked poultry were cut on the same butcher block with the same knives. Food handlers rarely washed their hands. Food was left at room temperature for two or three hours for breakfast and lunch buffets, then returned to the refrigerator. Leftovers were reworked and set out again for a midnight buffet. Once the problems were addressed, the number of *Salmonella* isolates declined, but on the eighth monitored cruise, there were still two *S. senftenberg* rectal isolates, and 9 percent of the passengers reported illness.

EIS officers boarded nine other cruise ships at random during January and February 1974, administering questionnaires. The diarrhea rate ranged from 1.9 percent to 10.2 percent of the passengers, averaging 5.7 percent — not much different from the *Statendam*'s record.

"We recommended that shipboard disease data be made public to put pressure on the cruise companies," Merson recalled. The

New York Times and *Miami Herald* ranked ships by illness records. Swiftly, the ships changed their food preparation and water storage practices, but cruise ship outbreaks have continued to plague tourists periodically.

Barry Levy's Minnesota Smorgasbord

Every year EIS officers assigned to state health departments investigated more than a thousand outbreaks. Barry Levy's experience illustrates the scope of problems such field officers encountered.

Twenty-nine-year-old Levy entered the Epidemic Intelligence Service in 1973. In his first eight weeks on the job in Minnesota, in August and September, he dealt with a smallpox importation scare (an Ethiopian who flew to Minneapolis for an operation); a typhoid case (a man who had recently visited Mexico); tuberculosis in a kidney transplant patient; a man who claimed to have leprosy (psychosomatic); a false cholera alarm; three cases of Rocky Mountain spotted fever; imported malaria in a Nigerian; dizziness in a girls' chorus; and telephone inquiries such as "Can rhubarb be poisonous?" and "Can a pet store legally sell tarantulas?"

In his first months, Levy also dealt with three major investigations, including a statewide *Shigella* epidemic that was ongoing when he arrived. When over a million asbestos fibers per liter were discovered in Duluth tap water, which came from Lake Superior, Levy was called in to do a retrospective study of gastrointestinal cancer in area residents. It was known that inhaling asbestos fibers could cause lung cancer and asbestosis, but what about drinking them? Levy could find no excess incidence, but the city's water was filtered to remove the fibers anyway.*

One Friday afternoon in mid-September, Levy got a call from a health officer in the town of Owatonna. Eight employees of a local insurance company had been hospitalized that morning. They had at-

---

*Levy knew that gastrointestinal cancer might develop only years later, but it appears that drinking asbestos-laden water is probably not a major health issue.

tended a company picnic on Tuesday night catered by Hoff's Bar, and some had also eaten at the bar's weekly smorgasbord the following night. Levy spent that weekend interviewing patients, tracking down others who attended the picnic and/or smorgasbord, and administering a questionnaire about what foods they had eaten.

He suspected *Salmonella*. (The lab later identified *S. schwarzengrund.*) Of the 173 people who ate at the picnic or smorgasbord, 125 became ill, yielding a 74 percent overall attack rate. The questionnaire results implicated potato salad, but fried chicken had also been served at both meals. Levy found that the bar owner had stored raw chicken in plastic pans in which he then prepared the potato salad. The bacteria from the raw poultry cross-contaminated the potato dish, then multiplied at room temperature for a few hours.

Levy calculated that the hospital expenses, visits to doctors, lost salaries and productivity of sick workers, economic impact on the restaurant, and cost of the investigation approached $30,000. The average cost of inspecting a Minnesota restaurant was $10.70. Levy's medical paper with these figures was summarized by EIS alum Larry Altman, a *New York Times* science reporter, and then *Time* magazine picked up the story.

In addition to his disease investigations, Levy wrote and distributed a monthly public health newsletter, initiated cervical and breast cancer screenings, offered training sessions, gave speeches, and appeared on local television and radio shows. When his boss retired in December 1974, Levy became the acting state epidemiologist, and he extended his service for a third year.

Northern Exposure

EIS officer Mickey Eisenberg was assigned to Alaska in 1973, where he became an expert in botulism due to the Eskimo taste for fermented meat. In the past, the fermentation process had usually been safe, because the traditional method involved digging a hole in the permafrost, putting in the raw meat, and covering it with grass, which allowed access to air. "With increasing availability of commercial products," Eisenberg wrote, "the use of convenience wrapping has increased, and plastic bags may provide a more perfect envelope for the creation of anaerobic conditions" required for the production of botulinum toxin.

Five Alaskan botulism outbreaks in the early 1970s were caused by food fermented in plastic bags. Four victims died, while others survived only on respirators. The EIS officer mounted a public information campaign about the dangers of plastic bag fermentation and botulism.

On Monday, February 3, 1975, Eisenberg learned that a Japan Air Lines Boeing 727 had landed in Copenhagen with a planeload of very sick Japanese employees of the Coca-Cola Company. They had won a sales contest and were on their way to Paris. The plane had stopped in Alaska en route from Japan. Of the 344 passengers, 196 collapsed with severe vomiting, diarrhea, and abdominal cramps.

The Danish labs found *Staphylococcus aureus* in passengers' vomitus and stool samples, as well as in uneaten portions of ham omelets that had been served ninety minutes before arrival in Copenhagen. The ham was loaded with toxins produced by the staph bacteria, which accounted for the very short incubation period. The breakfast omelets had been prepared in Anchorage by International Inflight Catering.

Eisenberg developed a food questionnaire that was translated into Japanese and sent to Copenhagen. Then he interviewed the Japanese catering personnel. Cook One had open staph sores on his right hand. With his bare hands, he had placed ham slices atop omelets, which were then inadequately refrigerated overnight for fifteen hours. On the airplane, they sat at room temperature for another seven hours and were then heated at 300 degrees Fahrenheit for fifteen minutes and served. By that time, they were filled with heat-resistant staph toxins. Cook One did not prepare all the ham omelets, though by reaching into a bucket of ham slices, he contaminated those used by Cook Two. Kenji Kuwabara, the fifty-two-year-old catering manager, committed suicide after learning that his cooks had been responsible for the illness.

Aviation regulations changed as a result of the outbreak. "Fortunately," Eisenberg wrote in his published report, "the cockpit crew did not eat the contaminated food." He suggested that in the future, the pilot and copilot should each eat different meals prepared by different cooks. The Federal Aviation Administration subsequently implemented that rule.

Forced Sterilizations

In July 1973 the Southern Poverty Law Center filed a suit in federal court in Montgomery, Alabama, in the name of two mildly retarded black sisters, ages twelve and fourteen, who had been sterilized after their illiterate mother signed a consent form with an X without understanding its import. The birth control clinic, funded by the U.S. Department of Health, Education, and Welfare, had actually sterilized eleven minors without parental consent. Shortly thereafter, a class action lawsuit was filed to ban the use of federal funds for any sterilization.

Twenty-six-year-old EIS officer Jason Weisfeld investigated and found that in 1972, nearly eight hundred women under the age of twenty-one had been sterilized in the United States. Most of them were black or welfare recipients in the South. "In local hospitals," he recalled, "some obstetricians were still performing tubal ligations on indigent women they felt had too many children on welfare."

With Carl Tyler, head of the CDC Family Planning Evaluation Unit, Weisfeld flew to Washington to brief HEW secretary Caspar Weinberger. The government settled the case out of court, and HEW eventually banned the use of federal funds to sterilize minors, mental incompetents, or anyone in an institution.

Dalkon Shield Deaths

Henry Kahn, an EIS officer in the Family Planning Evaluation Unit,* investigated the medical risks of IUDs compared to oral contra-

---

*First cousins Henry and Jimmy Kahn battled their way into the EIS after the FBI blocked their entrance due to Henry's antiwar activism and the blackballing of Jimmy's father as an alleged Communist.

ceptives, coming up with an ambitious plan to survey every obstetrician, gynecologist, and public health doctor in the country (and Puerto Rico) about their patients' IUD complications during the first six months of 1973. He sent out thirty-five thousand questionnaires, about half of which were returned. Kahn was ready to issue his report in June 1974.

Five IUD-related deaths were reported during the six-month period, which translated to an annual average of three deaths per million IUD users. The mortality rate for birth control pills was ten times higher, and the death rate for pregnant women was two hundred per million. But there appeared to be a problem with the Dalkon Shield, which caused 62 percent of the associated IUD hospitalizations, while it accounted for only 39 percent of all IUDs in use.

To ensure that the Dalkon Shield was not expelled, its four prongs lodged in the uterine wall, sometimes perforating it. Like all other IUDs, it had a tail string that passed through the cervix into the vagina, to allow women to check it and to aid removal. Unlike others, however, the Dalkon Shield string contained hundreds of fine nylon strands in a sheath, which acted as a wick to transport bacteria through capillary action from the vagina up into the uterus.

Just before Kahn's results appeared in the *MMWR*, a doctor published a report that four of his patients had died of infections contracted while pregnant and still wearing a Dalkon Shield. By August the FDA had been notified of seventeen pregnant women who died with an IUD in their uterus. Eleven of them wore Dalkon Shields, which were found to not only cause infections but also not reliably prevent pregnancy.

The manufacturer, the A.H. Robins Company, voluntarily withdrew the Dalkon Shield from the American market, while insisting that it was safe. Only in April 1975, amid snowballing lawsuits, did Robins take the product off the market worldwide. As a result of the Dalkon Shield disaster, the U.S. Congress passed the medical devices amendment, giving the FDA jurisdiction and making pretesting of IUDs and other medical devices mandatory.

A Safe Bet

New EIS officer Ward Cates took over abortion surveillance in 1974. He analyzed data from the Joint Program for the Study of Abortion, a large prospective cohort study of some eighty thousand women. He demonstrated that the impact of the 1973 *Roe v. Wade* decision had been to move abortions from the back alley to safer facilities, but that the number of births and abortions were about the same. "Legalization of abortion has been accompanied," he wrote, "by a sharp decline in abortion deaths — almost entirely due to the drop in illegal abortion deaths, from 39 in 1972 to just three in 1975." Antiabortion activists protested that the CDC was undercounting. "So we offered a bounty," Cates recalled: $100 to anyone who identified an abortion death not already in their database. "We paid out zero money."

Cates and EIS officer David Grimes also definitively shattered a harmful myth. Based on a misreading of data, it was standard practice to avoid performing abortions on women thirteen to fifteen weeks pregnant, because it was supposedly unsafe during that time. "Our findings clearly demonstrate that *any* delay increased the risk of complications to a pregnant woman who wishes an abortion," they wrote.

Perilous Plastic

In late January 1974 Houston-based officer Henry Falk got a call from Clark Heath about three chemical plant employees who had died of an extremely rare cancer, angiosarcoma of the liver. Falk was to fly to the B.F. Goodrich factory in Louisville, Kentucky, for a meeting the next day with officials from the National Institute of Occupational Safety and Health (NIOSH), which had just merged with the CDC.

Through employee medical records and intensive health screenings, Falk identified eight more with liver disease, two of whom had died. All eleven ill or deceased employees had worked for some time as "chemical helpers," who were lowered into a huge vat to clean it, chipping off the gunk that remained after polyvinyl chloride (PVC) was made. In the process, they released and inhaled trapped vinyl chloride monomer gas, the primary component of PVC.

There is no treatment for hepatic angiosarcoma. Victims usually die within six months of diagnosis. The eleven employees had on average spent twenty years working at the B.F. Goodrich plant. The disease was clearly dose-related to exposure to vinyl chloride monomer, but the incubation period was insidiously long. In February 1974 Falk visited three other PVC plants in Ohio, followed by a major investigation in a Firestone rubber plant in Pennsylvania. There had been angiosarcoma deaths in these plants as well. Many future cases were prevented by changes that made the process of making plastic safer.

The Texas Health Department then called Falk to ask him to help investigate cases of "meat-wrapper's asthma," a newly identified disease that afflicted those who spent their days cutting plastic wrap by pulling it across a hot wire, then enclosing meat in a Styrofoam dish. Falk joined Texas EIS officer Ben Portnoy in designing a case-control study.

Falk and Portnoy gave the questionnaire to 145 meat wrappers and to an equal number of meat cutters and checkout clerks as controls. About 10 percent of the meat wrappers had wheezing, shortness of breath, and chest pain, higher than the controls. The 17 meat wrappers who used mechanical cutters rather than fume-producing hot wires had no work-related respiratory tract symptoms.

Plastic wrap is 50 percent polyvinyl chloride, and melting it produces complex gases of chlorine, hydrochloric acid, and various allergenic substances. A resulting class action lawsuit helped to change industry standards so that the wrap was either chopped mechanically or a lower-temperature wire used, and fumes were vacuumed away.

"We helped 200,000 supermarket employees who were wrapping these things," Falk observed. His research in this area convinced him to stay with the CDC. "It would take a long time to treat that many people in a pediatric practice."

Parasites Are Us

When EIS officer Peter Schantz joined the Parasitic Diseases Division in 1974, he was already an expert in the field of zoonotic parasites —life-forms that can migrate from animals to humans. In August he was sent to investigate three cases of echinococcosis in Native American children. The life cycle of the tapeworm that causes this disease requires canines and sheep, originally bound together as predator and prey, but now as herd dogs and flocks. The tapeworm lives harmlessly in the dog, which excretes eggs that stick to grass. The sheep eats the eggs, which grow into round white hydatid cysts. After the sheep dies, a dog eats the sheep carcass along with the cysts, which then turn into tapeworms to begin the cycle anew.

When humans inadvertently ingested the eggs, they became victims. When the cysts grew large enough to cause pain, block organ functions, or rupture, the only cure at that time was surgery to cut out the cysts, which grow in the liver and lungs.*

Schantz's first stop was Tuba City, Arizona, where he examined a seven-year-old Navajo girl whose fever and cough led him to take a chest radiograph, which revealed four circular lesions in both of her lungs. She had three operations to remove the fluid-filled cysts, each over an inch in diameter. Liver scans revealed more cysts.

"The family often buys sheep, which are butchered in the back yard," Schantz reported. "Inedible portions of the carcass and diseased tissues are thrown in trash cans which are routinely scavenged by neighborhood dogs." The little girl had probably ingested tapeworm eggs after petting a dog with tapeworm eggs stuck to its coat.

The other two cases in New Mexico, a girl of the Santo Domingo Pueblo tribe and a Zuni boy, were similar and easily traced to dogs that ate diseased sheep. The boy's cyst was five inches in diameter, filled with green fluid. During Schantz's investigation, a fourth Santo Domingo boy was diagnosed. Reviewing medical records of seventeen hospitals serving the reservations, Schantz found ten additional echinococcosis cases from the previous five years, six of them Navajo children. He also learned of cases in Mormon shepherds in Utah and in Greek immigrants.†

---

*Today, chemotherapy can kill the cysts if detected early.
†Greek shepherds frequently fed their dogs sheep entrails. "Beware of Greeks bearing cysts," Schantz warned.

Schantz mounted an education program, which stopped transmission in Utah and helped considerably among the Zuni and Santo Domingo Pueblo tribe, who lived in stable communities. But he failed to reach many Navajo, who pursued a seminomadic lifestyle and often resisted advice from outsiders.

Dangerous Nurses

Nosocomial infections continued to afflict around 5 percent of hospitalized patients in the United States, costing about $1.5 billion a year. EIS officer Robert Haley launched the Study on the Efficacy of Nosocomial Infection Control (SENIC) in 1974. Years of study in more than three hundred acute-care facilities proved that proper infection surveillance/control efforts in hospitals reduced urinary tract infections, surgical wound infections, pneumonia, and bacteremia by 32 percent. It also showed that "most hospitals were failing to reduce any nosocomial infection rates and only a few had effective programs," Haley wrote.

Three successive hospital epidemics in 1974 and 1975 illustrated the uses and challenges of surveillance. Between June 16 and October 9, 1974, nine newborns at a community hospital in Elkins, West Virginia, were stricken with peritonitis. Three babies died. Doctors tentatively diagnosed the cases as neonatal necrotizing enterocolitis, an epidemic affliction of newborns whose cause remains a mystery. But the clinical symptoms were more typical of a perforated bowel.

When EIS officer Marcus Horwitz investigated, his case-control study looked at labor complications, infant weight, bassinet placement, and types of E. coli cultured from stools. There were no significant differences between cases and controls, so he conducted another study looking for an association between medical personnel and the sick babies. Only one nurse's aide had cared for the nine newborns who became ill. Horwitz suspected that routine rectal temperature taking had caused the problem, so he asked personnel on the ob-gyn service to demonstrate the procedure on Baby Alive dolls, which featured lifelike rectums. The nurse's aide who had cared for the sick babies pushed the thermometer nearly twice the maximum depth recommended to prevent perforation. The epidemic ceased when the neonatal unit switched to taking underarm temperatures.

The second outbreak took place in an Oklahoma City hospital in February and March of 1975, when seventeen major surgery patients developed Group A *Streptococcus* wound infections within forty-eight hours of their operations. Two died. EIS officer Walt Stamm suspected that there was a strep carrier in the operating room. Nurse A had assisted on twelve of the seventeen operations and had been working in an adjacent room during the surgery of four other patients. All cases occurred on days when she was at the hospital.

Stamm arranged for thirty-seven cultures to be taken from every part of Nurse A's body. Two vaginal swabs revealed a heavy growth of Group A strep. Stamm then placed four blood agar settling plates in the corners of a room, where he asked Nurse A to sit for twenty minutes, then exercise for ten minutes. Three of the settling plates developed strep colonies. She was treated with penicillin until her vaginal swabs tested negative.

The third outbreak took place in a Veterans Administration (VA) hospital in Ann Arbor, Michigan. During July and August 1975 an alarming number of cardiopulmonary arrests occurred in the coronary and intensive care units. The urine of three patients who arrested within fifteen minutes contained a steroidal neuromuscular blocking agent resembling curare. Often used with general anesthesia in surgery for muscle relaxation and as an aid to intubation or ventilation, it had not been prescribed for these patients. Suddenly, this was a criminal matter.

The administrator called the FBI as well as the CDC. EIS officer Mike Shasby joined the investigation. "We were sitting in a conference room at the VA hospital," he recalled, "and the FBI agents were telling me they weren't even sure there was a problem. I quietly plotted the incidence of cardiopulmonary arrests at the hospital over the past year. I showed them the graph, which suddenly spiked in August, and said, 'I think you've got a problem.'"

Shasby assembled a panel of nonhospital physicians to examine the records of the thirty-five patients who had arrests in July and

August. The doctors identified a subset of seventeen patients labeled "high suspicion," for whom the arrests were incompatible with their health problems. Six had died. All had been on intravenous drips. All but one had arrested during the 4 P.M.-to-midnight shift.

Only two nurses in the intensive care unit always worked that shift. One or both would seem to have been putting the blocking agent into the IV fluids. Motivation for the crimes was unclear. Euthanasia was unlikely, since most affected patients were not terminally ill. Several patients suffered multiple arrests and resuscitations. It may be that the perpetrators wanted to be perceived as saviors. What was particularly alarming was that routine hospital procedures did not identify the excess number of arrests until mid-August.

A jury found one nurse guilty of murder, but the conviction was overturned on appeal. Shasby's epidemiological evidence, though logically compelling, was dismissed as circumstantial. The same thing would happen in similar medical homicide cases investigated by EIS officers in ensuing years.

The Cleanest Water in the World

On June 13, 1975, Crater Lake National Park opened for the season. Advertised as having "the world's cleanest water," the Oregon lake lured some three thousand tourists each day during the summer. Some stayed overnight in the park's lodge. Four miles down the road was the park ranger station and a Youth Conservation Corps (YCC) program for high school students.

On June 25 five YCC leaders developed diarrhea, vomiting, and violent cramps, less than forty-eight hours after their arrival. YCC director Bruce Stubblefield and two more staff became ill that night. Because of the rapid onset and nearly universal attack rate, they suspected their illness came from the water. They discovered that the same illness was running through the lodge employees. A few days later the thirty YCC teen enrollees arrived, and they, too, soon became ill. Stubblefield had asked park officials to test the water, but they refused. So he clandestinely took water samples to the county health department.

Ralph Peyton, who ran the lodge, wrote a memo to his employees about the "Flu Bug," which he said was brought into the park by tourists. His memo suggested they take Kaopectate and "consume all of the liquids that you can handle."

Oregon state health officials finally invited the CDC to investigate, right in the middle of the July training course. Lyle Conrad called recent EIS grad Jeff Koplan, then assigned to the California State Health Department, and Koplan arrived at Crater Lake on Monday, July 7. He interviewed ill employees and called the CDC to request an EIS officer from the Enteric Diseases Branch. A preliminary questionnaire indicated a 90 percent attack rate in YCC and National Park Service employees. The following day Koplan discovered that while the lodge and rim facilities water appeared to be adequately treated, there was no detectable chlorine in the water supplying the YCC dorm or park service housing.

EIS officer Mark Rosenberg drove up to Crater Lake at midnight, having traveled twenty-three hours because he missed his connecting flight to Oregon. On Wednesday, July 9, Rosenberg and Koplan asked that six feet of snow be removed from the pump house at Munson Springs so that they could inspect the chlorination system. They found that the chlorine injection bypassed the water sent to the YCC and ranger stations. A second injector was installed to remedy that problem.

That night they met with eighty lodge employees and asked how many had been ill. All but five hands shot up. How many were still sick? Fifty. How many of those worked in food services? Thirty. Rosenberg and Koplan emphasized that no one who still had any gastrointestinal symptoms should be handling food. They asked that the employees fill out a questionnaire and submit to a blood drawing and rectal swab the following day.

Contaminated water was the likely source of the illness, Koplan and Rosenberg surmised, even though it was adequately chlorinated at the lodge. Sick restaurant employees were probably further contaminating the food. With thousands of tourists passing through the park every day, Koplan and Rosenberg concluded that the park should be closed.

No national park had ever before been closed due to illness. The following morning, Thursday, July 10, when they reported their conclusions to Gene Gangarosa and Philip Brachman, the bosses asked for more epidemiological data before taking such a drastic step. While Koplan collected questionnaires and conducted telephone surveys, Rosenberg began swabbing rear ends.

Meanwhile, the snow was melting quickly. Around 6:30 P.M., someone noticed an overflowing manhole cover above the sewage line. Rosenberg and Koplan dumped fluorescent dye into a manhole upstream from the one that was plugged and then watched as the green dye overflowed and ran down the hill. Soon afterward, the drinking water turned green. Early Friday morning, after a conference call with Gangarosa, Brachman, and CDC director David Sencer, the decision was made to close the park.*

The CDC lab identified enterotoxigenic *E. coli* in park water samples and the rectal swabs of victims. It is likely that one of the early visitors to Crater Lake had picked up the toxic *E. coli* in Mexico and deposited a diarrheal stool in a toilet at the lodge. Because of the clogged sewer line, the bacteria flowed under the snow into the water supply. "Water became increasingly contaminated as more ill persons added infectious fecal material to the obstructed sewer line," wrote Rosenberg and Koplan in their Epi-Aid report. The bacterial load had overwhelmed the water, even when it was properly chlorinated.

The epidemic caused illness in over two thousand staff and visitors, but its political repercussions were worse. Oregon senator Mark Hatfield held hearings on the outbreak in September 1975. Lodge owner Ralph Peyton had actively obstructed the CDC investigation, taking down warning signs and instructing his staff to cut out newspaper headlines about the outbreak so that guests would not be alarmed. In addition, employees were pressured into working while sick.

Yet Senator Hatfield did not go after Peyton, his Oregon constituent. Instead, he attacked CDC's Gene Gangarosa for delaying the park closing. Gangarosa tried to explain that he had wanted more informa-

*With a new water treatment system in place, Crater Lake was reopened on August 1, 1975.

tion to answer the "crucial question" of whether people were still becoming ill. Trying to explain the need for more epidemiological information, the CDC expert said, "A statistical sample is a numerator and denominator. And what you're talking about was numerator data, but what I wanted was an attack rate."

Hatfield lambasted him. "The house was on fire, and you had little interest in the fire," the senator said. "You were interested in how it started." He then excoriated the CDC, which "viewed the situation as a giant pastoral laboratory in which to conduct experiments" and to "practice its arcane statistical ritual."

And Ralph Peyton? He sued the National Park Service for failing to protect his investment by providing clean water to the lodge. He won a million-dollar judgment.

An Outbreak of Juvenile Arthritis

After his EIS graduation in July 1975, Allen Steere began a rheumatology fellowship at Yale. "I am not really being a traitor," he told his former CDC supervisor. "I believe that some rheumatic ailments are infectious diseases."

In November 1975 EIS officer David Snydman, the acting state epidemiologist for Connecticut, called Steere. Snydman had just heard about an unusual cluster of twelve juvenile rheumatoid arthritis cases in Old Lyme, a village of five thousand.

Juvenile rheumatoid arthritis was a rare disease supposed to affect one child in 100,000. Steere and Snydman contacted doctors, school nurses, local health officials, and mothers in Lyme and Old Lyme, looking for more cases.

They found a total of thirty-nine children and twelve adults who had suffered from arthritis since 1972, with a predominance of knee inflammations. Most cases began during the summer or early fall. Over half had had recurrent attacks. Blood and stool tests were negative for any known infectious agent. Although six families had multiple victims, they had contracted the condition in different years, which seemed to rule out airborne or person-to-person transmission. There was no common food, medication, immunization, or water source.

"The hit-or-miss pattern of onsets within families was most compatible with an arthropod-transmitted disease," Steere concluded. Arthropods, which include insects, spiders, mites, ticks, and crustaceans (to name a few), make excellent vectors for diseases.

One-quarter of the Connecticut patients reported an unusual expanding skin lesion that had appeared before the onset of arthritis. A Danish dermatologist at Yale told Steere that the lesions sounded like *erythema chronicum migrans,* a European condition thought to occur at the site of *Ixodes ricinus* tick bites, though no association with arthritis had been made. Suddenly the fact that all but three of the Connecticut families owned a dog or cat assumed significance.

Yet it was not the dog tick but the tiny deer tick (*Ixodes dammini*) that was the vector for the newly named Lyme disease. It took another six years before entomologist Willy Burgdorfer at Rocky Mountain Laboratories finally identified the responsible bacterium, which was duly christened *Borrelia burgdorferi.* It is a spirochete, a corkscrew-shaped microbe that, if untreated, can linger for years in the human body like the spirochete for syphilis, hiding from the immune system, and eventually affecting the brain, heart, and other organs.

For the next three decades, Steere would devote himself to studying the devious course of Lyme disease, as it spread throughout most of the country. It is now the most commonly reported arthropod-borne illness in the United States and Europe and is also found in Asia.

Why did it emerge as a public health problem only in the late twentieth century? "During the eighteenth and nineteenth centuries," Steere observed, "forests were destroyed in New England to make farms, and deer were hunted practically to extinction." But as farmland reverted to woods, the deer, now lacking predators, came back, along with their ticks. The suburban communities near the mouth of the Connecticut River were prime territory for Lyme disease. While deer are necessary for the tick, the spirochete life cycle requires two visits inside chipmunks or field mice, which also thrive in the suburban woodlands. Human beings as hosts are dead ends for the bacteria.

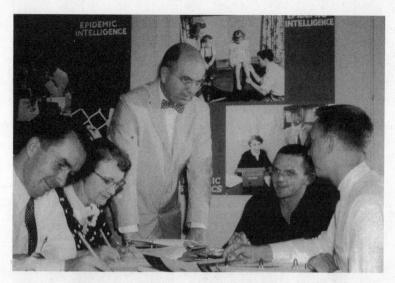

Alexander Langmuir, the founder and legendary chief of the Epidemic Intelligence Service, leans over recruits in a typically dominant pose. EIS officers Russ Alexander and Dorothy Califiore (one of the few female officers in 1955) are on the left.

Courtesy of Mary Jane Francis

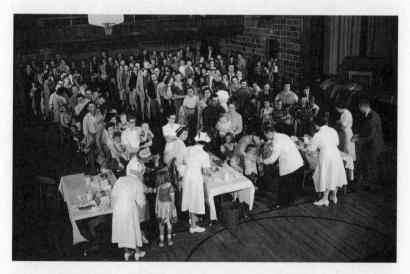

In April of 1955 the new killed-virus vaccine for polio, developed by Jonas Salk, was first given to U.S. children. Joy and optimism soon gave way to panic as the vaccine caused paralytic polio in some children. EIS officers traced the problem to live virus in some vaccines, primarily those made by Cutter Laboratories.

Courtesy of the March of Dimes Foundation

A corner of the EIS diploma shows an EIS officer "sliding down the epi curve to glory," a standing joke among epidemiologists who arrive just as an outbreak is burning itself out naturally, having run through the susceptible population. The EIS officer then takes credit for ending the epidemic.

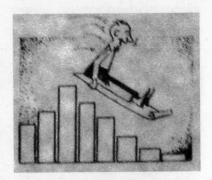

Courtesy of CDC

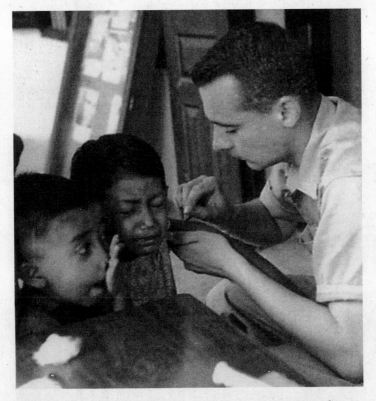

EIS officer Malcolm Page administers smallpox vaccine to apprehensive children in East Pakistan during the first major international EIS health expedition in 1958. "It is so difficult to travel through the villages and find the people," Page wrote. "Whenever we come in sight, the women run into hiding and just won't come out. . . . The children run into the jungle, climb trees." *Courtesy of Malcolm Page*

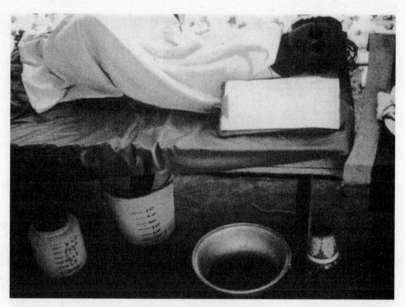

Cholera can kill within twenty-four hours by dehydration. In 1968 in Matlab, Bangladesh, a child lies on a cholera cot with a hole cut in the bottom to allow nearly continuous evacuation. EIS officers Barth Reller and Roger Rochat pioneered the use of oral rehydration therapy, which saved lives by replacing lost liquid and electrolytes — one of the greatest medical advances of the twentieth century.   *Courtesy of Barth Reller*

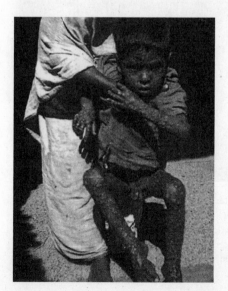

EIS officers took part in the final push to eradicate smallpox from India and Bangladesh in 1974 and 1975. This Indian boy suffers from the ancient disease that often killed the infected. The last wild case of smallpox occurred in Somalia in 1977. "It was almost a religious experience," EIS officer Walt Orenstein said. "It was so dramatic to see the disfigurement, the dead children, and to know you were getting rid of it."   *Courtesy of Richard Greenberg*

EIS officers have traveled by dogsled, helicopter, horseback, dugout canoe, and other unusual means. Here EIS officer Rick Greenberg (on left) rides an elephant in India in 1975 while pursuing smallpox. "Everything else in my life goes back to this moment in India, what we accomplished. It was a wonderful thing. You almost felt the earth should have stopped."

Courtesy of Richard Greenberg

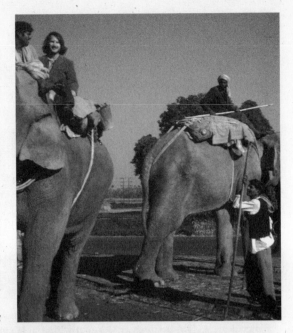

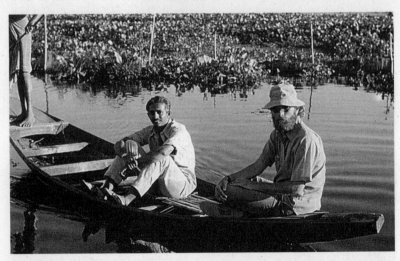

EIS officer Jeff Koplan (on right) takes to the waters of Bangladesh to help eradicate smallpox in 1975. He would later serve as director of the CDC. Sometimes he and other EIS officers forced vaccinations on unwilling people. Koplan explained that it was harmless, frequently vaccinating himself. If that did no good, "We chased and grabbed, and they got it anyway. But usually peer pressure from other villagers was enough."

Courtesy of CDC

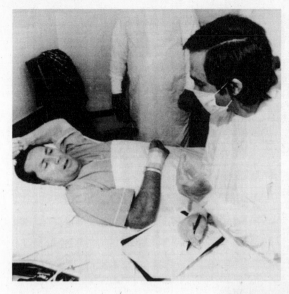

In 1976 a mysterious ailment struck down Legionnaires attending a convention in Philadelphia. At first it appeared that the dreaded swine flu had hit, but the culprit was finally identified as a new bacterium. Here EIS officer Steve Thacker questions a victim. "I turned around to look for the press," Thacker recalled, "and they weren't there." They were afraid to enter the room until the EIS officer reassured them.

Courtesy of AP Images

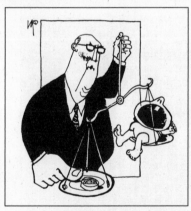

EIS officer Karen Starko's 1979 case-control study of children with lethal Reye's syndrome indicated that aspirin had caused the disease. Even after her findings were replicated, the aspirin industry successfully lobbied against warning labels for years, as this political cartoon indicates. Reye's syndrome has nearly disappeared now that aspirin is no longer given to children.

Cartoon by M. G. Lord, courtesy of The Nation

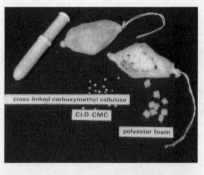

In 1980 EIS officers investigated women's deaths from toxic shock syndrome. Many were traced to use of the innovative Procter & Gamble Rely tampon, which resembled a bell-shaped teabag and swelled to completely fill the vagina, thus providing oxygen and a warm place for staph bacteria to multiply. The super-absorbent tampon "was a perfect little toxin factory," observed EIS officer Bruce Dan. *Courtesy of Bruce Dan*

Polio is the second major infectious disease targeted for eradication. Here EIS officer Kristy Murray administers an oral polio vaccine in Bangladesh in 2000. Polio is a more difficult enemy than smallpox, and success remains elusive.

Courtesy of Kristy Murray

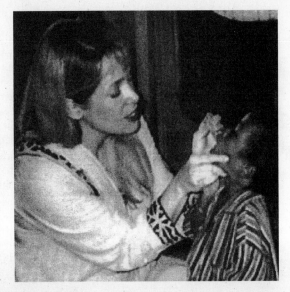

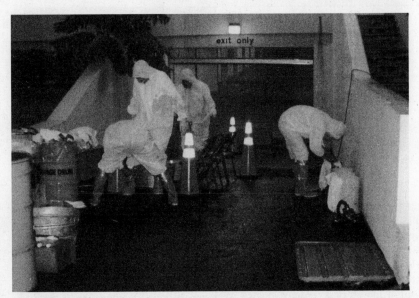

After a Florida photo editor died of inhalational anthrax in 2001, spores were found on his desk at American Media. EIS officers helped trace the bioterrorism that had spread through the mail in Florida; New York; Washington, D.C.; and New Jersey. Here FBI and CDC officials in protective suits prepare anthrax test samples for shipping outside the closed American Media offices.

Courtesy of Marc Traeger

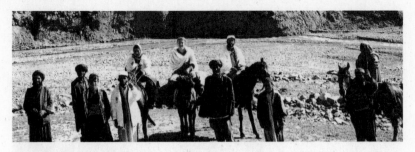

In 2002 EIS officer Linda Bartlett (center) rides into the remote mountains of Afghanistan, where she documented the highest rate of maternal mortality during childbirth ever recorded. Unattended women sometimes suffered from obstructed labor for days before dying, their babies undelivered. *Courtesy of Linda Bartlett*

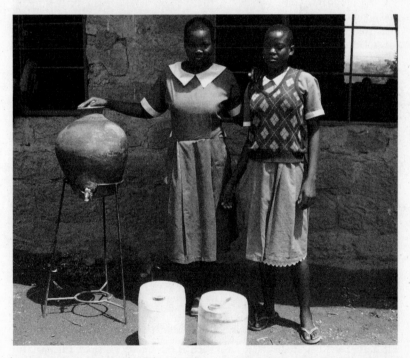

The Safe Water System (SWS), inspired by cholera investigations by EIS officers, features water containers with narrow tops to prevent hands from reaching into the water to recontaminate it after it has been disinfected with a mild bleach solution. Kenyan students pose with pots made by a local women's cooperative.

Courtesy of Ciara O'Reilly

In 2006 Senator Barack Obama visited Kenya, his father's native land, where he volunteered to be tested publicly for HIV to encourage Kenyan men to do the same. Here Obama walks with EIS alum Kayla Laserson. As president, Obama appointed EIS veteran Tom Frieden as the new CDC director.

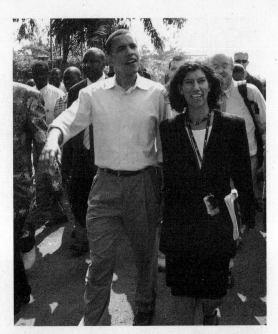

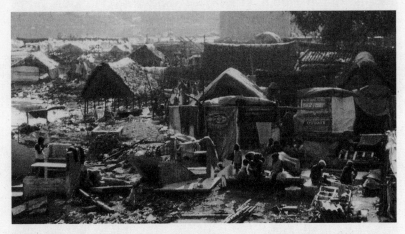

EIS alum Lee Riley studies slum areas such as this one in Saidapet, Chennai, India, where poverty and disease are bedfellows. As global warming raises sea levels, coastal slums in megacities will be inundated. "The most severe consequences of climate change will accrue to the poorest people in the poorest countries," writes EIS alum Mike St. Louis, "despite their own negligible contributions to greenhouse gas emissions." Malnutrition, unsafe water, and heat waves will increase.

11
TARGET ZERO

BY 1973 ONLY FOUR countries still reported major smallpox epidemics — India, Bangladesh, Pakistan, and Ethiopia. The most densely populated region, with the most smallpox, lay in the north of India along the Ganges River plain, including the states of Bihar and Uttar Pradesh.

EIS alum Bill Foege, head of the CDC Smallpox Eradication Program in Atlanta, was the chief proponent of the surveillance-containment strategy, which he had used successfully in West Africa.* In the spring of 1973 he attended an Asian smallpox planning session, where a discouraged Indian health minister said that his country was planning to push its eradication goal back to 1980. Foege assured him that if his government would only apply sufficient will, strategy, and resources, smallpox could be banished much sooner.

Swept away by his logic and charisma, members of the planning group agreed — but only if Foege himself would come to India. In August 1973 he moved to New Delhi with his family, leaving Mike Lane as head of the CDC smallpox program. Foege joined forces

---

*See pages 73–76, 101. In 1970, when Don Millar took over the CDC Bureau of State Services, Bill Foege became the head of the CDC smallpox effort.

with Nicole Grasset, a French epidemiologist, and M.I.D. Sharma, an Indian health official, both converts to the surveillance-containment strategy. He also recruited Don Francis, who, as an EIS officer, had headed the eradication effort in Sudan.

In October 1973 teams fanned out into the Indian countryside in a weeklong search for cases. "They went to a village, contacted the chief and schoolteachers, showed the smallpox recognition card, and asked if they had seen anyone recently with the disease," Foege said. "We found ten thousand new cases of smallpox. It was far beyond our ability to do containment."

The WHO teams conducted another search every month thereafter. Gradually, Foege and Francis improved the surveillance methodology. Their teams visited schools and asked children where they had seen smallpox. They went house to house. They walked through markets, beggar communities, and railroad stations, where many homeless people slept. Containment methods improved. "We would get a census of the village, who lived where," Foege said, "then go back late at night and find those who escaped previous visits. We adjusted, changing our tactics every month." Despite such efforts, smallpox continued to spread, particularly in Bihar, reaching a crisis point in May 1974. "In Bihar, we had 11,600 cases in just one week," Foege recalled.

At a meeting the following month, the Bihar minister of health ordered a return to mass vaccination. A young Indian physician protested. "When someone's house catches on fire, we put water on their house, not somewhere else." The minister agreed to give the surveillance-containment strategy a little more time.

Foege had recently discussed an idea with an Indian colleague. "It seems that an outside advisor has more credibility in India," he said. "I think if we get some international people here, locals will follow their lead." The colleague persuaded a top minister that the idea made sense. Epidemiologists from around the world were asked to come help with the smallpox crusade.

Many of those who responded were EIS officers and Public Health Advisors on ninety-day tours of duty. Using funds freed up by cutting the foreign quarantine budget — a bloated bureaucracy the CDC had taken over — CDC director David Sencer quietly paid for the program. "Dave Sencer is the unsung hero of smallpox eradication," Foege said. "He agreed to everything I asked."

"Don't Give Us Vaccinations — Give Us Food"

In mid-June 1974 the first wave of EIS officers arrived in India at the psychological low point of the entire campaign. They were given a three-day intensive course in the use of the bifurcated needle, surveillance containment, and Indian culture. Then the neophytes were sent off in a jeep with a driver and a paramedical Indian partner.

EIS officer Dan Blumenthal was assigned to the northern Bihar district of Samastipur, a thousand-square-mile area of rivers and rice paddies where a million and a half people lived in some 1,500 villages. There had been more than 4,000 cases of smallpox reported in the district since the beginning of 1974. When Blumenthal arrived, there were some 400 known active cases in 117 villages. But as he followed leads, he found many infected villages that had not been reported. Local health officers were underpaid and unmotivated. Many thought that the program was a waste of time because smallpox would never be eradicated.

"As the rains fell throughout July and August," Blumenthal observed, "the roads turned to mud, the rice paddies to lakes, and the lakes to floods." He borrowed an elephant when his jeep was mired in the mud. "When we finally got to the village, no one had been vaccinated, so we just vaccinated everyone we could find."

But finding people was not so easy. Most people were suspicious of the needle. Muslim women were not allowed to show themselves to strange men, though they might stick their arms out of a door to receive a vaccination. The majority of Indians were Hindus, many of whom worshipped Shitala Mata, the smallpox goddess with the power to cure or cause the disease. Vaccinations offended her.

Blumenthal vaccinated himself repeatedly to show that the procedure was harmless. He sought approval from the village headman.

Still, many people ran away, and some wouldn't allow their families to be vaccinated.

Smallpox wasn't the only problem afflicting Indians. "I saw kids with terrible malnutrition, people with huge goiters and rashes, people crippled by polio. Tetanus and cholera were major problems," Blumenthal remembered. "'Do you really want to help us?' people asked. 'Don't give us vaccinations — give us food.'

"At first, as I went from one outbreak to another, it felt like a rather purposeless adventure," he said. But smallpox transmission diminished naturally during the course of every rainy season, and as surveillance-containment efforts improved, the number of outbreaks diminished. "When I left the district at the end of my three-month assignment in early September," Blumenthal said, "the 117 outbreaks that were active when I arrived had been reduced to 34."

Steve Jones, a former EIS officer, was sent to the Bihar district of Muzaffarpur near Nepal. "The first few nights I lay there in this tiny bungalow with bugs all over me and geckos on the ceiling, thinking, *What the hell am I doing here?*"

But at the end of his first three months, he signed up again and ended up staying in India, then Bangladesh, for two years, helping to train other eradicators. "In five months, we went from a hundred infected villages in Muzaffarpur to very few. That was the addictive thing about smallpox eradication. There were no small steps."

One moonlit night, Jones investigated a case of possible smallpox in a small child. "It was obviously chicken pox," he recalled. "But the rule was that you vaccinated the household anyway," since one pox could be mistaken for the other. A young man in the house refused, but Jones held his arm and poked it with the bifurcated needle the requisite fifteen times. When Jones went outside, an angry crowd had gathered. "They thought we were robbers." He was clubbed over the head and was saved from being beaten to death only when his paramedical assistant threw himself over Jones's prone body. He realized that his overzealousness could backfire. "But I didn't use force a lot. And we were trying to accomplish this great thing. Smallpox was a killer."

The Second Wave

Late in August the second wave of EIS officers arrived in New Delhi. By that time, smallpox had been mostly contained in Uttar Pradesh, but there were still 2,600 active outbreaks in Bihar. Bill Foege gave a pep talk during one meeting.

"Now more than ever Bill thinks we can eradicate smallpox from the face of the earth," EIS officer David Pratt wrote in his diary. Pratt observed that "the epidemiologists at the meeting were from all over the world — Russia, Sweden, U.K., America, India and Burma. The unity of all these men [and women] in a common cause that transcends personal politics is refreshing and remarkable."

Pratt was responsible for the districts of Saran and Gopalganj. His diary recorded the swarms of mosquitoes coming through his netting at night, the floods, his driver stealing gasoline, his thoughts on mortality as he watched a Hindu cremation. Mostly, though, he wrote about his attempts to get Indian health officers to do their jobs.

SEPTEMBER 21, 1974: *Some of these guys are incredibly lazy. . . . They don't consider it negligent to wait a week before confirming a possible smallpox outbreak.*

SEPTEMBER 22, 1974: *We visited four tolas [neighborhoods]. Thirteen cases of smallpox were found. . . . We heard that cases [had gone] to a folk doctor. We checked with him. . . . Bottles of powder, paint and paste applied to leprosy, cutaneous TB and smallpox. High level quackery! We vaccinated him and his assistant.*

OCTOBER 4, 1974: *Unless you are shown otherwise you can assume that everyone is corrupt and takes bribes. . . . Doctors frequently lie to me.*

OCTOBER 7, 1974: *I really don't know how to express the sense of frustration. [This doctor] knows the problem, knows the methods to rectify it and won't do it. . . . I had my first failure to vaccinate a resistant woman. She would not listen to reason. . . . Finally, her husband got very agitated, started screaming and threw me out,*

*saying that I had insulted his house and that I had no right being
there (true). I really felt bad about that one.*

Despite his frustrations, Pratt witnessed smallpox cases gradually
dwindle. By the time he left in late November, there were no known
cases in his districts.

Elsewhere in Bihar, EIS officers Bob Fontaine and Wilbert Jordan
split the troubled Katihar District between them. "I went to villages
of aboriginal tribal people who used bows and arrows," Fontaine recalled. "With the chief, I had to smoke this overpowering tobacco
rolled up like a cheap cigar. Once we gained his confidence, he would
organize everyone for the vaccinations."

An African American born in rural Arkansas, Jordan grew up with
overt racism and was particularly disturbed by the Indian caste system. "If I sent someone into a village, and a Brahman said there was
no smallpox, he meant that there was no smallpox in the Brahman
section," Jordan recalled, even though among the Muslims or un-
touchables there would be many cases. "I had to hire different outreach workers—a Muslim, Brahman, and two tribal [untouchable]
doctors."

In what he describes as his "worst experience in India," at a state
dinner Jordan sat across from a tribal doctor who was served on a tin
plate while everyone else ate from expensive china. Jordan objected.
"I was told I was making a scene. We were there as guests of the government and were not there to change policies. It made me mad at the
white epidemiologists because they were able to adapt more easily to
the caste system. I had marched in Arkansas, and they expected me to
accept this?"

Being black was an advantage in Indian villages, though. "I was
more popular than any superstar. People would stare at Bill Foege,
this tall, blond-haired white guy, but I got more stares than he did."
Jordan also attracted attention by dancing. "In my head, I'd hear the
Impressions singing, 'People get ready, there's a train a-coming.' I'd
grab a kid and start dancing with him, and we'd dance and vaccinate.
My workers thought I was crazy, but that's how we got it done."

Jordan's approach didn't always work. In one village, a father refused to have his eleven children vaccinated. "When we came back two months later, nine had died of smallpox," he said.

When Fontaine and Jordan arrived in Katihar, there were 160 infected villages. By the time they left in December, there were only one or two. Six-foot-tall Jordan had lost 60 pounds, down to 134. An American lab identified seventeen kinds of parasites in his stool.

EIS officer Jason Weisfeld worked in three districts with relatively low transmission, which meant constant travel. "We ran from outbreak to outbreak twenty hours a day, living out of the jeep. . . . After discussing it with community elders, we often immunized villagers in the middle of the night, adding an element of surprise."

Even those who worshipped the smallpox goddess could be persuaded much of the time. "When they saw the infections, blindness, and death caused by smallpox, they didn't refuse other assistance," he said. Indian holy men influenced Weisfeld to begin a lifelong spiritual quest.

Endgame in India

By the time the third wave of EIS officers arrived in early December 1974, there was hope that smallpox might be banished from Asia within the next few months. Pakistan had detected its last case in November, leaving only India and Bangladesh on the continent, plus a few imported cases in Nepal.

A 50-rupee reward ($5.50) was introduced for anyone reporting a new smallpox case, and four local guards were hired for each smallpox-affected house (two during the day, two at night), to make sure that everyone who entered was vaccinated. The number of outbreaks had fallen steadily during the autumn, but with the end of the monsoons and the beginning of winter, rapid smallpox transmission could be expected.

EIS officer Rick Greenberg, assigned to the Rohtas district in eastern Bihar, dutifully instructed his block medical officers to fill in their containment books, to post guards outside houses, and to vaccinate everyone in surrounding areas. But smallpox kept spreading.

Greenberg said, "I naively believed that people would do what they said they would." After a few weeks, Bill Foege sent Steve Jones to train him.

Jones taught Greenberg to make unannounced spot checks. *Trust no one. Hire your own people and fire them if they don't perform.* It worked. "I hired people to verify that the work was being done, and then I hired people to spy on my spies." By the end of his three months, Greenberg got to announce to a cheering state assembly that Rohtas was free of smallpox.

EIS officer Walt Orenstein was assigned to the Gonda district of Uttar Pradesh, particularly the village of Paraspur, where smallpox had come roaring back. Rewards were pushed to 100 rupees for new cases.

After Paraspur was brought under control, Orenstein was transferred to Aligarh to stanch an outbreak there. In addition to routine house-to-house searches, he set up special teams to search for extra cases in the beggar community and at train and bus stations. It appeared smallpox might be gone, when Orenstein heard of a new case: a seven-month-old girl had died. The father had hidden his son's smallpox from Orenstein's vaccination team, and the baby had caught it from her older brother. She was the last case in Uttar Pradesh.

"I saw this terrible disease disappear before my eyes by using a vaccine in an epidemiologically defined strategy," he said. "It was an epiphany." Orenstein returned to the United States intent on employing a similar strategy to eliminate measles transmission there.

The day after Christmas 1974, EIS officer Mary Guinan joined Orenstein in Uttar Pradesh. Guinan, a medical doctor with a chemistry degree, had been at Johns Hopkins when she heard about the smallpox eradication program. "I wanted a chance to be part of this historic thing, ridding the world of smallpox."

She was the only female physician in her EIS class. "At Tuesday seminars they would call for smallpox volunteers," she recalled, "so I would ask to go. *No, India doesn't want women.* I pointed out that Indira Gandhi was the prime minister. I was persistent, and finally they let me go."

She arrived nearly a month into the third wave, assigned to Lakhimpur Kheri, a remote northern district in the foothills of the Himalayas, where smallpox was supposed to be gone but a suspect case had been reported. She found herself sleeping in an abandoned hospital full of rats gnawing at the door. "I sat up all night shining the flashlight to scare them away." Her jeep wouldn't cross the three rivers intersecting her district. She was relieved when a wealthy raja loaned her an elephant for a few weeks. "Elephants swim, it's incredible," she remarked.

In Lakhimpur Kheri, Guinan ran into all the usual problems, plus a new one. The Indian government was vigorously pressing for family planning. Rumors spread that the smallpox vaccination scar was a secret marker for those who would be sterilized. But she persisted, and the outbreak waned.

Guinan left in mid-April, her job in Uttar Pradesh done. "I petitioned to stay longer, but they wouldn't let me. Smallpox wasn't quite gone from India. It was close enough to smell it. It was intoxicating."

Bill Foege also returned with his family to the CDC in April 1975, confident that smallpox would soon be gone from Asia. The last case in India was identified in May. But in neighboring Bangladesh, outbreaks continued.

Hanging On in Bangladesh

EIS alum Stan Foster had been battling smallpox in Bangladesh since 1972.* In July 1973 EIS officer Jeff Koplan arrived to help Foster, taking charge of smallpox eradication in southern Bangladesh.

"Tomether akhane Bashunto Rugee ache?" the EIS officer asked schoolchildren, which in Bengali meant "Have you seen smallpox?" Then he showed them the grotesque diseased features on a smallpox identification card. "The kids would babble and point, and we'd ask the teacher if we could borrow little Mohammed for the afternoon." And so it went, tracing cases, sending containment teams.

Some people were afraid and ran away. Koplan explained that it

---

*See pages 113–114.

was harmless, frequently vaccinating himself. If that did no good, "we chased and grabbed, and they got it anyway. But usually peer pressure from other villagers was enough. We would meet with a religious elder, get approval, explain that smallpox was a threat to everyone."

Stan Music was doing the same thing in northwestern Bangladesh. He, too, arrived in July 1973, fresh from two years as an EIS officer in Florida. "There is one helluva lot of smallpox here," he wrote to a friend, "about 2,000 cases a week (most of them imported and most in my area)."

At first, Music and his teams launched what he called "almost military style attacks" on villages. "Women and children were often pulled out from under beds, from behind doors, from within latrines," he wrote. Music was frustrated by the lack of good surveillance information. "We learned very quickly that we couldn't trust the routine claims of freedom from smallpox."

In September 1973, in a remote village, Music found "one little boy, barely two years old, [who] was in the final agony of hemorrhagic smallpox." In that same village, there was a home where the husband refused to have his family vaccinated. "I broke the door down and vaccinated — with a struggle — every member of the family, including the man. He was very angry. We just couldn't let people get smallpox and die so needlessly."

By October 1974 only ninety-one infected villages remained in the country. But severe floods destroyed much of the harvest, and famine struck Bangladesh in November and December 1974. Refugees flooded the cities, and in the crowded conditions, smallpox flared up. Then many people departed for their native villages for the Eid al-Adha festival on December 22.

By the end of January, 572 villages had been reinfected. In mid-February the government ordered the bulldozing of all urban slums throughout Bangladesh, a disastrous program, since the slum dwellers seeded smallpox wherever they went. The Bangladesh secretary of health and the local WHO representative reacted to the new epidemics by suggesting a return to mass vaccination and abandonment of surveillance-containment efforts. "I thought we had lost the global program," Stan Foster said. "I wanted to quit, to go bury my head somewhere." At this nadir, Alexander Langmuir arrived as a consultant. "You should stay and fight it out," he advised Foster. "But either the WHO rep has to go or you do." Within a week the WHO director was reassigned to another country.

Another emergency influx of international epidemiologists arrived. Steve Jones and Don Francis brought much-needed expertise from India, including the system of four house guards and rewards for new case identification. House-to-house searches began for the first time, and up to twelve locals were hired to help vaccinate in each infected village.

Bangladesh, slightly smaller than the state of Iowa, contained some 80 million people in 1975. Yet by July, there were only forty-five outbreaks in the entire country. Only fifteen outbreaks were reported in August, and then the last case appeared to have been identified in September.

On November 15, 1975, Foster received three telegrams. The first two congratulated him on eliminating smallpox from Bangladesh. The third began: "ONE ACTIVE SMALLPOX CASE DETECTED." It was on Bhola Island in the Bay of Bengal. Rahima Banu, a three-year-old girl, survived, and she proved to be the last case of naturally transmitted *Variola major* on Earth.*

In October 1977 Ali Maow Maalin, in Somalia, was the last endemic case of smallpox (*Variola minor*) in the world.

The Legacy of Smallpox Eradication

Epidemic Intelligence Service officers always relied heavily on people around them, and nowhere was that truer than in their smallpox

---

*The last case of *Variola major* occurred in Birmingham, England, in 1978, due to a laboratory leak, so it was not naturally occurring. Smallpox virus was subsequently limited only to freezers at the CDC and in the Soviet Union. But the Soviets secretly experimented with their smallpox, and some virus may now be in unknown locations, possibly in the possession of terrorists.

eradication efforts. Epidemiologists from all over the world deserve credit for the success of the effort, but the greatest heroes were the Indians and Bengalis who devoted themselves to the cause.

It was not always easy for EIS officers to return to normal American life after the intensity of smallpox eradication. The urgency of their task and the immediacy of the results were addictive, and it gave them a perspective on what really mattered. "It was a very humbling experience," Wilbert Jordan recalled. "It made me appreciate what I had. I made myself a vow that if I ever got back to America and heard myself complaining, I would kick myself in the ass."

But it was also jarring to return and be treated like a regular person. "I was a superstar in India," Jordan said. Wynn Hemmert had reverse culture shock when he came home to his wife and two small children. "I was sort of a sick stranger for a while. My wife looked at me, obviously thinking, *What happened to you?*"

Mostly, though, they came back with an overwhelming feeling of pride and accomplishment. "It was almost a religious experience," Walt Orenstein said. "It was so dramatic to see the disfigurement, the dead children, and to know you were getting rid of it." For Rick Greenberg, "everything else in my life goes back to this moment in India, what we accomplished. It was a wonderful thing. You almost felt the Earth should have stopped."

Many veterans of the smallpox eradication crusade went on to become leaders in the world of public health. They brought a self-confident, can-do attitude, a refusal to accept that anything was impossible, a sublime impatience with stodgy bureaucracy or indifference to suffering. "We were cocky and arrogant, we smallpox warriors," Stan Music said. "We became tough to deal with sometimes. We knew you could overcome any obstacle if you just pushed hard enough."

Sometimes that pushiness in India and Bangladesh amounted to intimidation and coercion. "We overstepped," Steve Jones admitted. But the crusaders were, after all, trying to save lives, trying to rid the world of an ancient scourge.

A few years later Bill Foege called smallpox eradication "an incarnation of Gandhian ideals," which led to "non-violent social change [and] a better world."

D.A. Henderson summarized his approach to supervising field epidemiologists: "Give them running room, some support, and some backup. Ask them questions, make them think about what they are doing, but by God give them the room to move, then you have great things happen."

Don Francis, writing back to his colleagues about his 1973 smallpox eradication efforts in Sudan, mentioned the qualifications an EIS officer should have. "I think what the EIS course teaches us all is how to fly by the seat of our pants and come out on top. Just give all graduates a bit of baling wire, a piece of bubble gum, and a slide rule, and send them off."

In addition, Francis noted, officers should know how to repair Land Rovers and learn foreign languages. "Tolerance must be part of the curriculum" — tolerance for eating raw camel's liver, incredible heat, horrible roads, and cultural differences. Add to that "the ability to enjoy something in all this chaos," including scenes of great beauty, wonderful people, and "finally seeing one of the most wicked diseases disappear from the faces of children."

12
THE YEAR OF LIVING DANGEROUSLY

EIGHTEEN-YEAR-OLD Private David Lewis, in basic training at Fort Dix, New Jersey, felt lousy on a five-mile evening march on February 4, 1976. As he struggled to keep up, he gasped for breath, then collapsed. He died two hours later at the base hospital. A flu bug was taking its toll at Fort Dix. Lewis's flu had led to viral pneumonia.

The New Jersey state lab found that most throat swabs from sick soldiers detected the A/Victoria virus, the new H3N2 Type A strain, named for the Australian state where it had first been isolated. But the lab could not identify the flu virus from the throat swab of David Lewis or several others. Swabs were sent to the CDC in Atlanta. Late on February 12 CDC lab chief Walt Dowdle got the results. The dead soldier and three others had been infected with swine flu, H1N1, which normally afflicted only pigs.

Dowdle was stunned. He knew that the pandemic of 1918, which had killed at least 20 million worldwide, including more than 500,000 in the United States, had probably been caused by a similar virus. By the late 1920s the H1N1 virus had mutated to become less harmful in humans, then disappeared in 1957. No one knew exactly what had caused the 1918 pandemic, since no whole viral samples had been saved. But antibodies in the blood of survivors reacted with swine flu virus, which meant that they must be closely related. Virologists thought that humans must have passed the virus on to pigs during the pandemic, where it had survived since then.

In the United States, flu had hit twice in 1918. Some type of influenza appeared in March, causing a mild three-day illness. After spreading quickly in many countries, it vanished by summer. But in September, flu returned to the United States, having become a killer. It roared through several military camps, including Fort Dix, and then ripped through Philadelphia in October. Could this 1976 strain be the harbinger of another pandemic?

Dowdle immediately called CDC director David Sencer about the swine flu at Fort Dix. Sencer convened an emergency meeting of important immunization officials at the CDC for Saturday, February 14. By happenstance, famed virologist Ed Kilbourne Sr. had written an editorial in the *New York Times* on Friday, citing a theory of recycling pandemic strains and warning that swine flu was due to hit.

During the Saturday meeting, which included many EIS veterans, plans were developed to confirm the swine flu isolates, to look for further evidence of its spread, and to begin preparations for a swine flu vaccine. The official record of the meeting ended ominously: "The real question is—is this the beginning of the next pandemic? Will we expect widespread outbreaks of swine influenza in the U.S. next fall?"

Responsibility for influenza surveillance fell to former EIS officer Mike Hattwick, the head of the viral Respiratory and Special Pathogens Branch. An eight-year-old Wisconsin boy had contracted flu in October of 1975, and the Wisconsin state lab had sent the child's sera to the CDC, which found it was swine flu—merely interesting at the time, but now it seemed urgent.

Hattwick called Michigan-based EIS officer Mike Shasby and dispatched EIS officer Rick O'Brien from his Atlanta branch. On February 18, 1976, Shasby arrived in Sheboygan, Wisconsin, to meet the boy and his family on their hog farm, taking blood samples from the six children and their parents. He slogged into the frigid pens to bleed the pigs. O'Brien soon joined him. They visited other Sheboygan hog farms, bleeding more people and pigs. They also took blood from the boy's classmates, local slaughterhouse workers, volunteers at the county courthouse, patients at a hospital, and residents of a nursing home.

Serological tests revealed that the hogs on the first farm had swine flu antibodies. So did the boy's father and four siblings, even though none of them had become ill. None of the boy's classmates had antibodies. Most of the nursing home residents did, but that was to be expected, since they had lived through the 1918 pandemic and its aftermath.

Shasby and O'Brien concluded that people could indeed catch flu from swine, but that person-to-person transmission was unlikely to have occurred in Sheboygan. Each family member had probably caught it directly from the pigs. Otherwise, it should have spread in the school and elsewhere.

Meanwhile, EIS officers joined state health officials in taking blood samples from civilians living near Fort Dix. They found no evidence of swine flu. Army medical investigators looked back at sera taken from soldiers hospitalized at the fort in January and February. They identified 8 recruits whose illness had been caused by swine flu virus, bringing the total to 12 cases. When they bled 308 fellow platoon members of the original 4 cases, 68 (22 percent) tested positive for swine flu antibodies. The investigators planned a wider sample of Fort Dix recruits.

On February 27 Sencer and other public health officials met at FDA headquarters in Washington. Harry Meyer of the FDA Bureau of Biologics reported that vaccine manufacturers were working with swine flu seed virus, gearing up for a trial run with experimental vaccine. Hattwick reviewed the ongoing A/Victoria influenza epidemic. Excess mortality was looking sizable, comparable to the Hong Kong flu pandemic of 1968 that killed some thirty thousand people in the United States. So far, only one death could be attributed to swine flu.

In the middle of the meeting, a doctor called from Charlottesville, Virginia, to report that two hospitalized patients had swine flu antibodies. EIS officers Jim Veazey (based in Virginia) and Charles

Hoke from Hattwick's branch investigated and discovered that one patient had been feeding pigs for two weeks before her illness. The other had no known swine contact but had recently purchased home-slaughtered pork sausage, though he had not yet eaten it. They could find no evidence of ongoing transmission in either case.

By the first week of March the army had collected sera from 1,321 Fort Dix soldiers, of whom 273 tested positive for swine flu antibodies. The CDC projected that there were around 500 soldiers with subclinical infections at Fort Dix. None of the soldiers could recall any recent contact with pigs. It appeared that human-to-human transmission of swine flu had taken place.

The Swine Flu Campaign

On Wednesday, March 10, 1976, CDC director David Sencer convened a special meeting of the Advisory Committee on Immunization Practices (ACIP), along with other expert consultants. The group concurred that "it is likely that other [unrecognized] outbreaks are currently in progress or will be in the future." As far as anyone knew, there had never before been such a major antigenic shift without a resulting pandemic. It was agreed that "the production of vaccine must proceed and that a plan for vaccine administration be developed."

On March 24 President Gerald Ford dramatically announced "that unless we take effective counteractions, there could be an epidemic of this dangerous disease next fall and winter." Ford asked Congress to appropriate $135 million for enough vaccine to immunize everyone in the United States.

As the campaign ratcheted up in April, ACIP member and EIS alum Russ Alexander wrote to Sencer, "I strongly recommend some hesitation before beginning vaccine administration programs. . . . There still seems to be time to be cautious if there is no further evidence of significant swine flu outbreaks by September."

In mid-May Ron Hattis sent the CDC his lengthy paper, "The Swine Flu Scare: War Against a Phantom Epidemic?" As an EIS officer, Hattis had investigated rubella outbreaks on military bases that failed to expand far in the civilian population. He concluded that something similar may have occurred at Fort Dix. Like Alexander, Hattis urged that swine flu vaccine simply be stockpiled.

A CDC swine flu steering committee voted to reject the stockpile option, arguing that in the event of a swine flu epidemic, there would be insufficient time to immunize millions of people.

Field trials over the summer indicated that the vaccine worked for adults but was not potent in children. Only 2 percent of recipients developed adverse reactions such as fever, but insurance companies refused to cover the unprecedented program. Unless Congress agreed to indemnify the drug companies, there would be no insurance, and without insurance, no immunization.

A Deadly Veterans' Convention

On Monday, August 2, the members of the EIS class of 1976 reported for their first day of duty. At 8:45 A.M., new EIS officer Bob Craven's phone rang in his cubicle in the war room for the National Influenza Immunization Program. "Okay, so it's apparently pneumonia. Four dead? Twenty-six more are ill?" His voice rose with every phrase. "And they were all at the convention?" Craven was taking notes furiously. "Please get details and call back as soon as you can."

As Craven hung up, he banged on the cubicle partition. "This is it!" he yelled to his neighbor Phil Graitcer. "Swine flu." The caller was a doctor from the Veterans Administration Medical Center in Philadelphia. He had just learned about a disease afflicting Pennsylvania American Legion members who had attended their annual convention, held July 21 through 24 in the City of Brotherly Love.

Graitcer tried to call EIS classmate Jim Beecham, who had been assigned to the Pennsylvania State Health Department in Harrisburg. Busy. Busy. Busy. Finally he got through. Beecham said he was already fielding calls about the Legionnaires' illness and deaths.

David Sencer and other top CDC brass got a briefing. Within hours the first three EIS officers were flying to Pennsylvania. Graitcer reported to Philadelphia to work with EIS alum Bob Sharrar, the city epidemiologist, and John Harris, who had just moved to Philadelphia for a third-year EIS extension. Craven landed in Pittsburgh. Ted Tsai, the new EIS officer in the bacterial Special Pathogens Branch, headed to Harrisburg to join Beecham.

Sencer called a 7 P.M. meeting. The first priority was to rule swine flu in or out. Whatever it was, three first-year EIS officers couldn't handle it alone. To take charge in the field, Sencer tapped David Fraser, who had investigated Lassa fever in Sierra Leone as an EIS officer* and now headed bacterial Special Pathogens.

On Tuesday, August 3, Fraser flew to Harrisburg, while six field officers in nearby states drove to cities across Pennsylvania. Walt Orenstein arrived in Philadelphia to lead the CDC group there. Public health nurses searched their district hospitals for new Legionnaire cases. Obituary columns in local newspapers alerted the team to additional convention-related deaths. Beecham and Tsai compiled a list of 115 suspected cases, including 20 deaths. Three victims lived within ten miles of Fort Dix.

In the afternoon, the state lab called Graitcer to report on serum tests of Legionnaire victims' blood samples. They had tested positive for swine flu antibodies. Most victims were over fifty, though, so they were likely to have swine flu antibodies anyway. More definitive tests were necessary, and the results wouldn't be ready for a couple of days.

By Wednesday there were twenty EIS officers visiting hospitals across the state to interview Legionnaires. Many patients were on respirators in intensive care units and could not speak, but others could answer questions.

In Chambersburg, EIS officer Steve Thacker donned a surgical mask, gown, and gloves to talk to Legionnaire Thomas Payne, forty-eight, who had spiked a 108-degree fever but miraculously survived. Thacker went down his list of questions. Had Payne stayed at the Bellevue-Stratford, the grand old Philadelphia hotel on Broad Street that served as headquarters for the convention? When did he first feel ill? Had he attended the testimonial dinner? Did he eat the

---

*See pages 123–125.

Go-Getter's breakfast? Had he participated in the parade down Broad Street? Did he go to any of the hospitality rooms? What did he drink there? The final question must have seemed strange: "Did you have any contact with pigs?" No, he had not associated with swine.

In panic mode, the formerly deadlocked congressional health subcommittee moved to break the impasse over insurance, voting to make the government liable for injury or death claims resulting from swine flu vaccination. A few days later the legislation passed, clearing the way for vaccination to begin.

Exhausted EIS officers returned from the field. Few patterns emerged from the compiled questionnaire results, other than time spent at the Bellevue-Stratford. The disease appeared to have a five- or six-day incubation period, and fatalities occurred about a week after onset. Most of those who died were older, many of them heavy smokers and drinkers. First symptoms were achy muscles, malaise, and a slight headache, followed by a rapidly rising temperature, chills, and often abdominal pain, vomiting, and diarrhea. Breathing became labored, accompanied by a dry cough. Chest X-rays revealed patchy pneumonia. Autopsies found bloody froth in the lungs.

Lab scientists tried to identify an infectious agent from lung tissue. Bacteria were thought to have been ruled out within the first two days, along with fungi and rickettsia. Viruses took longer to identify, since they had to multiply in fertilized eggs. Finally, on Thursday morning, August 5, the injected eggs were ready. They revealed no evidence of swine flu or any other virus. "I think all of us can breathe a sigh of relief that this is not flu," Sencer told journalists. There was no evidence of secondary spread to family members or other contacts, and fewer illnesses and deaths were reported each day. The epicurve was forming into the classic bell shape of a common-source outbreak.

But what *was* the common source? Sencer said that lab work would continue, that "infection of some kind cannot be ruled out completely," but that the emphasis in the search had shifted toward toxic chemicals, either natural or man-made.

The Mystery Deepens

Phil Graitcer and other EIS officers pursued every possible lead. A garbage strike had left mounds of refuse on the streets. Could rats be spreading the disease? If the Bellevue-Stratford had something to do with it, why weren't hotel employees ill and dying? The only employee who had recently recovered from a flu-like illness was the twenty-six-year-old air-conditioning repairman, who refused to allow his blood to be drawn for tests.

The Legionnaires had used up the hotel's ice supply within an hour of their arrival in Philadelphia, so they brought in bagged ice. Graitcer found the ice manufacturer, inspected the plant, and secured water specimens, but could find nothing wrong. He collected Merit cigarettes given as free samples to the Legionnaires and sent them back to the CDC. He learned that high-class hookers had serviced some Legionnaires and wondered whether it could be a sexually transmitted disease. But he could not locate the prostitutes.

The media swarmed all over the story. Everyone from respected scientists to crackpots contributed their theories. With more than three thousand calls an hour flooding the CDC telephone lines, even director David Sencer helped answer the phones. *A military truck from Fort Detrick leaked lethal biowarfare germs. A left-wing group was trial-testing a poison they intended to use at the upcoming Republican National Convention. The plague was a warning from Martians that they didn't appreciate our Viking space probe. It was a Mormon plot.*

EIS officer Mitch Cohen took his share of bizarre calls, so, when someone called to say that he had come down with a similar pneumonia two years before at an Odd Fellows convention, Cohen could be forgiven for thinking that the caller was indeed just another odd fellow. "It was in September 1974," the man continued, "at the Bellevue-Stratford. I know a lot of others who caught it, too. One of them died." The man's claim turned out to be true. Cohen and fellow EIS officer Bill Terranova eventually found twenty cases, including three deaths, among those who had attended the 1974 convention. The incubation period and symptoms were strikingly similar to the

Legionnaires' disease, as virtually everyone now called the mysterious malady. It appeared that the Bellevue-Stratford had hosted a sporadic environmental microbe or toxin that became active only in certain conditions in late summer.

Friction and Frustration

After a week in Harrisburg David Fraser was certain that the key to the mystery lay somewhere in or near the Bellevue-Stratford Hotel. On Wednesday, August 11, Fraser moved his entire operation to Philadelphia. The team stayed in the Bellevue-Stratford, ostensibly as a sign of support for the beleaguered hotel, but he was also using himself and his EIS officers as guinea pigs.

Meanwhile, John Harris, Phil Graitcer, and EIS officer Carlos Lopez were plotting an epi-curve for non-Legionnaire pneumonia that had occurred near the hotel. Andrew Hornack, a three-hundred-pound bus driver, had driven a Pittsburgh high school band to march in the Legionnaires' parade on July 23. He had stood on the sidewalk in front of the Bellevue-Stratford only briefly to watch the students. Hornack died of what the EIS officers now named Broad Street pneumonia. The epi-curve of such illnesses nearly matched that of the sick Legionnaires. Fraser thought the bump in city pneumonias was an artifact of publicity — there probably weren't any more cases than usual, just more being brought to their attention. Harris thought that Fraser's official case definition — someone had to have entered the Bellevue-Stratford — ignored possible spread into the city. In addition, a nun and priest, who had stayed at the Bellevue-Stratford while attending the International Eucharistic Congress of Catholics, had come down with the illness.

Results from a case-control study (the first of several) had implicated the main lobby of the Bellevue-Stratford as the area most victims had in common. Friday, July 23, was the time of heaviest exposure. Fraser thought that the disease was probably airborne. After all, it primarily affected the lungs.

With George Mallison, CDC's veteran environmental investigator, EIS officer David Heymann crawled through the Bellevue-Stratford's complicated system of air-conditioning ducts, collecting dust samples. On the roof, Mallison found a possible cross-connection between the potable water supply and the water in the cooling tower. He also studied Philadelphia weather. There had been a temperature inversion from July 22 to 24, driving warm air down. The usual westerly wind had temporarily turned around to the east at the same time, and a two-week drought was broken by an afternoon shower on July 23, the day most Legionnaires were apparently exposed.

On Monday, August 16, two weeks after the investigation had begun, there was still no answer. Another case-control questionnaire was prepared and distributed, and a few days later the EIS officers scattered back to their regular assignments.

In Atlanta, Fraser and Ted Tsai analyzed all of the data. They identified 180 victims, 29 of whom had died. Most had attended the Legionnaires' convention, while seven were at the Eucharistic Congress held August 1 to 8, and three at the candle-makers' and magicians' conventions held at the Bellevue-Stratford just before the American Legion meeting.

The media and politicians turned on the CDC for its failure to solve the mystery, while Fraser and Sencer were grilled at congressional hearings. And in the wake of all the negative publicity, the Bellevue-Stratford closed.

More Deaths in Pennsylvania

On October 1, 1976, the first swine flu immunizations were given to the elderly and ill in Boston and Indianapolis. Within the first ten days, more than 2 million Americans were immunized.

On Monday, October 11, three elderly Pittsburgh residents died after being vaccinated in the same clinic on the same day in the same hour. They had all received the same lot of Parke-Davis vaccine. Within days thirteen states suspended their swine flu programs and demand fell dramatically elsewhere.

Phil Graitcer and Bob Craven visited the clinic to investigate and learned that around 10:30 A.M. on October 11, a sixty-four-year-old woman with a history of angina had complained of feeling dizzy after her shot. An ambulance arrived, sirens blaring, but by that time the woman felt okay. Then at 10:55 A.M. seventy-five-year-old Julia Bucci, who had been previously diagnosed with arteriosclerosis, said that she felt weak just after receiving her vaccination. The ambulance was called back, and she was taken away. She died of a heart attack an hour later. At 11:10 A.M. an eighty-three-year-old woman who had sat near Bucci in the waiting area summoned a policeman and said she felt that she was going to collapse. A rescue vehicle was summoned for the third time to take her to the hospital, where she recovered quickly.

At 11:15 A.M. seventy-one-year-old Charles Gabig, who had witnessed all of this, was vaccinated. Overweight, with a history of heart problems, he died of acute myocardial infarction two hours later. Ella Michael, seventy-four, who had heart disease and emphysema, was vaccinated at 11:25 A.M., after asking a clinic nurse what was wrong with the patient being taken out on a stretcher. She died later that day of a heart attack.

Laboratory analysis found nothing wrong with the Parke-Davis vaccine, and there had been no adverse reactions from the fourteen thousand other injections. Graitcer and Craven concluded that "the anxiety provoked by seeing medical emergency procedures being performed may have precipitated these deaths." In other words, three older people with preexisting heart problems had probably worried themselves to death.

The swine flu program slowly revived. The CDC explained that coincidental deaths after vaccination — particularly of the sick or elderly — were bound to occur. By October 15 there had been thirty-five such deaths, each investigated by an EIS officer.

Terror in Africa

EIS officer Joel Breman had just attended the autopsy of a Detroit man who had died of a heart attack shortly after inoculation with the swine flu vaccine when he received a phone call. Breman listened, his brow furrowing. "A new African disease? One hundred percent mortality? Wow. I see. Let me talk it over with my family."

He was not eager to leave his wife and two children. On the other hand, the mysterious disease now ravaging rural Zaire and southern Sudan might be the biggest challenge of his career. So, on the evening of Friday, October 15, 1976, Breman was on an airplane crossing the Atlantic, sharing stories and bourbon with Karl Johnson from the CDC Bureau of Laboratories. Between the two men sat another EIS officer, who said little. The CDC men stopped at the World Health Organization in Geneva on their way to Africa, both out of courtesy and to get any information they could. The reticent EIS officer, terrified, decided to return to Atlanta.

By chance, on their midnight connecting flight to Kinshasa, Breman and Johnson sat near Bill Close, an American doctor who was the personal physician to Mobutu Sese Seko, the dictatorial president of Zaire. Close promised to help in any way he could.

Arriving at 6:30 A.M. on Monday, October 18, Breman and Johnson were whisked directly to the Belgian Medical Mission, where a meeting of international health officials was in progress. Breman was told that the epidemic had begun in the village of Yambuku, about six hundred miles to the northeast. A Catholic mission hospital run by Belgian nuns had been its epicenter. Eleven of seventeen hospital staff were dead. A Belgian nursing sister, brought to a Kinshasa hospital, had died of hemorrhagic fever on September 30. A nun who had cared for her had died October 14, and now Mayinga, a Zairian nurse, was suffering from the disease. They had given her convalescent serum brought from South Africa from Marburg survivors,* hoping that it might help. As far as anyone knew, Mayinga was the only such case there in the capital of Kinshasa.

The entire Bumba zone, where the outbreak had occurred, was now quarantined. There was an airplane waiting to fly a team to the city of Bumba, from which they would drive to Yambuku to find and stifle the epidemic.

Good, thought Breman. *They seem organized, and they have a plan.* The health commissioner stopped, with an air of expectation. In the

---

*Serum is the part of blood that contains antibodies. Marburg virus, which causes another hemorrhagic disease, was identified during a 1967 outbreak in Marburg, Germany.

tense silence, all eyes turned to Breman and Johnson, and Breman realized that *they* were the intended team. The hungry, sleep-deprived CDC men were supposed to hop directly on a plane to track down the deadly virus. They politely refused, explaining that Johnson would remain in Kinshasa to set up a laboratory. That afternoon they visited the hospital to examine the ailing Mayinga.

The following morning Breman and a team of four other doctors — two Belgians, one Zairian, one other American — flew on President Mobutu's airplane to Bumba. The plane was expected to return in four days. After sleeping at the Catholic mission, the team took the bumpy, muddy road to Yambuku.

At the mission they found only three Belgian nuns and an elderly priest. The rest of the staff and patients had fled or died. "We were scared out of our wits," Breman recalled. "We didn't know if we would get it." Over a bottle of Johnnie Walker, the sisters told them that the first known case was a teacher at the mission school, who had developed a fever shortly after returning from a mission tour to the north in late August. A nursing sister gave him a shot of chloroquine, believing that he had malaria. A few days later his diarrhea turned bloody, and he died on September 8.

Nine other hemorrhagic cases occurred during the first week of September. All had received treatment for other diseases at the outpatient clinic. Then the first nun, a midwife, died. Other medical staff and patients also succumbed. The surviving nuns and the priest had not directly cared for patients.

Breman realized that the disease might have been spread by hospital procedures. The next day the doctors split into four teams to visit nearby villages, with the nuns and a local missionary acting as interpreters. Breman was relieved to find that, while many had died, most villagers remained well, having escaped the disease.

Over the next three days, the teams visited sixty-seven villages, forty-three of which had been infected. Eight villages still had active cases. In the first rough estimate of suspected patients, 353 cases were recorded, of whom 325 had died already. After a weeklong incubation period, victims developed excruciating headaches and fever, followed by diarrhea and exhaustion. Patients were vomiting and excreting blood by the fourth day. Many bled from the nose, ears, and vagina. Patients generally died a week after their first symptoms appeared.

While the mortality rate was incredibly high, transmissibility appeared to be relatively low. Pregnant women seemed to be particularly susceptible, and when they delivered stillborn, premature infants, they apparently transmitted the disease to their caretakers. Those who washed and prepared bodies for burial often contracted the disease. The epidemic had peaked in the last week of September.

One evening, masked, gowned, and sweating profusely from humidity, heat, and fear, Breman toured the eerily silent Yambuku Mission Hospital, with its 120 empty beds. The facility had treated more than six thousand people a month. Most came for outpatient injections, including pregnant women who wanted vitamin shots. Mere pills were not considered to be as potent as medicine delivered by a magical needle. There, in the delivery room, he found a vaginal speculum, scalpel, and a syringe on a tray. Carefully, he placed them in a plastic bag.

Breman learned that five syringes and needles had been issued every morning to the outpatient staff and prenatal clinic. Used throughout the day, they were rinsed in a pan of warm water between patients, but boiled only at night — a perfect way to spread a blood-borne disease.

After three days the team drove back to Bumba, but no airplane arrived. The Catholic mission radio could not reach Kinshasa. Two days later Breman was summoned to the Protestant mission, where he was relieved to hear the voice of EIS alum Joe McCormick over their shortwave radio. The president's airplane was unavailable, McCormick explained, because Mobutu had flown his family to Europe to avoid the epidemic. The team had to arrange for another flight.

On October 27 an airplane finally arrived. The doctors boarded with two Zairians who had miraculously survived the disease and from whose blood a serum could be prepared that might treat future patients. Mayinga, the nurse, had died. She proved to be the last case in Kinshasa.

The team had been unable to verify the source of the epidemic, its reservoir, intermediate hosts, or possible vectors. But at least they could name the virus. "We would like," said Johnson, in a tape recording he and Breman made for their colleagues in the United States, "to propose the name *Ebola,* taken from a small river that flows just to the north of Yambuku."

Ebola in Sudan

On October 30 Joe McCormick was airlifted with a Land Rover to Kisangani, Zaire, near the Sudanese border. In southern Sudan, another Ebola outbreak had preceded Yambuku's by a few weeks. McCormick's task was to find the link between the two.

Without authorization or proper papers, he crossed into Sudan to reach the town of Nzara, where the Ebola epidemic had begun. He entered the hospital, where he found only one doctor. "The patients, the nurses, all of them are running away," he told McCormick. Seven of thirteen patients had died of the new disease.

The first patient had worked at the local cotton factory, as had many subsequent victims. Visiting the factory, McCormick looked up and saw that the high ceiling was festooned with bats. He wondered if they might be the Ebola reservoir.

McCormick knew that EIS alum Don Francis was part of a WHO team designated to investigate the south Sudanese outbreak, so he left him a note, detailing what he had discovered. He then covered the difficult five hundred miles to Yambuku, within northern Zaire. He found no evidence of Ebola anywhere along the route. Convinced that the outbreaks in Sudan and Zaire were not connected, McCormick returned to Kinshasa.

Hours after he left, Francis arrived and read the note. Investigating further, he discovered that one of the cotton factory victims had belonged to a local sex club, where transmission took place. "When the owner of the club got sick," Francis said, "he had enough money to go to the teaching hospital in Maridi."

In Nzara, the epidemic died out, but at the larger Maridi hospital, it exploded. When Francis and his colleagues arrived in early November, the head doctor and sixty-one nurses had come down with Ebola, and thirty-three had died. The disease had spread widely in the town. The epidemic was stopped when disposable protective gear was distributed to hospital staff and proper isolation techniques were employed. The last case in Sudan was admitted to the Maridi hospital on November 25.

To get specimens, Francis conducted an autopsy on a patient who had just died, carrying the body outside because hospital staff wanted nothing to do with it. "As I sat on the ground cutting open the body, I wore a respirator, protective gown, and double gloves," he recalled, "but it started to rain, and my clothing stuck to my skin. In retrospect, it was not smart." The liver was enlarged, and blood poured from it when cut, but the other organs appeared normal.

"The toxicity of this disease was unbelievable," Francis said. "Even those who recovered lost half their body weight, and then they peeled. We had people who peeled so extensively that they shed a cast of their feet, calluses, toenails, and all."

The Sudanese Ebola outbreak affected 284 people, killing 53 percent of them. The final patient tally in Zaire was 318 and the death count 280, yielding an incredible 88 percent mortality rate. The Zaire and Sudan strains were later proven to be genetically distinct.

The reservoir for Ebola remained a mystery. In humans, it was a dead end, since it killed so quickly and efficiently, and it required close contact with blood or urine to spread. Small epidemics had probably gone unnoticed in remote villages. It was only when hospitals and their needles amplified Ebola spread (and when white people died) that it attracted worldwide attention.

As Joel Breman returned to Yambuku on November 10 for comprehensive surveillance of the now-contained outbreak, along with a collection of blood samples to check for antibodies, he pondered a worst-case scenario. *If Ebola ever adapts to humans,* he thought, *so that it gets into the respiratory tract and has efficient airborne transmission, it could lead to the extinction of the human race.*

An Ascending Paralysis

The Ebola epidemic received scant attention in the United States compared to the unsolved Legionnaires' mystery and the ongoing swine flu drama. On November 29 EIS officer Henry Retailliau reported that he had tabulated 103 deaths following swine flu vaccination, but that they matched patterns in the general population. "A death from Guillain-Barré one month after vaccination has been reported," he mentioned, but otherwise most died from heart problems.

Within a few days, however, eight more Guillain-Barré syndrome cases were reported. No one knew what caused the neurological disorder, named after two French doctors who identified it in 1916. Frequently, it is preceded by an acute respiratory illness. Beginning with numbness in the legs, paralysis creeps up the body, affecting the arms and occasionally the face. Most people recover quickly, but some suffer permanent nerve damage, and about 5 percent die. Since Guillain-Barré was rare, national reporting was not mandatory, so it was hard to know what level was abnormal.

EIS alum Larry Schonberger was put in charge of the investigation. As active surveillance identified more cases, Schonberger noted that they were clustering in the second or third week following vaccination. On Monday, December 13, he presented the facts to CDC leaders. His data indicated that vaccinated people had twice the risk of developing the syndrome as the unvaccinated. From his home on Martha's Vineyard, Alexander Langmuir advised, "Just keep your eye on it. It looks suspicious now, but it might just disappear."

The next day Schonberger got a call from the New Jersey state epidemiologist, EIS alum Ron Altman, who reported that his state's cases were probably being undercounted, since the vaccination program had started two weeks late there.

At 2 A.M. Schonberger awoke to a realization. "My god, I have it!" His long division to determine risk had used the number of persons vaccinated and unvaccinated as denominators. Instead, he decided to use "person time" in the denominator, adjusting for the time period during which someone was or was not vaccinated. By this time, Wednesday, December 15, a total of ninety-four cases of Guillain-Barré syndrome had been found in fourteen states, with four deaths. Fifty-one had been vaccinated within three weeks of the onset of paralysis.

When Schonberger recalculated the figures using person time, he found that vaccinated people had more than seven times the risk of developing the syndrome as the unvaccinated. These figures were convincing, and the CDC suspended the swine flu vaccination program on December 16.*

Finally, a Solution

Cleaning up his lab in preparation for the new year, Joe McDade decided to reexamine a Legionnaire outbreak slide he had made by smearing a section of guinea pig spleen over the glass. Thirty-six-year-old McDade had been at the CDC for only a year. In the late 1960s he had worked at Fort Detrick, specializing in Q fever, a rickettsial disease considered ideal for biological warfare because it was debilitating, usually nonlethal, and had no secondary spread.

Rickettsia are smaller than normal bacteria and will not grow on regular agar plates, so McDade had ground up lung specimens from dead Legionnaires and injected them in guinea pigs, looking for Q fever. When the guinea pigs sickened, he sacrificed them and made slides, using an unusual stain that worked on rickettsia. He saw a few bacteria on the slides, but he figured they were contaminants. He also injected guinea pig spleen into fertile eggs. To eliminate contaminating bacteria, he added antibiotics. Nothing grew.

Now on December 27, he took his time reexamining a slide, looking at a hundred separate microscopic fields. After a half hour, he came across a large cluster of bacteria, indicating real growth, not mere contamination. *Hmmm.* He decided to inject sick guinea pig spleen into fertile eggs again, but without antibiotics this time. After three days the egg embryos died. They were teeming with rod-shaped bacteria and reacted strongly to antibodies in Legionnaires' convalescent serum.

---

*While vaccination with the swine flu vaccine was associated with contracting Guillain-Barré syndrome, subsequent influenza vaccines have not been implicated.

McDade had solved the mystery of Legionnaires' disease. It was caused by an "exceedingly fastidious" bacterium, later christened *Legionella pneumophila*. It grew only in fluid with high concentrations of iron and the amino acid cysteine. Fortunately, it responded well to erythromycin and tetracycline, common antibiotics.

When McDade reported his preliminary findings, John Bennett suggested testing them against specimens from the 1965 St. Elizabeths Hospital outbreak. The antibodies reacted strongly to the *Legionella* bacteria. A few weeks later Pontiac fever specimens were reexamined. They, too, contained Legionnaire antibodies.*

Innocence Lost

The year 1976 marked a turning point for the Epidemic Intelligence Service as it reached its twenty-fifth anniversary. Up until then, the CDC had largely flown under the political radar. That began to change with Senator Mark Hatfield's 1975 fury at the CDC for failing to close Crater Lake earlier. With swine flu, the CDC was lambasted for making the opposite mistake — acting too quickly to avert what turned out to be a phantom outbreak.

During the swine flu campaign, an unprecedented 47 million Americans were vaccinated, proving that mass immunization campaigns were doable. Even the Guillain-Barré disaster showed that the influenza surveillance system worked. As Lyle Conrad observed later in the year, however, the focus on swine flu had diverted resources from other immunization programs. Measles cases shot up 64 percent over the previous year.

The Legionnaires' outbreak had not been a shining hour for the CDC disease detectives either. Before McDade's laboratory breakthrough, the official conclusion was that the disease was probably airborne, with the Bellevue-Stratford lobby implicated, but the final Epi-Aid report incorrectly stated that "several possible sites of exposure outside the hotel (sidewalk . . . etc.) were not associated with illness."

---

*See pages 69, 97–99. It was not clear why the Pontiac fever version of *Legionella* was more contagious yet less lethal. The bacterium was most deadly to older people in poor health, such as the hard-drinking, chain-smoking veterans.

McDade's lab test proved that the so-called Broad Street pneumonias were indeed caused by the same *Legionella* bacterium.

As subsequent EIS investigations found, the *Legionella* bacteria were widely distributed in nature, but they proliferated and were aerosolized in human-engineered environments such as cooling towers, showerheads, and sprinklers. The bacteria had probably multiplied in the cooling tower on the Bellevue-Stratford roof, flowed down the front of the building during the brief wind shift and temperature inversion, then washed into the lobby and/or had been sucked into the air-conditioning system.

The terrifying Ebola virus came from somewhere in the rain forest but probably was not new. It killed hundreds of people primarily because victims were injected with unsterilized needles. At the same time, preventable infectious diseases such as measles, tetanus, tuberculosis, and malaria were still devastating the developing world. As the human population expanded and pushed into new environments, nature was likely to come up with more surprises, and with the global village shrinking, diseases would spread more quickly. Finally, 1976 reminded public health experts that nature was difficult to second-guess. Swine flu did not necessarily return in predictable cycles.* "Will the program's failure damage the credibility of future immunization programs?" asked Larry Altman in the *New York Times*. Measles and diphtheria vaccinations were already at dangerously low levels in the United States. What would happen in the next few years?

---

*Ironically, H1N1 flu (related to swine flu) appeared in China in the fall of 1977 and swept the world. It was identical to a 1950 ancestor of the strain that had disappeared in 1957, so it affected only those without antibodies, who were twenty years old or younger. Virologists concluded that it had escaped from a laboratory freezer. It is still circulating at low levels.

13

SUPERWOMEN (AND MEN)
OF THE LATE SEVENTIES

ON FEBRUARY 7, 1977, David Sencer was publicly fired by incoming HEW secretary Joseph Califano, who insisted that it had nothing to do with the swine flu campaign, but no one believed that. Califano appointed Bill Foege as the new CDC director. EIS alum Foege, who had pushed the surveillance-containment method for smallpox eradication, promised to continue Sencer's emphasis on scientific rigor and integrity. "We expect to be tougher than our critics," he said. "And if you look at the last year, that might require some imagination."

The July 1977 EIS training class included five female officers, part of a wave of smart, self-confident women who would enter the program in the next few years. Two years later the EIS skit at the end of their training would feature numbers called "Superwoman" and "What If Women Ran the CDC." There was a reason for broader recruitment efforts: physicians no longer needed to avoid the draft. Most who chose the EIS now did so because they were already interested in public health.

New EIS administrator Mary Moreman actively recruited men and women in medical schools and teaching hospitals, where she could count on EIS alums to refer good candidates. She also started a program for senior medical and veterinary students to work with EIS officers during an eight-week elective — another effective recruiting strategy.

The chronically underfunded EIS program continued to evolve and grow, somehow scraping by "after fits and starts complicated by the budgetary crisis in HEW and the lack of a continuing resolution to cover CDC's budget this fiscal year," as a 1977 issue of the *EIS Bulletin* stated.

In April 1977 Secretary Califano announced that in the next two years, 90 percent of the country's children would be immunized against diphtheria, pertussis, tetanus, polio, measles, rubella, and mumps. EIS alum Alan Hinman returned to the CDC to take charge of the Immunization Division and to coordinate the enormous effort. By 1980 all fifty states would mandate proof of childhood immunization as a school entry requirement unless parents objected. Thus, the abrupt abandonment of swine flu immunization did not, as some had feared, hurt future vaccination efforts.

At the global level, EIS alum Rafe Henderson (with the CDC still paying his salary) moved to Geneva in 1977 to jump-start the World Health Organization's Expanded Program on Immunization (EPI), the successor to the successful smallpox eradication effort. While other diseases might not be quickly eradicated, at least the mortality from measles (a killer in Africa), tetanus, and other childhood infections could be reduced. In July 1977 EIS officer David Heymann moved with his family to Cameroon to implement the EPI program there.

The Expanded Program on Immunization aimed to reach 80 percent of the world's children with standard childhood vaccines by 1990. CDC director Bill Foege stressed that saving lives in the developing world required two things — adequate vaccination and safe water. He moved to reset priorities for the CDC, seeking input from EIS officers and employees. A CDC "Red Book Committee," created in December 1977, came up with a list of health problems that went well beyond the traditional focus on infectious diseases. Cancer, cardiovascular disease, alcohol use, environmental hazards, motor vehicle accidents, smoking, violence, and unwanted pregnancy made the list.

Claire Broome and Vaccine Efficacy

In August 1977 freshman EIS officer Claire Broome, assigned to the bacterial Special Pathogens Branch, investigated an increase in pertussis cases at Grady Memorial Hospital's emergency room, which served Atlanta's impoverished African American population.

The disease, caused by the bacterium *Bordetella pertussis,* is nicknamed whooping cough, since in its paroxysmal stage it causes a severe hacking cough followed by a sharp, high-pitched intake of breath. It can kill infants, and in the Atlanta outbreak, 39 percent of the 115 cases were under the age of one. Fortunately, only five (all unvaccinated) were severe cases, and none died. In Broome's Epi-Aid, she suggested that vaccination rates (three doses by six months of age) be increased and that laws mandating vaccination before school entry be enforced.

Vaccine efficacy became Broome's primary interest. In 1977 a new vaccine against *Streptococcus pneumoniae* had been licensed after South African clinical trials. The vaccine protected against fourteen of some ninety known serotypes of *S. pneumoniae,* but no one knew how well it would work in the U.S. population.

Broome set up a surveillance system to track which serotypes were causing disease in the United States to identify any shifts that might indicate that the vaccine must be modified. Then she began to get requests from physicians for serotyping vaccinated patients who had come down with pneumococcal pneumonia. "In a true *aha* moment," she recalled, "I realized that I was staring at data that could tell me how well the vaccine worked." If it were 100 percent efficacious, then none of the vaccinated patients would have any of the fourteen serotypes in the vaccine.

Using an algebraic formula to compare the strains causing disease in the unvaccinated versus the vaccinated, she could estimate vaccine efficacy without resorting to a huge, expensive field trial. Broome's method (still in use) showed that the vaccine worked only half the time. That figure has been gradually improved over the years.

The Devious Transmission Routes of Hep B

In 1977 there was still no effective vaccine for hepatitis B. The blood-borne pathogen, which could linger in the body and cause long-term liver damage, was spread when blood or semen from one victim entered another person's bloodstream.

EIS officer Steve Hadler went to Elbert County in northeast Georgia in August 1977 for an outbreak of hepatitis B among injecting drug users. He uncovered sixteen cases, young whites aged fifteen to twenty-four, that had occurred over the previous ten months — twelve men and four women. Nine had been hospitalized. Hepatitis B had spread at first among habitual male drug users, and then through shared needles at two large parties. In his report, Hadler concluded that the best way to combat future outbreaks was to educate high school students about the hazards of needle sharing.

In September 1977 Hadler investigated a New Orleans dialysis center where seventeen patients and one staff member had contracted hepatitis B over the last year. His case-control study failed to pinpoint the problem, though he observed breaks in sterile technique when staff neglected to change gloves between each patient and shared hemostats and clamps between dialysis stations.

EIS alum Jim Maynard, director of the Phoenix CDC lab where Hadler was based, realized that the homosexual community would be perfect for field-testing the new hepatitis B vaccine made by Merck. A man with hepatitis could infect a woman during sex, but anal intercourse, during which the lining of the colon could easily be abraded, was a more effective mode of transmission. In 1978 Maynard recruited EIS alum Don Francis to organize the trials. Hadler spent much of his last EIS year working with homosexual subjects, getting baseline data on hepatitis B rates before starting the trials.

The Last Diet They Would Ever Need

The FDA learned of eleven women who died after drastic weight loss. All had read *The Last Chance Diet: When Everything Else Has Failed*, by Pennsylvania osteopath Robert Linn. Published in the fall of 1976, the book soared to the bestseller list. Was something wrong with the liquid protein diet? Was there product contamination?

On Tuesday, November 1, 1977, FDA official Richard Swanson called EIS officer Harold Sours. On Thursday Sours received basic information on the patients and their location. Swanson asked for a report by the following Tuesday, when the FDA had already announced it would hold a press conference.

Sours called state-based EIS officers, asking them to get victims' medical records. He requested anything about diets or starvation from the CDC librarian. Over the weekend he flew to Minnesota, where several women had died. On Monday he flew to Cleveland, where a man attending a Case Western Reserve diet clinic had perished. Then he returned to Atlanta, got a few hours' sleep, and caught an early morning plane to Washington, D.C., just in time for the press conference.

On the various airplanes, Sours read a book written by Jewish doctors trapped in the Warsaw Ghetto during World War II. "They described the same EKG patterns and voltage decreases I was seeing in these medical charts," he said. "I concluded that these dieters were probably dying of starvation, not from a contaminated product."

At the press conference, he reviewed the eleven cases and stated his preliminary conclusions. Within the next few months Sours turned up a total of fifty-eight diet-related deaths, but he narrowed his investigation to seventeen that fit a distinctive pattern. With the exception of one man, all were women between the ages of twenty-three and fifty-one who had died of cardiac arrhythmias after following Linn's diet advice. None had heart problems before the weight loss. They had subsisted on three hundred calories a day in what Sours termed a "supplemented fasting diet." That meant drinking a liquid dietary supplement — basically gelatin, containing collagen, a protein component of connective tissue.

The deceased dieters were from ten states and the Canadian province of Ontario. Sours recognized a sad pattern in the cases. Typical was a thirty-three-year-old woman, who had worked as a lab technician for a doctor. She stood five four and weighed 247 pounds. In

March 1977, over the objections of her employer and her private phy-sician, she went on the diet, supplemented by multivitamins. Her anx-ious doctor examined her as she lost 90 pounds over seven months. Her vital signs and potassium levels remained normal. Near the end of October she fainted twice at work and was admitted to the hospital. The next day she had several episodes of ventricular fibrillation and, despite treatment, died that night.

Sours concluded that the problem was systematic self-starvation. The FDA had hired a polling firm to conduct a national random tele-phone survey to determine how many young to middle-aged white women had gone on the liquid protein diet for two months or longer. From this data, Sours estimated a rate of 59 annual deaths per 100,000 dieters.

Since Linn's liquid protein supplement was a food product, ban-ning it would be like outlawing cottage cheese. The issue was how it was used. By the time 1978 commenced, the fad diet had crashed, along with sales of the supplements, due to adverse publicity and cau-tionary statements from the FDA.*

Lambs to Slaughter

EIS officer David Morens boarded a plane for Cairo on November 2, 1977. He had been tapped to look into what might be a dengue out-break. Just before he departed, a Yale lab identified it as Rift Valley fe-ver (RVF), first found in 1931 in Kenya. Mostly it was known to affect sheep, with a few incidental cases in humans. The virus had never be-fore been found in Egypt.

Once he landed, Morens learned that human cases had occurred in villages along the Nile River Delta, afflicting as many as 100,000 people. After enduring fever, shaking chills, headaches, and aching joints, most victims recovered, but 1 percent or more hemorrhaged internally and died of liver failure or shock. Farmers at first denied any

---

*One victim's husband sued Robert Linn and his publisher, but the courts ruled that even deadly diet advice was protected by the First Amendment's freedom of speech provision. In 1984 the FDA mandated warning labels on protein supplements with fewer than four hun-dred calories.

illness among their sheep, afraid to decrease the value of their flocks just when lambs were in demand for an Islamic holy feast.

Morens eventually concluded that the Rift Valley virus had probably been introduced to Egyptian sheep by smuggled Ethiopian camels. The disease was spread to humans primarily by *Culex pipiens* mosquitoes, as well as by direct contact with sheep blood during lambing or slaughter. In one instance, the virus was aerosolized as wind kicked up blood-soaked dust and six people who inhaled it were sickened.

The U.S. Army Medical Research Institute of Infectious Diseases (USAMRIID, the former Fort Detrick biowarfare facility) delivered three thousand doses of an unlicensed vaccine for RVF, but the epidemic came to an end primarily when the mosquito season ceased in December. The EIS officer estimated that several hundred people had died among a population that had never been exposed to the virus and therefore had developed no immunity.

Environmental Hazards

In the late 1970s EIS officers were confronted with alarming potential environmental hazards, but proving harm was difficult. EIS officer Dale Morse, for instance, could not demonstrate the deleterious health effects from arsenic or PCBs in well water in Alaska, Arizona, and Mississippi, or from lead in drinking water in Bennington, Vermont, near a battery plant.

In 1977 Morse investigated carnations and chrysanthemums imported from South America. Plant inspectors and florists in several states complained of sporadic headaches, skin irritation, watery eyes, and decreased feeling in the extremities. Pesticide residue on the flowers, which could be absorbed through the skin, varied from undetectable traces up to 4,751 parts per million. Morse recommended that imported food regulations be extended to cover ornamentals as well.

On December 8, 1977, a farmhand cleaning manure in a calf barn near Eau Claire, Wisconsin, collapsed and died, killed by breathing hydrogen sulfide produced by stirrers in the liquid manure system. Morse concluded that the barn was inadequately ventilated and that a westerly wind blew through the only open door, preventing dispersal of the toxic gas. He recommended better ventilation, education, and surveillance.

A few months later EIS officer Roger Glass investigated two similar work-related deaths aboard a Louisiana shrimp boat in the Gulf of Mexico. On July 19, 1978, a crewman descended into the hold to pack freshly caught shrimp on ice and fell into a coma. When the captain rushed to resuscitate him, he, too, was overcome, as was a second crewman. The captain regained consciousness long enough to crawl out of the hold, but the two crewmen died.

Glass found that since 1970 there had been two similar incidents aboard shrimp boats holding more than a week's catch in hot summer weather. He identified a total of twenty-four cases of asphyxiation during that period on commercial fishing vessels, twenty-one of which were fatal.

The Louisiana shrimpers had been at sea for eleven days, and though they used plenty of ice and the catch appeared to be in good shape, Glass concluded that the shrimp had gradually decayed, depleting the oxygen. He recommended purging the atmosphere of the hold before descending into it and using respirators as standard shipboard equipment.

Poisoned Land, Sick Buildings

In December 1978 Clyde Foster, the mayor of Triana, Alabama (population six hundred), called the CDC, asking for an evaluation of DDT levels in his citizens, nearly all African Americans. From 1947 until 1971, the Olin Corporation had produced DDT nearby. Thousands of tons of plant waste had been dumped into a tributary of Indian Creek, which flowed into the Tennessee River at Triana.

EIS officer Kay Kreiss tested fish from the creek, finding up to 450 parts per million of DDE, a DDT-related compound, compared to the FDA's limit of 5 parts per million for interstate commerce. Kreiss then conducted a study of all six hundred Triana residents. The average town DDT levels were five times higher than the national geometric mean, and the amount increased with age, independent of fish consumption. Experts had thought that DDT reached a steady state in which excretion matched intake, but Kreiss found that it simply accumulated over time. "No acute health effects of DDT exposure were demonstrated," she concluded, but noted that there might be unrecognized long-term impacts.

Along with the Love Canal dioxin scandal in Niagara Falls, New York, revelations about Triana's DDT led to the passage of 1980 Superfund legislation to clean up severely polluted locales.

In the spring of 1979 Kreiss met with five state-based EIS officers who had contacted her in the previous months about a new phenomenon dubbed sick building syndrome. During the energy crisis of the late 1970s, many new office buildings were hermetically sealed, with central air-conditioning recirculating some of the filtered air. Employees began to complain of headache, fatigue, inability to wear contact lenses, and burning nose and throat.

Investigators from the National Institute for Occupational Safety and Health had tested for chemical fumes and, failing to identify any obvious problem, dismissed the complaints as mass hysteria. "I didn't buy that," Kreiss recalled. "Psychosomatic complaints often involve fainting or hyperventilating. They are usually episodic line-of-sight phenomena. These sick building symptoms didn't match, and they were continuous." She believed that stale air with too much carbon dioxide may have caused the problems. Subsequent research confirmed her suspicions. "Later work also showed that building-related symptoms were associated with air-conditioning of any kind (warmth, humidification, air cooling)," she said, "probably because they contribute to dampness," in conjunction with absorptive materials such as carpets that act as receptacles for irritants and microorganisms.

Take Aspirin and Drink Plenty of Fluids

In December 1978 a flu epidemic hit Phoenix. The day after Christmas EIS officer Karen Starko, working at the Arizona Department of Health Services, got a call from EIS alum John Sullivan-Bolyai, who was doing his pediatric residency in Phoenix. He had learned of seven cases of Reye's syndrome in children in three Phoenix hospitals and thought she might want to investigate this cluster.

Starko visited several of the children — five girls, two boys — in the hospital. They were in comas, on life support, holes drilled in their skulls to relieve the pressure. Within days, two were dead. These had all been healthy, normal children who apparently had had routine bouts of influenza, according to their parents. After a day or two, the kids were out of bed, feeling better. Suddenly they began to vomit relentlessly, then became sleepy, delirious, or combative, and finally fell into a coma.

Starko initiated a case-control study in January 1979, choosing as controls sixteen of the victims' elementary school classmates who had come down with flu and recovered uneventfully. Her questionnaire focused on the week prior to illness, asking about symptoms, medications, type of home heating, pets, and immunizations. In February she began to analyze the results, but figuring out what was in the various medications proved to be a challenge. There were decongestants, gum, lozenges, and Pepto-Bismol, as well as aspirin (acetylsalicylic acid) and Tylenol (acetaminophen). After research and several visits to drugstores to study labels, Starko compiled her results.

Aspirin. All seven children who developed Reye's syndrome had taken aspirin (salicylates) in one form or another, compared to half of the controls, and in heavier doses.

Starko did some research. She found that EIS officer David Reynolds had investigated eleven fatal cases of Reye's syndrome in Oklahoma from October 1968 through June 1970. EIS alum Calvin Linnemann had reported in 1974 on twenty-four Ohio children with Reye's syndrome. All of the victims in both studies had taken aspirin. Starko brought her data to Larry Schonberger in Viral Diseases, but he said, "Gee, I think previous EIS officers looked at aspirin before in some studies and it was dismissed." Stunned, she asked him to find the paper that ruled out aspirin.

A few weeks later Schonberger reported to Starko that he had reviewed studies by EIS officers Tom Glick (1967–1969) and Larry Corey (1973–1975). More than half of the victims in Glick's study had taken aspirin, and he had not looked at specific brand-name medications. Corey had studied hundreds of cases during a nationwide influenza B epidemic, and 78 percent had taken aspirin. Schonberger had also looked at the medical records of the baby with Reye's syndrome from his EIS days. She had been given aspirin.*

Starko's Arizona case-control study was compelling, but with only seven cases, it hardly constituted proof. Schonberger advised Gene Hurwitz, his EIS officer already working on a Reye's case-control study in Ohio, to focus on aspirin use. Michigan-based EIS officer Ron Waldman, working on his own study, did the same.

One missing piece nagged at Starko — the unusual pathology findings of cerebral edema combined with tiny fat drops within liver cells. Perhaps salicylate poisoning produced something similar. Her supervisor Lyle Conrad suggested she write to the Armed Forces Institute of Pathology in Washington, D.C., and within two weeks, on September 24, 1979, she received details of eleven cases of "acute salicylism in infants and children." All had "small cytoplasmic fat vesicles." Starko's hands trembled as she read the letter. "I wanted to scream," she recalled. "This was it!" Seven of those cases had antecedent upper respiratory infections. In other words, they were probably Reye's syndrome cases.[†]

As Hurwitz and Waldman worked on their larger studies, Starko submitted her paper to *Lancet*. It was rejected. Frustrated, she called her supervisor, Lyle Conrad, and said, "I really think CDC should publicize this issue before another Reye's syndrome winter season." Her results were subsequently tacked onto an *MMWR* summary article in July 1980. "Further investigations are needed to more clearly define the possible role of salicylate use and toxins in the pathogenesis of Reye syndrome," it concluded.

Four months later the *MMWR* followed up with verification: ninety-five of ninety-eight victims in the Ohio case-control study and

---

*See pages 118–119.

[†]Starko believes that Reye's syndrome *is* simply salicylate toxicity. Fever and dehydration caused by flu or chicken pox, in conjunction with an immature metabolism, make aspirin more potent in young persons, rendering them more susceptible to salicylate's toxic effects. The few cases of non-aspirin-related Reye's syndrome are, she thinks, due to inborn genetic factors.

all but one of the twenty-five Michigan patients had taken aspirin. "Parents should be advised to use caution when administering salicylates to treat children with viral illnesses," the article concluded. The following month, Starko's study was finally published in *Pediatrics*.

In June the surgeon general issued an advisory and the FDA proposed a warning label on aspirin. The aspirin industry demanded more studies and successfully delayed a warning label on medication containing salicylates until 1986.* From 1981 through 1985, more than 1,000 U.S. children contracted Reye's syndrome, with 291 deaths. Up to a third of the survivors probably suffered permanent brain damage.

Publicity about the hazards of aspirin, including that generated by the EIS officers, gradually reduced its use for children, so that Reye's cases in the United States fell from a peak of 555 in 1980 to 36 in 1987, and finally to just 2 cases in 1997, by which time most children's medication no longer contained aspirin.

Sterilization and Abortion Surveillance

In January 1979 EIS officer Michael Rosenberg watched a rural surgeon perform a tubal ligation on a woman in a dusty Bangladesh office. When he was done, two assistants lifted the drugged woman from the table, laid her on the floor in a corner, and turned their attention to the next operation.

In densely populated Bangladesh, abortions were technically illegal, but desperate women sought the operations anyway, resulting in an estimated 7,800 deaths a year. Consequently, women lined up for sterilizations. But an alarming number died following the tubal ligations, which is why Rosenberg was observing the operations. "Whenever a patient would moan in pain," he recalled, "assistants would simply administer another few cc's of Valium. Tiny women, ninety-five pounds, were getting doses five to ten times what we might have given to a three-hundred-pound man in the United States."

---

*In support of the drug makers, EIS alum Heinz Eichenwald, the chairman of the Committee on the Care of Children, wrote on February 28, 1983, of "the concern of many pediatricians that their ability to use an important treatment modality [aspirin] would be impeded by unwarranted fear." He dismissed the case-control studies.

Clearly, some women were dying of Valium overdoses. Over the next two years Rosenberg helped institute a training program in the use of anesthetics and put a surveillance program in place to monitor safety.

After HEW secretary Joe Califano, a devout Catholic, slashed federal funding for abortions in August 1977, EIS officers Ann Marie Kimball and Julian Gold went to McAllen, Texas, near the Mexican border, to investigate a cluster of nine hospitalizations following illegal abortions. Hispanic women with little money were seeking abortions from *parteras,* lay midwives. Some crossed the border to Reynosa, Mexico, where pharmacies offered injections supposed to terminate pregnancies. One twenty-seven-year-old victim had previously obtained a legal abortion using Medicaid funds. Now pregnant again, she tried the Reynosa injection, which failed, then resorted to an inexpensive lay midwife. She subsequently developed septic shock and died with heart and kidney failure.

In December 1978 Gold investigated an unusual abortion-related death in Colorado. Even though Colorado had replaced the federal funding cut by Califano, three young women had taken pennyroyal oil as a supposedly natural way to induce abortions. Two took a quarter ounce and got horribly sick within two hours, but recovered. The third, an eighteen-year-old student, took a full ounce. She died of multiple complications from a poisoned liver. The terrible irony was that she wasn't pregnant after all.

The FDA did not regulate herbal remedies, so Gold and his supervisors, Ward Cates and Carl Tyler, sought media coverage from national wire services, herb trade-association magazines, women's health-center newsletters, and medical journals. They also convinced the pennyroyal oil distributor to discontinue the dangerous product's sale.*

Saving Babies in the Birth Defects Branch

Late in 1977 EIS officer Peter Layde began to look at pilot programs that screened babies for congenital hypothyroidism (thyroid hormone

---

*Pennyroyal oil is again widely available, advertised primarily for aromatherapy.

deficiency). Untreated, this condition, which afflicts approximately one in six thousand children, results in stunted physical and mental growth (cretinism). In its early stages, hypothyroidism was difficult to diagnose. After a year or so, when the condition became obvious and treatment usually began, it could prevent physical deformities, but not brain damage. If caught near birth, however, with regular thyroid hormone replacement children could grow up normally. "It was considered too costly to test routinely for such a rare condition," Layde said.

He spent most of his EIS years studying the problem and published his results in the *Journal of the American Medical Association* in May 1979. The average cost to screen one infant was $1.55, so to find the one in six thousand would cost $9,300. Treatment for life would cost another $2,500, for a total of $11,800 per case. For each untreated case, Layde estimated that special education and institutionalization would run around $92,000, and the net productivity lost from a healthy child would add another $14,000, so routine screening would save society about $94,000 per case. Layde's paper had a major impact, with every state implementing the screening program for congenital hypothyroidism. Approximately a thousand children per year were thereby spared mental retardation.

On Friday, July 27, 1979, pediatrician José Cordero got a call on his first day on duty after the EIS training course. A Memphis doctor was reporting three cases of what appeared to be Bartter syndrome, a rare genetic disorder in which children's kidneys cannot reabsorb potassium or chloride. The condition produces metabolic alkalosis (blood not sufficiently acidic) with resultant muscle cramping, weakness, constipation, and failure to grow. These three babies had all the symptoms, but the doctor said they had quickly recovered with potassium and chloride supplements.

"During my residency I had treated a child with Bartter's," Cordero recalled, "and even with high supplemental doses, he did not recover quickly. I suspected this was something else." All three Tennessee babies were lactose intolerant and were drinking Neo-Mull-Soy, an infant formula. Cordero suspected that the formula contained insufficient nutrients. Over the weekend he and fellow EIS officer Frank

Greenberg called every pediatric nephrology (kidney-related) training program in the United States. By Monday night they had found
thirty-one additional suspect cases, twenty-six of whom were known
to be taking Neo-Mull-Soy.

On Tuesday Cordero called the FDA and Syntex, the California
manufacturer. On Thursday the company, which sold a tenth of the
country's soy-based formulas, voluntarily took all of its infant formula
off the market and sent a Mailgram to pediatricians notifying them of
the problem. As a direct result of the investigation, the Infant Formula
Act of 1980 was passed, specifying a safe level of needed nutrients, including chloride.

Polio and the Amish

In January 1979 a young Amish woman in Franklin County, Pennsylvania, contracted polio. The lab revealed that this woman had wild
type 1 polio, and her community setting was ominous. The Amish
deeply distrusted any government program, and few had been immunized. One case of wild polio meant that the virus was probably already widespread in her community, since only one in two hundred
infections is symptomatic.

EIS officer Marjorie Pollack reviewed her notes from the spring of
1978, when she had kept tabs on a large polio outbreak in a Dutch Re-
formed community in the Netherlands. It, too, was type 1, and when
some asymptomatic members visited Canada, they spread it among
fellow church members there. Then she learned that an Amish family, which had lived near one such Ontario community, had moved to
Pennsylvania later in 1978. The epidemiological link was forged.

The molecular fingerprints of the Dutch, Canadian, and American strains were identical. In April two more paralytic cases occurred
among the Pennsylvania Amish, and it became easier to persuade
them to accept vaccination. As many Amish lined up to receive oral
polio vaccine drops on their tongues in May and June, more contracted polio — in Pennsylvania, Iowa, Wisconsin, Missouri, and Canada — for a total of seventeen cases. By July 1, 70 percent of the nation's

Amish had received at least one dose of OPV, and there were no more cases. The last wild polio outbreak in the United States was over.

Crawling among the Khmer Rouge

On Sunday morning, October 28, 1979, EIS officer Rick Goodman was in Kuala Lumpur, Malaysia, screening Vietnamese boat people seeking asylum in the United States. Three other EIS officers were doing the same thing at other staging areas around Southeast Asia.

At 1 A.M. the phone rang. "Rick, you've got to pack up and fly to Bangkok immediately." It was Philip Brachman calling from Atlanta. The Vietnamese had invaded Cambodia and overthrown the murderous Khmer Rouge regime of Pol Pot. Nearly 400,000 Cambodian refugees — persecutors and persecuted — had fled. About 30,000 had been transported to a hastily constructed refugee camp near Sa Kaeo, Thailand, twenty miles from the border.

When Goodman and two other EIS officers arrived the following day, they found ten large canvas hospital tents in the corner of a hastily bulldozed field surrounded by barbed wire. Each tent held a thousand sick Cambodians (or Kampucheans, as they had relabeled themselves). Goodman crawled from patient to patient on the dirt floor of his assigned tent. On their chests with a Magic Marker he wrote quick notations — M for malaria, F for fever, D for dead. He recorded clinical information on separate cards for each patient.

In fleeing, many who had never been exposed to malaria had traveled through mosquito-infested areas. Some were in the throes of seizures from terminal cerebral malaria. Others suffered from malnutrition, pneumonia, diarrhea, dehydration, anemia, fractures, skin diseases, and lice infestation. "Everyone was incredibly sick except a few teens and young adults wearing plaid clothing," he recalled. These former Khmer Rouge soldiers, who had probably committed atrocities during the war, removed the corpses.

Gradually some order emerged. Plywood hospital cots and antibiotics arrived along with intravenous drips for the severely dehydrated. Stripped to his waist in the heat, Goodman delivered babies, born as nearby children were dying. Yet over the course of a week, those who didn't die began to regain strength after being treated for malaria and given nourishing food.

At the end of the week, Goodman returned to Kuala Lumpur, as Roger Glass, Ward Cates, Phil Nieburg, and Connie Davis arrived to take over for three months. Glass, who had recently finished his EIS stint, had just begun working on diarrheal diseases in Bangladesh when he and his wife, Barbara Stoll (a pediatrician), were summoned. Cates, another EIS veteran, came from the CDC Family Planning unit in Atlanta. Nieburg and Davis were current EIS officers.

Goodman had helped establish primary care and basic organization. Glass and his colleagues set about doing public health surveillance. What was the mortality rate? What resources were needed for what diseases? They gathered death information daily from the medical staff and learned that cerebral malaria was the leading killer. "We put sixty-two malaria patients in a single ward with an Israeli chief resident, giving them IV quinine in proper doses with rehydration," Glass recalled. None died.

The few remaining children under five had severe anemia, malnutrition, and malaria. "We took blood from journalists and volunteers," Glass said, "and an Australian blood banker typed the blood." By transfusing the children, they replenished their red blood cells and saved their lives. When a bacterial meningitis outbreak began, they gave sulfadiazine to people living in adjacent tents, stopping its spread within ten days. They set up regular tuberculosis treatment for those with chronic cough and fever and initiated a measles vaccination program for children at the highest risk.

Within four days of their arrival, the CDC crew had produced a full report on how to stop mortality in the camp with key interventions. The head of the International Committee of the Red Cross, who had initially been irritated with their keeping records instead of pitching in to help, was converted to belief in the value of epidemiology. The mortality rate dropped from 9.1 deaths per 10,000 per day during the first week to 0.7 deaths by the fifth week. At two other refugee camps — Kamput and Khao-I-Dang — the same surveillance and treatment techniques were employed.

By the time EIS officers Susan Holck and Stephen Preblud relieved Glass and his colleagues three months later, organized systems were in place in the camps, but measles and polio outbreaks necessitated mass vaccination programs. Cholera broke out among the million refugees in transitory border camps near the Thai-Cambodia border. "We closed contaminated wells, got new ones dug. We provided oral rehydration solution and some IV drips and got control of it," Holck recalled.

She was dismayed to find that no one had considered offering contraceptives to the women. Many starving women had stopped menstruating by the time they entered the camps, but with proper nourishment, they had become fertile again and were getting pregnant. "I couldn't imagine raising children in that environment," Holck said. She arranged for birth control pills and Depo-Provera injections for those who wanted them.

14
BUDGET WARS AND NEW PLAGUES

ON SUNDAY, JANUARY 13, 1980, Andy Dean, the Minnesota state epidemiologist (EIS 1974–1976), called Jeff Davis, his Wisconsin counterpart (EIS 1973–1975). "I've just seen two previously healthy young women who nearly died, and I know of three others. First they started vomiting—"

Davis interrupted him. "Then they developed severe diarrhea, a high fever, and a bright red rash. Then they went into shock. Their kidneys and livers began to fail, and they became severely dehydrated. As they got better, the skin on their hands and feet peeled off in whole sheets."

"Yes. Exactly. What is it, Jeff?"

"My EIS officer and I have interviewed three cases here in Wisconsin, and I've found four more that occurred since last July. Six of them were menstruating. It's called toxic shock syndrome. It's probably caused by a staphylococcal strain that produces a toxin, but no one has isolated it yet."

After he hung up, Dean called the CDC, where EIS officer Kathy Shands was assigned to monitor the problem. As spring progressed, Shands learned of new toxic shock cases across the country. Of fifty-five cases thus far reported to the CDC, fifty-two had been in young women, most of whom were menstruating and had staph infections. Seven had died.

After Shands wrote an initial report for the *MMWR,* and the *Washington Post* then ran a front-page article, more than one hundred more cases flooded in, and state-based EIS officers began active surveillance. Shands formed a Toxic Shock Syndrome Task Force, recruiting fellow EIS officers George Schmid, Debby Blum, and Bruce Dan. By this time, Jeff Davis had nearly completed a case-control study in Wisconsin that implicated tampons.

The four members of the TSS Task Force did their own study, asking fifty-two patients in twenty states to name an age-matched friend as a control. Within a week they had found and questioned all of them on the telephone, asking intimate questions about marital status, sex frequency, intercourse during menstruation, use of tampons or pads, brands used, menstrual patterns, what medications they had taken, and more. They also contacted the major U.S. tampon manufacturers, asking for materials used, manufacturing practices, and marketing history. They learned that new, more absorbent brands of tampons had replaced the standard rayon or cotton with polyacrylate fibers, polyester foam, and various forms of cellulose.

The case-control study failed to implicate any medication or activity other than tampon use. All of the TSS cases used tampons, compared to forty-four out of the fifty-two controls. Tampons were thus implicated, but not by much.

The second *MMWR* article appeared on June 27, 1980. "No particular brand of tampon is associated with unusually high risk," Shands wrote. Still, she knew that Procter & Gamble's new Rely tampon was overrepresented, though not with statistical significance. The article resulted in a media frenzy, and the young officers began to consult directly with CDC director Bill Foege and the surgeon general.

Over the Labor Day weekend the EIS officers conducted a second case-control study, using fifty new TSS cases and requesting three friends as controls for each case. To make sure that brand information was accurate, they asked patients and controls to read the labels from their tampon packages to them over the phone.

In this study, 71 percent of the cases used only one tampon brand, Rely, compared to 26 percent of the controls. Procter & Gamble had rolled out Rely nationally throughout 1978, claiming that it "even absorbs the worry." When the EIS officers presented their prepublication finds, a P&G executive asked, "You realize what this means to P&G? What if you're wrong?" Bruce Dan shot back, "What if *you're* wrong? What if it were your daughter?"

The results were published in the *MMWR* on September 19, 1980. Under pressure from the FDA, on September 22 P&G announced that it was "voluntarily" withdrawing Rely from the market.

That was two weeks too late for Pat Kehm, a twenty-five-year-old Iowa mother who died of toxic shock syndrome on September 6 after wearing a Rely tampon. Her husband sued the manufacturer, and his lawyer discovered that, despite mounting evidence that its tampons were implicated, P&G had mailed free samples of Rely to 2 million households during the summer of 1980 and told its sales force not to initiate discussions of toxic shock with physicians.

Over the next year, the TSS Task Force and other researchers continued to work on the mystery. Why was Rely so dangerous? Studies showed that approximately one out of every ten women harbored staph in their vaginas, and 1 percent or so had the strain that produced the staph toxin, which was finally identified in 1981, with help from Dan and Shands. The Rely tampon resembled a bell-shaped tea bag, swelling to completely fill the vaginal canal. Staph bacteria require oxygen and a warm place to multiply, and the tampon provided both. Rely also contained Pluronic L92, a slippery chemical used to ease work with fibers. The chemical turned out to promote staph growth. The superabsorbent tampon "was a perfect little toxin factory," observed Bruce Dan.

Toxic shock did not cease with the disappearance of Rely. Other highly absorbent tampons also produced the syndrome, and in addition toxic shock occurred in nonmenstruating women as well as in men, as EIS officer Art Reingold documented. A fourteen-year-old boy contracted TSS after he hurt his foot falling off his bike, and a woman came down with it after giving birth. Other cases were associated with mastitis, bursitis, burns, and insect bites. Soldiers in training at Fort Dix got "toxic sock syndrome" from infected blisters.

Yet tampons would continue to be associated with many toxic shock cases, even after the FDA finally mandated warning labels in 1982. By 1984 more than twenty-five hundred cases of toxic shock syndrome had been documented in the United States.

Trying to Stay in Control

In 1980 the CDC investigated health effects from the Love Canal toxic waste dump in Niagara Falls, New York, as well as chemical contamination in Woburn, Massachusetts. In neither case could the investigators prove that people suffered damage from their exposures. Over the previous four years, EIS alum Glyn Caldwell had sought information on military veterans who were used as human guinea pigs during the 1957 "Smoky" hydrogen bomb test in Nevada. In 1980 he reported finding 9 cases of leukemia among them where 3.5 were expected, though that did not prove causation.

As Caldwell later observed, investigating environmental contamination was a complicated, time-consuming, and often thankless task, with "strident calls to close down the presumed offending dump, plant, or industrial area" and "extravagant speculation linking the known exposure to any and all diseases." Careful scientific studies were often perceived as evidence of "foot dragging, if not incompetence."

This generalization could also apply to the investigation of the effects of the defoliant Agent Orange, widely used during the Vietnam War. In 1980 Dave Erickson and Godfrey Oakley of the CDC Birth Defects Division were gearing up for a congressionally mandated study to determine if the children of Vietnam veterans had unusual numbers of birth defects due to their fathers' exposure to Agent Orange. Erickson invited pediatrician Joe Mulinare, just accepted into the EIS, to help plan the study and also assigned him to look at neural tube defects.

A British paper in *Lancet* had suggested that vitamin supplements taken before conception might prevent spina bifida and anenceph-aly. The occurrence of these two neural tube defects had been declin-ing slightly over the last decade, possibly from improved nutrition or fewer exposures to harmful chemicals. Mulinare looked back at the last five years of Atlanta birth defects data. He found that for white mothers, multivitamin consumption did seem to be correlated with fewer neural tube defects.

In the Agent Orange questionnaire, Mulinare included queries about mothers' vitamin consumption before and during the first weeks of pregnancy, along with 120 other risk factors. This survey would produce a massive data set in a few years.* The investigation of exposure to Agent Orange showed no increased risk of fathering ba-bies with birth defects.

Volcanoes and Heat Waves

On May 18, 1980, Mount St. Helens erupted in Washington State, kill-ing fifty-seven people and spewing tons of lava and ash into the air, followed by a second eruption on June 12. With the help of eight EIS colleagues, Peter Baxter set up hospital surveillance, which showed a threefold increase in emergency room visits for asthma and bronchi-tis. There was little to be done other than to recommend that people wear masks.

The eruptions had other indirect consequences, as EIS officers Marty Blaser and Bruce Weniger discovered in August 1980, when they went to Red Lodge, Montana, to investigate a citywide diarrhea outbreak. They found that *Giardia,* a protozoan parasite typically car-ried by beavers, dogs, and muskrats, was the primary culprit. Cysts had been washed into the unfiltered water supply by two episodes of unusually heavy water runoff when dark ash from Mount St. Helens settled on the snow of the Rockies, in conjunction with sunny, hot weather in May and June.

---

*Meanwhile, there were widely publicized fears that Bendectin, an antinausea medication for pregnant women, caused birth defects. EIS officer José Cordero's investigation cleared the drug, but it was forced off the market anyway amid mounting hysteria and lawsuits.

Expanded Mandate, Exported Expertise

In the fall of 1980 Marty Blaser blazed an EIS trail in violence epidemiology. Over the previous year, twenty-two African American boys had been murdered in Atlanta. When Blaser read that the stumped police were consulting a psychic, he decided that EIS officers could do at least as well. With Bruce Weniger and others, Blaser conducted a case-control study of the victims, finding that they tended to run errands for money and were frequently alone on the streets or in shopping centers. Just as the EIS officers were completing their study, the police caught the killer, and the murders ceased.

To better reflect the broadening CDC mandate, Bill Foege instituted a long-planned reorganization late in 1980, changing to the plural Centers for Disease Control, made up of the Center for Prevention Services, Center for Environmental Health, Center for Health Promotion and Education, and Center for Infectious Diseases, among others. While Philip Brachman remained the head of the Epidemiology Program Office (EPO), he would no longer be completely in charge of EIS officers, who were assigned to various centers.

In 1980 the first official EIS clone, called a Field Epidemiology Training Program (FETP), commenced in Thailand, with EIS alum David Brandling-Bennett as its first advisor, still paid by the CDC.* After training, recruits were assigned to different departments in the Thai Ministry of Public Health, where Brandling-Bennett visited each trainee at least weekly. The EIS-like recruits investigated outbreaks of hepatitis, cholera, and foodborne diseases. In the ensuing years, other FETP programs would begin in other countries, using essentially the same model.

Reaganomics

Ronald Reagan's inauguration on January 20, 1981, signaled a crisis for the CDC. The conservative Republican had declared war on government expenditure. Various reductions in force were rumored, with

---

*In 1975 a Canadian EIS-like program had begun with input from EIS alums, but without a resident CDC advisor.

budgets slashed. Three days after taking office, President Reagan met with antiabortion leaders. On their list of demands was the firing of EIS alum Ward Cates, chief of the CDC Abortion Surveillance Branch. In defending the reasoning for abortion, Cates had written an article comparing penicillin as a treatment for syphilis to abortion as a solution for unwanted pregnancy. "My intention was to show how safe abortion was," he recalled ruefully, "but many saw me as saying that pregnancy was a disease." Cates was reassigned to work on sexually transmitted diseases.

Spanish Toxic Oil

An epidemic broke out in Spain in the first week of May 1981. By the end of the year, it would put over 13,000 people in the hospital, killing 314 of them. It was first recognized in Madrid, where 140 people sought help for respiratory distress within a week. Patients did not respond to antibiotics and soon developed eosinophilia, a condition with an abnormally high number of a type of white blood cells, often associated with an allergic reaction.

The Spanish government appealed to the CDC, which assigned the case to EIS alum José Rigau, a Puerto Rican. Madrid was too large for a quick study, so Rigau chose the town of Las Navas del Marqués, about fifty miles away, with only two hospitals and four thousand people. Although the disease often afflicted members of the same household, it had not spread in schools, barracks, or hospitals, so Rigau focused on the home.

In early June he completed an initial case-control study of 27 case households and 108 control homes without disease. The only item used more frequently in the case than control households was a brand of shampoo, but it was found in only 8 case families.

As Rigau was mulling over the results, he heard a rumor that olive oil sold on the street might be involved. He resurveyed and found that all 27 case families had consumed unlabeled cooking oil bought from itinerant salesmen versus 30 of the 108 control households. He discovered that one salesman had sold oil to every case household. The same man had also sold shampoo to some of them.

To protect its native olive oil industry, Spain permitted only the importation of denatured rapeseed oil — contaminated by aniline 652, a benzene derivative — for use in metal working. Spanish businesses had been buying the cheap oil, refining it to remove the aniline, and selling it to distributors, who in turn mixed it with other cheap oils and animal fat and sold it to itinerant salesmen in five-kilo cans as cooking oil. But this batch of illegal oil still contained aniline.

The newly labeled Spanish toxic oil syndrome caused severe neurological illness in many victims and paralyzed, then killed those who had consumed (or inhaled or touched) the most oil.

The Graveyard of Epidemiologists

Wally Schlech arrived on July 17, 1981, in Halifax, Nova Scotia, to investigate an outbreak of listeriosis, a disease called the "graveyard of epidemiologists" because no one had ever traced its mode of transmission.

The bacillus *Listeria monocytogenes* is common in soil, water, and vegetation and causes brain swelling in cows, sheep, and other ruminants. Because the animals stagger as if chasing their tails, it is known as the "circling disease." Listeriosis is not often a serious problem for adult humans unless they are already ill or their immune systems are compromised. Pregnant women normally survive it with only a high fever, but it is deadly to their fetuses.

The epidemic had begun in March. By the time it stopped a few months later, it had affected forty-one people in the Maritime provinces, including thirty-four babies, sixteen of whom died, along with two adult deaths. It was the largest listeriosis outbreak ever recorded in humans.

Schlech conducted an initial case-control study, matching four healthy babies to each case infant, and four age- and sex-matched adult controls to each adult case. He asked about exposure to other cases of listeriosis or to wild or domestic animals. He questioned them about gardening, hiking, and other outdoor activities. Finally, he asked them to recall what, in general, they had eaten over the last few months. The results were inconclusive.

When an elderly man visiting from Ontario—an outlier—was hospitalized, the EIS officer interviewed him and his wife, then examined the contents of their refrigerator, including bananas, coleslaw, and radishes. Reinterviews revealed that many more cases than controls had eaten coleslaw; when Schlech nudged patients' memories, they all recalled having eaten coleslaw. A few days later the lab found the virulent strain of *Listeria* that had caused the outbreak in the elderly man's coleslaw.

Schlech tracked the slaw to a regional manufacturer who purchased cabbage from many local farmers and several wholesalers. He called regional large-animal veterinarians and found that a farmer's sheep had died of listeriosis in March on Prince Edward Island. When Schlech visited the organic farm, he discovered that the owner fertilized his cabbage with raw sheep manure (standard practice is to age or steam the manure). After the October harvest, he had put the cabbage in a cold storage shed for the winter. *Listeria* grow in the cold and so probably proliferated in the cabbage over the winter. The farmer then sold the vegetables to the coleslaw manufacturer.

At last, *Listeria* could no longer be called "the graveyard of epidemiologists," but was instead the springboard for Schlech's career. Upon graduation from the EIS, he took a position at Dalhousie University in Nova Scotia, becoming a leading authority on listeriosis. The bacillus was subsequently tracked to other foods such as milk, soft cheese, and undercooked chicken.

The Disease of the Century

EIS officer Wayne Shandera, assigned to the Los Angeles Health Department, had heard office rumors about some mysterious new illness in the gay community. Then, in December 1980, a pathologist from Los Angeles County Hospital called to say he had recently seen six men with very unusual lymphadenopathy (swollen lymph nodes). *I wonder if they're gay?* Shandera thought. He phoned them at their homes but could find no common thread. One man admitted to being gay and another said he injected drugs, but that was all.

Two months later UCLA immunologist Mike Gottlieb called about a patient, a previously healthy thirty-year-old gay man, with *Pneumocystis carinii* pneumonia (PCP), a fungal infection that normally afflicts only those with damaged immune systems, such as cancer chemotherapy patients or organ transplant recipients. It was weird.

In April Gottlieb called again. Now he had seen three young men with PCP, and he knew of another. All were gay, and one had already died. This was an outbreak. Could Shandera help write it up for the *MMWR*? Sure, he said. After he hung up, the EIS officer looked through the messages on his desk. Among them was notification of a fifth PCP case, a deceased gay attorney. Later that day Shandera visited one of Gottlieb's young men. He was thin, wasted, and sallow. He had foamy white oral yeast infections and very few helper T cells, key parts of the immune system.

Shandera and Gottlieb wrote up the cases, publishing a summary in the May issue of the Los Angeles County Health Department's newsletter and submitting a fuller description to Mike Gregg, the *MMWR* editor, for the June 5, 1981, issue.

Visiting the Hollywood Gay Men's Clinic, Shandera conducted interviews with a subset of patients with swollen lymph nodes, using other clients as controls. He found no significant difference in the use of antibiotics or in the level of cytomegalovirus (CMV, a herpes virus) infection, which was nearly universal in homosexuals. "I thought maybe there was a killer CMV strain causing all of this," he said.

The KSOI Task Force

Steven Phillips read Shandera's *MMWR* article about gay PCP cases in Los Angeles. Phillips, nearing the end of his EIS service at the New York City Health Department, had identified four PCP cases at Bellevue and two in other hospitals. The EIS officer notified the CDC. Here was evidence of another cluster.

Alvin Friedman-Kien, a dermatology professor at New York University, also read Shandera's *MMWR* report. For two years he had been seeing gay men with purplish blotches on their skin from Kaposi's sarcoma. He notified the CDC. Calls to San Francisco revealed that the unusual cancer was common among homosexual men there as well.

No one could figure out why these young gay men were coming down with such rare diseases. Kaposi's sarcoma, for instance, normally afflicted elderly Italians, Polish Jews, and a subset of Africans. It appeared that these homosexuals were subject to opportunistic infections that usually preyed on those whose immune systems were weakened by some other underlying cause.

Hurriedly, the CDC put together a Kaposi's Sarcoma and Opportunistic Infections (KSOI) Task Force, headed by Jim Curran of the VD Control Division, assisted by EIS officer Harold Jaffe, an STD veteran, and EIS alum Mary Guinan, a herpes expert. Curran also recruited EIS officers from other groups, including Alex Kelter from Chronic Diseases and Harry Haverkos from Parasitic Diseases, to set up a national surveillance system.

Haverkos surveyed eighteen major metropolitan areas in the United States. In each city, field EIS officers scoured hospital records and called physicians, gay health clinics, and the heads of four hospital departments — pathology, oncology, dermatology, and infectious diseases — looking for KSOI cases. No increased incidence of Kaposi's sarcoma was noted until 1980. Since the CDC was the only source of pentamidine, a drug used to treat *P. carinii* pneumonia, Haverkos also looked at the history of that drug's usage to treat adults with no known underlying disorder. Such pentamidine requests had begun in July 1980 and snowballed during 1981.

This was apparently a new syndrome, and its incidence was growing rapidly. Haverkos also learned of gay men suffering from cerebral toxoplasmosis (a parasitic infection), cryptococcal meningitis, herpes simplex, shingles, Burkitt's lymphoma, and the *Cryptosporidium* protozoa that caused prolonged diarrhea. Many callers complained of swollen lymph nodes, fatigue, and night sweats. They didn't fit the stringent case definition (opportunistic infections or Kaposi's sarcoma), but Haverkos recorded them anyway.

In October 1981 the task force began to conduct a case-control study of gay KSOI victims in New York City and California. The teams interviewed a total of 50 gay KSOI patients (39 with Kaposi's sarcoma, 8 with PCP, and 3 with both), age-matched with 120 homosexual controls. The original idea had been to find four controls for each case — two from an STD clinic, one referred by a private doctor, and one gay friend who had never been a sexual partner — but it proved almost impossible to find gay friends who had not once been lovers as well.

The twenty-page case-control questionnaire covered educational level, income, recent travel, prescription medicine and illicit drug use, ancestry, previous illnesses, and a detailed sexual history, including favored practices and positions. The PCP patients usually had a more virulent illness that killed sooner. The Kaposi's victims, on the other hand, often still looked healthy other than a few purple bruises. "They were all eager to help," said EIS officer Martha Rogers, who worked on the New York City study, "wanting to know what was going on. They were all losing friends and lovers."

EIS officer Polly Thomas, who worked with Rogers, described herself as a wholesome, ingénue type. Her first interviewee sold bathtub-made street poppers, amyl or butyl nitrite inhalants designed to enhance orgasms and loosen anal sphincters. Well educated and funny, he told her all about his sexual practices, then, observing her wide-eyed reaction, said, "This is the first interview you've done, right?" A few months later his death certificate came across her desk.

In San Francisco, a large former football player fainted on top of EIS alum Mary Guinan as she was drawing his blood. "I was trying to get the tourniquet off his arm and stuck myself with the needle. There was blood all over both of us." She roused him (she doesn't recall whether he was a case or control), cleaned them both up, and went on to the next interview.*

The major difference between cases and controls turned out to be the number of sex partners. Controls had sex with about twenty-five

---

*A few years later, when Guinan developed a purple lesion on her arm, she panicked, recalling the needlestick and concluding that she had Kaposi's sarcoma. But the bruises disappeared.

men a year, while the median annual number of sex partners for cases was sixty-one. Cases were also more likely to have exposure to feces through fisting (inserting a balled fist into the rectum) or rimming (licking around and inside the anus) and had more syphilis, non-B hepatitis, and diarrheal parasites. While 96 percent of both groups had tried poppers, cases had used more of them over their lifetimes. The patients with KSOI met sex partners twice as frequently in bathhouses for anonymous sexual encounters.

No incriminating microbe could be identified in the cases. In September 1981 many thought that a toxin might be causing the disease. "I expected it to be like toxic shock syndrome or Legionnaires' disease," Rogers said, "kind of a spectacular blip, but then we'd figure out the cause and it would be over."

By the beginning of 1982, the task force had identified 159 KSOI cases, mostly in homosexual men, but also in injecting drug users. Although fifteen states, the District of Columbia, and two foreign countries reported cases, more than three-quarters of the patients were from New York City, San Francisco, or Los Angeles.

Patient Zero

Interviewing local cases and lovers of those who had died, Dave Auerbach, the EIS officer who replaced Wayne Shandera in Los Angeles, realized that a web of sexual relations connected many of them. And he kept hearing about Gaetan Dugas, an attractive French Canadian airline steward who apparently often flew in for sexual encounters. Auerbach called the CDC, and sociologist Bill Darrow came out to help.

With Auerbach, Darrow traced a cluster that spread beyond Los Angeles. Of the first nineteen cases identified in Southern California, eleven had died, but Darrow and Auerbach were able to find nine who had had sexual contact with one or more other patients within five years of the onset of symptoms.

They also found and interviewed Dugas, who bragged of his conquests, estimating that he had sex with about 250 men each year. In December 1979 he had developed swollen lymph nodes, and in May

1980 was diagnosed with Kaposi's sarcoma. Dugas could name 72 of his sexual partners from 1979 through 1981. Four were from Southern California and 4 from New York City. Ultimately, Auerbach and Darrow were able to link 40 patients in ten cities by sexual contact. In their article, they published a chart showing the spiderweb of sexual contacts, with "Patient 0" (Dugas) in its center.

The cluster strongly implied an infectious agent that could be transmitted sexually by semen or blood with a fairly long incubation period. One man spotted his Kaposi's sarcoma lesion thirteen months after he had slept with Dugas.

While Auerbach worked on the Los Angeles cluster, EIS officer Bess Miller reviewed the records of fifty-seven gay men in Atlanta, New York City, and San Francisco with lymphadenopathy but no KSOI. Miller reported her findings in the May 1982 *MMWR*. Immunologic evaluation of eight subjects revealed depressed helper T cell counts. Nearly half of the Kaposi's sarcoma patients and a quarter of those with PCP had a history of swollen lymph nodes before onset. "Since the initiation of this study, one patient with lymphadenopathy has developed Kaposi's sarcoma," she reported.

The Four Hs and a Disease Christening

As 1982 progressed, it became evident that this was not simply a "gay plague." In New York City, Polly Thomas interviewed heroin addicts with the syndrome who told her about sharing needles. They were clearly not all closet homosexuals.

EIS officer John Hanrahan interviewed seven young men in New York state correctional facilities with PCP who admitted to intravenous drug use before they were incarcerated, but who insisted they had not been victims of homosexual prison rape and had not taken drugs since. One man had been imprisoned for thirty-six months, indicating at least a three-year incubation period.

Polly Thomas interviewed a woman in a New Jersey hospital, the wife of an addict, who said that she didn't inject drugs. Other evidence of heterosexual transmission soon accumulated.

Then Haitian immigrants began to sicken and die of the syndrome.

"The first few Haitians I interviewed told me that they had been paid to have sex with American gays on vacation in Port-au-Prince," Thomas said. "They were simply destitute, not gay themselves. Then they would marry and infect their wives." But subsequent Haitians insisted they were purely heterosexual.

In early July Harry Haverkos interviewed an Ohio hemophiliac patient, the third who had come down with the new syndrome. He was neither gay nor a drug user, and he wasn't Haitian. Haverkos concluded that he must have gotten it from contaminated Factor VIII, a clotting agent concentrated from thousands of blood donors. This meant that the disease was probably caused by a virus transmitted through donated blood. In that case, the nation's blood supply was imperiled. Now there was a four-H club of victims — homosexuals, heroin addicts, Haitians, and hemophiliacs.

On July 27, 1982, Jim Curran and others from the CDC presented their evidence at a Washington, D.C., meeting that included representatives from the blood industry, hemophiliacs, gay activists, the FDA, and the NIH. Curran pushed for donor deferral guidelines, asking the high-risk groups (gays, drug users, and Haitians) not to donate blood. The hemophiliac groups, protective of Factor VIII, refused to believe the data. Gay community leaders protested that their civil rights would be violated if homosexuals were singled out and not allowed to donate blood. And blood bankers worried about adequate supply. No action was taken, other than finally to give the new immunological disease a name: acquired immune deficiency syndrome, or AIDS.

AIDS: Not Going Away

AIDS cases were proliferating. Five more hemophiliacs contracted the disease. Polly Thomas got reports of babies in New York City who appeared to have AIDS, indicating that it could be transmitted in the womb. On October 28, 1982, the CDC reported that 691 Americans had contracted AIDS, and 278 of them were dead. Outside the United

States, 52 cases had been reported in fifteen other countries, mostly in Western Europe.

On October 30 a San Francisco baby who had received extensive blood transfusions at birth died of AIDS. EIS officer Dave Auerbach found that one of the donors had been diagnosed with AIDS. Auerbach visited the deceased blood donor's brother, who gave him a small black address book containing the name of a doctor who saw mostly gay patients. Auerbach asked the doctor to pull the dead man's file, which included treatment for rectal gonorrhea. Here was the smoking gun — AIDS was being transmitted by transfusion.

The media had virtually ignored AIDS. The victims were stigmatized minorities — gays, drug addicts, Haitian immigrants. Only when it became clear that AIDS was killing babies, getting into the blood supply, and spreading heterosexually did the media pay attention. On December 10, 1982, the *New York Times* reported the case of the transfused San Francisco baby, but it was only the third story that it ran on AIDS the entire year — and this was the premier newspaper in New York City, one of the epicenters of the AIDS epidemic.

That December the CDC received reports of ninety-two new AIDS cases, bringing the total close to nine hundred cases in the United States. The number of reported cases seemed to be doubling every six months, and the known cases were probably just the tip of a huge iceberg, especially if the incubation period was measured in years rather than months. The AIDS story was just beginning.

Big Mac Attack

In February 1982 field EIS officer Steve Helgerson, based at the Oregon Health Department, was tracking an epidemic of bloody diarrhea in Medford, Oregon. It began with fierce abdominal cramps, followed by watery diarrhea, then gushes of bright red blood. Stool cultures were negative for *Salmonella, Shigella, Campylobacter,* and parasites, and victims had little or no fever. Antibiotics appeared to make things worse.

EIS officer Lee Riley, in the Enteric Diseases Branch, flew to Oregon. As he and Helgerson drove down to Medford, they tossed around ideas including the notion that the illness could have been caused by a poison or chemical, because of the lack of fever. They conducted a case-control study with twenty-five cases and forty-seven matched neighborhood controls. All but one of the cases remembered eating at a McDonald's within two weeks of getting sick versus only thirteen controls. Most of the cases had eaten a Big Mac.

With rehydration, hospitalized patients usually recovered within a week, and the outbreak petered out. Riley headed back to Atlanta. At the April 1982 EIS conference, he presented a report tentatively concluding that an unidentified pathogen had somehow gotten into the rehydrated onions. It couldn't have been the hamburgers, he thought, since McDonald's cooked them enough to kill any bacteria.

Then in early June 1982, an identical outbreak occurred in Traverse City, Michigan. Again, most victims had eaten Big Macs. Michigan-based EIS officer Robert Remis suspected the hamburgers. On a busy Friday night he measured the grill temperature and found that, as frozen hamburgers were continually clunked down, the grill surface was cooling. The burgers were not being thoroughly cooked.

Soon afterward, the CDC labs isolated a rare serotype, *Escherichia coli* O157:H7, from Oregon and Michigan patients' stool samples. Remis visited the Greeley, Colorado, slaughterhouse that had supplied the hamburger meat to McDonald's, where he watched as four hundred cows an hour were stunned, killed, bled, and eviscerated. "As they moved along, blood and feces were everywhere," he recalled.

Joined by Lee Riley, Remis went to McDonald's huge Ohio processing plant, where patties were made and frozen. In contrast to the Colorado slaughterhouse, it was an impressively clean, efficient operation. The EIS officers discovered that McDonald's kept frozen samples from each lot, and the CDC labs subsequently isolated *E. coli* O157 from the lot that had gone to both Oregon and Michigan. The ground beef had probably been contaminated by cattle manure before coming to the plant.

Although some other types of *E. coli* can also cause diarrhea, most varieties actually help digest food, synthesize vitamins, and guard against dangerous microbes. This mutated strain's Shiga toxin attacks the lining of the intestine without causing a fever. Antibiotics kill bacteria but leave the Shiga toxin to do its damage. Resistant to acid, salt, and chlorine, it is able to live for weeks in moist environments. It can survive freezing as well as heat up to 160 degrees Fahrenheit. And because of the American penchant for fast food, it was likely to strike again.

By late September, seven Sacramento children had come down with hemolytic uremic syndrome (HUS), which can result in kidney failure, internal bleeding, severe anemia, and brain damage. The cause of HUS, a condition first identified in 1955, remained a mystery. EIS officer Martha Rogers thought that HUS might be similar to Reye's syndrome, so she asked about medications taken during the illness as well as about allergies, family history of renal disease, travel, and food history. The only thing that stood out was eating at a fast-food chain, though it wasn't statistically significant. Later, EIS officers would prove that when the *E. coli* O157 toxin gets into the bloodstream, it causes HUS, which kills about 5 percent of its victims.

The Violence Epidemic

It was ironic that new infectious diseases — toxic shock syndrome, AIDS, and *E. coli* O157 — were cropping up in the early 1980s just as the CDC was trying to shift its focus to chronic diseases and human habits. The March 12, 1982, issue of the *MMWR* published the first table of "Potential Years of Life Lost," ranking what killed people at younger ages (excluding infant mortality). By far the leading cause was "accidents and adverse effects," mostly from motor vehicles, followed by cancer and heart disease. In fourth place was the category of suicides and homicides. Fifth was liver disease, due primarily to alcoholism. The first infectious diseases appeared seventh on the list: pneumonia and influenza.

At the EIS conference the following month, several EIS officers presented pioneering studies of violence. Janine Jason mined FBI data, finding that family members or acquaintances were involved in 76 percent of homicides that weren't associated with another crime such as robbery. Jason brought CDC attention to child abuse, both physical and sexual. Poverty, single-parent homes, and low education were primary risk factors, she found, and stepfathers were more likely than natural fathers to commit incest. Because of multiple, overlapping reporting systems between child protective services and the police, child homicides were vastly underreported, she concluded.

EIS officer Brandon Centerwall presented a correlation between television viewing and the "homicide epidemic in the United States." The murder rate had doubled between 1955 and 1970, at the same time that TV sets had invaded homes. "The homicide rates increased later for blacks than for whites [and] later for persons in rural areas," Centerwall observed, perhaps because African Americans and rural populations delayed purchase of televisions.

He also studied Atlanta murder statistics to determine why there was a higher homicide rate for blacks. "Homicide rates were a direct linear function of residential overcrowding," he reported. "There is no evidence in this study that Atlanta blacks have any greater cultural predisposition for homicide than do Atlanta whites under equivalent socioeconomic circumstances."

In July 1982 Carl Tyler recruited Jim Mercy, the first Ph.D. sociologist to become an EIS officer, grooming him to spearhead the new focus on violence epidemiology. Mercy studied gang warfare in Los Angeles. While there, he investigated the deaths of twenty men over the past decade from LAPD-administered choke holds intended to subdue suspects by temporarily putting pressure on the carotid artery. His confidential study resulted in the choke hold being halted.

In the November 12, 1982, *MMWR,* Mercy wrote: "From 1976 to 1979, 47 percent of all homicides were precipitated by an argument, 1 percent involved a gang fight. . . . In 1981, 50 percent of homicides were committed with handguns, 13 percent with rifles or shotguns." In an editorial note, he called for "public health and intervention strategies," but preventing human violence would prove far more challenging than battling microbes.

III

COMPLEX CHALLENGES

(1982–PRESENT)

15

ENTERING THE COMPUTER AGE

ON FEBRUARY 20, 1983, EIS officer Scott Holmberg flew to Minnesota to investigate a particularly virulent *Salmonella* outbreak. The majority of the ten victims had taken antibiotics a day or two before onset, and six had been hospitalized. State health officials feared that the antibiotics might be contaminated.

Holmberg deduced that the antibiotics were fine, but they had precipitated the illness. This *Salmonella newport* strain proved to be resistant to penicillin, amoxicillin, ampicillin, carbenicillin, and tetracycline. The patients had somehow acquired the *Salmonella*, which didn't bother them until they took antibiotics for some other ailment. Then, with other competing organisms knocked out, the resistant *Salmonella* had proliferated.

Holmberg's case-control study was inconclusive. He sent a request to all state epidemiologists to report any cases of multiresistant *S. newport*. On March 30 he got a call from South Dakota about four cases. A mother and her infant daughter, who lived on a dairy farm, had taken amoxicillin for sore throats in mid-December, then developed diarrhea. In February their male cousin-by-marriage on another dairy farm had followed the same pattern. The fourth case was a sixty-nine-year-old man who had been hospitalized in December after a farm accident and had an anal exam with the same sigmoidoscope just used on the sick mother. He thus acquired the *S. newport,* was given a host of antibiotics, and died.

Holmberg learned that an uncle who raised cattle had given steaks and hamburger to both families. All 105 of his beef cows had been slaughtered in mid-January. A dairy calf that had strayed onto the beef farm had died, and a USDA lab had identified *S. newport* in the remains. Identical plasmids were found in the dead calf and in the cases in South Dakota and Minnesota.

Holmberg reviewed the food histories he had taken in Minnesota. All cases had eaten hamburger. The uncle told Holmberg that he always threw in a handful of tetracycline per ton of feed to promote growth and prevent disease in his livestock. Holmberg was able to trace the uncle's beef from the slaughterhouse to the specific supermarkets where the Minnesota patients shopped. Eventually, he found a total of eighteen cases in four states, though there were probably many more people who ate the hamburger but hadn't taken antibiotics, and who were consequently either asymptomatic or only mildly ill.

This outbreak was proof that resistant organisms developed in animals fed antimicrobials (primarily to fatten them faster) and then caused disease in humans. Holmberg documented that the fatality rate for people infected with drug-resistant *Salmonella* was twenty-one times greater than for regular strains. His investigation spurred FDA hearings and calls for a federal ban on adding antibiotics to animal feed. Although some breeders voluntarily stopped the practice, there is still no regulation in place. "If you want to buy antibiotics for yourself," Holmberg observed, "you need a prescription, but not if you go to the feed store."*

Problem Here ➞

At the end of 1982 EIS alum Carl Tyler took over from Philip Brachman as the director of the CDC Epidemiology Program Office. EIS

---

*Two years later EIS officer Caroline Ryan investigated a multidrug-resistant *Salmonella* outbreak with more than sixteen thousand confirmed cases, traced to improperly pasteurized milk in a Chicago dairy plant. Many victims had taken antibiotics a few days before falling ill.

alum Jim Mason became the new CDC director in September 1983 after Bill Foege resigned. Mason, a devout Mormon and the father of seven, and Tyler, the champion of abortion rights, would serve uneasily together for the next six years.

Regardless of the politics of the top dogs in the CDC, EIS officers continued to make discoveries and travel the globe. Rob Tauxe, a medical doctor with a master's in public health, joined the Enterics Branch in 1983. In mid-August he investigated a *Campylobacter* epidemic at the University of Georgia. Tauxe and his colleagues traced the epidemic to undercooked chicken, barbecued by inexperienced male college students, eager to chow down with a couple of beers.

In October Tauxe conducted a national survey of college health services and discovered that *Campylobacter,* only recently recognized as an important pathogen, was isolated from student stool samples at least ten times as frequently as any other bacterium. Several illness clusters were connected to chicken consumption. "A disease outbreak is a sign that something has gone wrong," Tauxe observed. "It's like a giant arrow pointing, *PROBLEM HERE!*"

In January 1984 EIS alum José Rigau called from Puerto Rico about a baby with salmonellosis whose father had bought a pet turtle. In 1975 the FDA had banned the sale of these reptiles in the United States, including territories such as Puerto Rico.* Tauxe discovered that some forty-eight thousand pet turtles labeled "for export only" had nonetheless been shipped to Puerto Rico in the past two years.

Every turtle Tauxe collected from eighteen pet shops yielded the bacteria. The EIS officer tracked the shipments back to one Louisiana turtle-raising pond. The illegal exports to Puerto Rico were halted, but an estimated 4 million turtles had been legally exported to other countries.

The Guru and the Salad Bars

On September 26, 1984, the Oregon state epidemiologist called the CDC about sixty cases of *Salmonella typhimurium* associated with

---

*See pages 110–111.

several restaurants in The Dalles, a city of 10,500 along Interstate 84 bordering the Columbia River. EIS officer Tom Török, stationed in New Mexico, flew to Oregon, and was joined the next day by EIS officer Bob Wise out of Atlanta.

Wise set up a data management system to make sense of the 751 cases eventually identified, along with the many variables associated with each one. Many travelers off the interstate had stopped for food only once, so it was deduced that the first sick customers ate on Wednesday, September 12, at the Portage Inn. Two days later Arlo's Restaurant also must have served something replete with *Salmonella*. The cases petered out, but suddenly, other people began to sicken. Their illness was traced to something they consumed sometime from September 21 to 23, at the Portage Inn, Arlo's, and eight other restaurants in The Dalles.

Török's case-control studies implicated salad bars as the source of disease. Since the epidemic seemed to be limited to The Dalles, Török reasoned that the contaminated item was probably produced locally. It couldn't be the water, since no residential cases had been reported. But the two restaurants in the first wave shared no common food sources.

He searched in vain for an event that linked those who worked for the ten restaurants. The Portage Inn had catered nineteen banquets concurrent with the outbreak period. The same staff had prepared salad bars for the banquets, yet no attendees had gotten sick. Perhaps customers had inadvertently or intentionally carried the bacteria from salad bar to salad bar?

The Dalles was the county seat of Wasco County, where in 1981 the guru Bhagwan Shree Rajneesh had purchased a ranch, attracting thousands of followers seeking enlightenment along with sex and drugs. Relations with neighbors had quickly soured. Török and Wise had heard accusatory rumors. But there was no obvious motive for deliberate contamination, nor had anyone claimed responsibility for the outbreak along with an ultimatum or threat.

After three weeks Török returned to New Mexico to deal with bubonic plague cases. EIS officer Rob Tauxe flew out to continue the baffling investigation. He, too, came up blank.

A year later the Rajneeshee cult collapsed, as Ma Anand Sheela (Sheela Silverman), who had run the compound, and medical director Ma Anand Puja (Diane Onang) resigned and fled to Europe. The Bhagwan accused them of various crimes, including sabotage of the salad bars. A vial of *Salmonella typhimurium* with the same plasmid fingerprint as the outbreak strain was found in Puja's medical laboratory. She had purchased it legally, since it was routinely used around the country to train technicians in identifying bacteria.

Puja, a nurse practitioner, had grown the *S. typhimurium* in large-scale production, then, with other cult members, sprinkled the brownish liquid repeatedly on items in local salad bars. FBI investigators interviewed an associate who said that Puja had "delighted in death, poisons, and the idea of carrying out various plots." The salad bar contaminations were meant as a test run before putting *Salmonella* into the town's water supply to disable voters who might revoke the cult's tax-free status.

EPO director Carl Tyler refused to allow Török and Tauxe to publish their article on the investigation, afraid that it would provoke copycat events, as the Tylenol-cyanide poisonings had in 1982.

A decade later, in the wake of the 1995 sarin gas attacks by the Aum Shinrikyo cult in the Tokyo subways, Török and Tauxe were finally allowed to publish their paper on the salad bar contamination, the first major bioterrorism event in the United States.

Interminable Diarrhea

In July 1984 EIS officer Kristine MacDonald went to Brainerd, Minnesota, where more than a hundred residents had contracted seemingly interminable diarrhea. For most victims, the affliction had already lasted nine months. In her report, MacDonald described a typical case, an otherwise healthy seventy-seven-year-old man who defecated up to twenty times a day and lost twenty pounds during the first month of illness. "Nine months after onset of illness," MacDonald wrote, "the patient had gained weight and had less urgency, but was still having six to eight watery stools per day."

A case-control study implicated raw milk from a local dairy. The CDC labs tested the milk and stool samples. Nothing. "Brainerd diarrhea may well prove to be the latest of the newly recognized syndromes caused by an infectious agent," MacDonald concluded.

In 1987 the chronic diarrhea struck in rural Illinois. EIS officers Sue Trock and Julie Parsonnet traced the outbreak to untreated well water from a local restaurant, but again, no infective agent could be identified. Despite extensive investigations in many subsequent outbreaks, no one has yet solved the mystery of Brainerd diarrhea.

Child-Killing Rotavirus

EIS alum Roger Glass returned to the CDC in 1986 to specialize in diarrhea caused by viruses. His lab helped to document that Norwalk virus (norovirus) often caused otherwise unexplained cruise ship outbreaks regularly investigated by EIS officers. Because the tiny virus can apparently float through the air, it is particularly difficult to control. Fortunately, the illness it causes is relatively mild and brief.

But Glass was concerned with a far more dangerous virus. Working at the Cholera Research Lab in Bangladesh in 1979 through 1980, he had identified rotavirus as a major cause of diarrhea and death in infants. Rotavirus, so named because it resembles a spoked wheel under an electron microscope, was discovered in 1973. Nearly all children on Earth are infected with the virus in their first four years of life. If they survive, they develop lifelong immunity.

Glass recruited EIS officer Mei-Shang Ho to document the impact of rotavirus in the United States, where it primarily struck infants in the winter. For a recent six-year period, Ho extracted data on children under five years of age from the National Hospital Discharge Survey. She found that over 200,000 such children were hospitalized each year with diarrhea, with a prominent peak occurring in October through April. These excess winter cases accounted for a third of the annual total and mostly affected children four months to two years old. In other words, rotavirus probably accounted for at least 70,000 annual hospitalizations.

Then Mei-Shang Ho looked at ten years of mortality data from the National Center for Health Statistics. Only 9 percent of the childhood diarrheal deaths listed an agent such as *Shigella* or amoeba. More than five hundred deaths per year among children under five were caused by "diarrhea of nonspecific etiology," mostly during the winter months — i.e., probably rotavirus. Overall, black infants were four times more likely to die of diarrhea than whites, but in the South it was much worse, with Mississippi's black children dying at a rate ten times higher than whites.

Ho found that the mothers of the dead black children in Mississippi were often teenage high school dropouts who had not received good prenatal care and who probably didn't seek prompt treatment for their children. Ho and Glass called for special outreach to such mothers, teaching them to use oral rehydration solution and encouraging them to bring in diarrheic children for prompt medical attention.

Rotavirus took its worst toll in the developing world. An estimated 3 to 5 billion cases of diarrhea occurred every year in Asia, Africa, and Latin America, killing 5 to 10 million. Several candidate vaccines were being developed, but it would take nearly three decades before a rotavirus vaccine was finally licensed.

The High Priestess of *E. Coli*

Having learned that the probable cause of hemolytic uremic syndrome was *E. coli* O157:H7, EIS officer Patty Griffin began to call pediatric nephrologists around the country, proposing a study to look for the bacteria in the stools of HUS patients. This study would prove O157's crucial role as *the* primary cause of hemolytic uremic syndrome.

In October 1986 Griffin flew to Walla Walla, Washington, where she joined Olympia-based EIS officer Steve Ostroff, tracking a large *E. coli* O157 outbreak to the ground beef at Taco Time, a fast-food restaurant. They identified thirty-seven cases, two of whom died.

Griffin and Ostroff traced the meat back to dairy farms in southwest Washington. They found O157 in the stools of six cows from four different farms, but not with the same plasmid profile as the outbreak strain. While the lethal *E. coli* strain was rare, it was evolving, and with hamburger meat ground from a mix of hundreds of old dairy cows and the worst cuts of beef, even one tainted cow could infect an entire lot. The EIS officers concluded that the outbreak had probably been statewide but that most cases had gone unrecognized.

During his remaining EIS time, Ostroff set up routine surveillance for *E. coli* O157 in Washington, and that state became the first to make *E. coli* O157 a reportable disease. Griffin went on to become the CDC expert on the disease, earning her the informal title of "high priestess of *E. coli*."

The Eternal Freshman

EIS officer Mike St. Louis was dubbed the "eternal freshman" for his unquenchable enthusiasm. His primary EIS work was to explore why *Salmonella enteritidis* epidemics kept occurring, particularly in the northeastern United States. In June 1986 St. Louis investigated a multistate *S. enteritidis* outbreak associated with frozen lasagna, jumbo stuffed pasta shells, manicotti, and ravioli made by Rotanelli Foods at a production plant in New Rochelle, New York. St. Louis traced the problem to raw eggs in the cheese stuffing. The products were labeled "Fully cooked. Just heat and serve," but many people did not heat the food sufficiently to kill bacteria. The company subsequently changed the label and switched to pasteurized liquid eggs.

By the spring of 1987 the CDC had been alerted to sixty-five *S. enteritidis* outbreaks in the northeast in the prior two years, most traceable to raw or inadequately cooked grade A eggs. St. Louis looked back at the 1973–1984 register of *Salmonella* outbreaks, searching for egg ingredients. He compiled impressive statistics linking *S. enteritidis* with eggs.

EIS officers had made the egg-*Salmonella* link twenty-five years before,* but past outbreaks had been traced to fecal contamination

---

*See pages 46–48.

of cracked or soiled eggs. The modern Rotanelli plant had purchased unblemished large white eggs and then disinfected their exteriors. St. Louis buried himself in poultry research and found a 1944 article in the *British Medical Journal* stating that *S. enteritidis* could persist in the ovaries of chickens. Could the hens actually be depositing bacteria *inside* the intact eggs they laid? He published the suggestion in the *Journal of the American Medical Association,* raising a storm of protest from the egg industry.

Illinois-based EIS officer Sue Trock incubated whole eggs from an implicated farm, washed and flame-sterilized them, then cracked and cultured them. She found an abundance of *S. enteritidis.* Until then, eggs had been considered perfectly packaged natural products requiring no refrigeration. Illinois was the first state to demand chilled eggs (to prevent bacterial proliferation), even in transport, and the FDA soon followed suit.

AIDS in Africa

The number of AIDS cases skyrocketed from around a thousand identified cases at the beginning of 1983 to a million by the end of the decade, by which time an estimated 10 million people were infected worldwide. Half of them lived in Africa.

In October 1983 EIS alum Joe McCormick, head of viral Special Pathogens at CDC, and colleagues documented thirty-eight AIDS cases in the end stages of the disease in two hospitals in Kinshasa, Zaire's capital, with about the same number of male and female victims. Ten died during the three weeks of the study. One was a twenty-one-year-old woman who, desperate for money, had worked as a prostitute. When he returned from Zaire, McCormick warned that AIDS in Africa was being spread by heterosexual contact. But U.S. Assistant Secretary of Health Ed Brandt refused to believe it, asking, "Have you considered other vectors, like mosquitoes?" McCormick decided to establish an AIDS research project in Kinshasa.

In 1984 virologists were zeroing in on what was ultimately named the human immunodeficiency virus (HIV), which caused AIDS. The following year, when tests for HIV antibodies became available, Mc-

Cormick decided to test the blood samples he and his colleagues had collected from villagers in Yambuku, Zaire, during the first Ebola outbreak in 1976.* Five of the 659 frozen specimens (0.8 percent) were HIV-positive.

In November 1985 he dispatched Special Pathogens EIS officer Don Forthal to Yambuku to look for those five villagers. Because few people left the stable rural village, Forthal was quickly able to learn that three had died after wasting away with AIDS-like symptoms. He secured blood samples from the two survivors, both of whom were still HIV-positive. The woman appeared healthy, but the man had a low helper T cell count.

McCormick sent Belgian EIS officer Kevin De Cock to Zaire in September 1986. In the Yambuku area, De Cock took blood samples in the same villages from which the 1976 specimens had been taken, seeking to produce comparable results. Of the 389 sera he secured, three were HIV-positive — precisely the same 0.8 percent rate as a decade before.

It appeared likely that a few AIDS cases may have occurred for years in rural areas. But with the end of colonial rule and the rise of dictators, slaughter, and rape, people fled to the cities, where many women resorted to prostitution. Multiple sex partners spread AIDS, as did the widespread use of nonsterile syringes in hospitals and clinics. Around the same time, EIS alum André Nahmias, a professor at Emory University, tested 672 blood samples taken in 1959 in Kinshasa (then called Léopoldville) for genetics research. One sample, the oldest yet found, was HIV-positive.

Researchers subsequently identified a closely related chimpanzee virus, dubbed simian immunodeficiency virus (SIVcpz), which does not kill chimps. Genetic detectives, looking at the various mutations, have concluded that the virus jumped from chimps to humans around 1930, somewhere in or near the Congo region.

From 1960 to 1975, Zaire imported thousands of Haitians as contract laborers. When they returned to Haiti, a few might have car-

---

*See pages 170–174.

ried the virus. During the 1970s Haiti became a cheap erotic destination for gay pleasure seekers. It is possible that sexual tourists brought AIDS back to North America with them.

In 1968 a gay St. Louis teenage boy died of Kaposi's sarcoma and cytomegalovirus. His frozen serum was found to contain HIV, proving that AIDS was already in the United States at least as far back as the 1960s. It may have returned with World War II soldiers from the African campaign, but that is pure speculation.

Yellow Fever

Kevin De Cock returned to Atlanta on Sunday, November 30, 1986. Four days later he flew back to Africa to investigate a yellow fever epidemic in Nigeria. The yellow fever virus is transmitted by mosquitoes. After an incubation period of a few days, victims develop fever, muscle ache, and headache. Many recover, but in others, the virus invades multiple organs, including the liver. In most parts of the world, sanitation efforts had stymied the disease, and in 1937 an effective vaccine was developed.

At one point, there was hope that yellow fever could be eradicated, until it was discovered that humans were not its only reservoir. In tropical regions, monkeys carry the virus, causing periodic outbreaks of jungle (sylvan) yellow fever when mosquitoes bite monkeys, then humans. It was such an outbreak that De Cock investigated, along with CDC virologist Tom Monath and others.

The epidemic epicenter was the Oju area of Benue state in south-central Nigeria, where isolated villages and family compounds were set amid elephant grass and locust bean trees. There were limited health-care facilities. A local school had been converted to a make-shift sick bay. Nearby were freshly dug graves.

The first yellow fever deaths had occurred in July with the onset of the rainy season, but they had only come to the Nigerian government's attention in October at the epidemic's peak. A mass vaccination campaign was mounted in November and December, but it failed to reach a quarter of the population, and much of the vaccine was impotent because of improper refrigeration.

The CDC team went to see the Benue state military governor and urged him to employ the military to mount an effective vaccine campaign, which got under way in January. By that time the dry season was beginning, and the *Aedes africanus* mosquitoes that carried the virus were disappearing, though the next generation might also carry the virus.

When De Cock left at the end of December, he estimated that 9,800 people had contracted yellow fever with jaundice and that 5,600 had died — and that was just in Oju, so that the total in the region was considerably higher. He feared that someone from Benue state might carry the virus to a more urban region, where *Aedes aegypti* mosquitoes would serve as the vector for a yellow fever epidemic that required no monkeys. In March 1987 that is just what happened in the city of Ogbomosho, three hundred miles to the west. A third yellow fever epidemic broke out to the north in Mariga in September 1987. In total, yellow fever had killed some 35,000 Nigerians — and the media ignored it.

"A safe and effective vaccine against yellow fever has been available for 50 years," De Cock wrote in frustration, "but the disease continues to occur in Africa and South America." He suggested the inclusion of yellow fever vaccine in the Expanded Program on Immunization (EPI), but such adoption was painfully slow, country by country, and more than a million Nigerians would die of yellow fever from 1984 to 1994.

AIDS Denial and Paranoia

During the 1980s in the United States, the number of diagnosed AIDS cases doubled every six months. On January 4, 1983, blood bankers at a CDC meeting had refused to acknowledge transfusion-associated AIDS. EIS alum Don Francis pounded the table in frustration. "Tell us a number you need," he said. "If we have twenty, forty, a hundred cases — will you believe it then?"* Tests of AIDS patients' blood

---

*The CDC helped end AIDS transmission to hemophiliacs in late 1984 by proving that heat-treating the clotting Factor VIII killed HIV.

had shown that the vast majority contained antibodies to hepatitis B. There was no AIDS test yet, but why not look for hep B antibodies as a proxy measure?

The blood bankers and regulatory agencies refused to consider his suggestion, but in March the FDA agreed to ask high-risk individuals to refrain from donating blood on an honor system. Mandatory testing and name-based reporting were politically unacceptable and might have driven cases underground. Frank discussion of sexual practices and AIDS education were restricted by conservative legislators.

By July 1983 EIS officer Harry Haverkos had documented ten AIDS cases from blood transfusions and was astonished that the FDA and blood bankers remained skeptical.

Ken Castro, assigned full-time to the AIDS Activity Unit in July 1983, traveled extensively to investigate AIDS cases with "no identifiable risk" — i.e., not gays, drug users, hemophiliacs, Haitians, or anyone who had sexual relations with those at high risk. About 4 percent of AIDS cases had no identifiable risk. Castro suspected that those cases were hiding something. "Black and Hispanic men had machismo and found it hard to admit having sex with men," he said. White Southern Baptists had similar issues.

When a lab technician in Humboldt, Texas, got AIDS, it appeared that a worst-case nightmare might have come true — AIDS acquisition in a laboratory. The patient was on a ventilator and could not speak. When he recovered somewhat, he called Castro to admit that, although married with two children, he had occasionally had casual encounters with gay men.

In San Francisco, Castro interviewed a father and son who both had AIDS. The son was openly gay. Could this be the first case of interfamilial transmission? The father denied any drug use or homosexual activity, but his business partner confided to Castro that they had sex with young men when traveling to Middle Eastern countries.

Castro conducted a special investigation of Haitians, concluding that those with AIDS were more likely to have had multiple sex partners, and that heterosexual transmission was primarily involved. "We ended up removing Haitians as an official risk group, since we traced their AIDS to behavioral factors," he said.

AIDS in Belle Glade

In April 1985 the CDC hosted the first international AIDS conference in Atlanta. Two doctors from Belle Glade, Florida, created a sensation with a study suggesting that AIDS was transmitted there by mosquitoes. Although the CDC experts were sure that mosquitoes did not carry the AIDS virus, it was crucial to prove that insects could not transmit the disease. On May 13, 1985, Ken Castro left for Florida.

The tropical region drew migrant workers from the United States and the Caribbean. Castro found thirty-one AIDS victims, all adults living in a congested slum area, most of whom were Haitians, drug users, prostitutes, or homosexuals. If mosquitoes were spreading the disease, they apparently didn't fly to the wealthier parts of town, nor did they bite children or the elderly.

Although Castro's preliminary report was convincing, he needed more evidence. From February through September 1986, he and his team conducted a door-to-door survey. They uncovered a total of seventy-nine AIDS cases, including three babies born to HIV-positive mothers. They also found thirty HIV-positive residents who had not yet developed AIDS.

The cases occurred in two overlapping clusters of homosexuals and drug users, connected by two bisexual male heroin addicts. Castro's study, published in *Science*, emphatically disproved the theory of mosquito-transmitted AIDS. However, he could do little to stop AIDS in Belle Glade or elsewhere, other than to urge education, counseling, and voluntary testing.

Testing for an Incurable Disease

Just before EIS officer John Ward joined the AIDS Activity Unit in July 1984, the identification of the human immunodeficiency virus (HIV) was announced. By February 1985 two AIDS blood tests had been developed — an enzyme-linked immunosorbent assay (ELISA) and the more time-consuming but definitive Western blot.

Ward and others fanned out across the country to host community meetings, explain how the tests worked, and field questions. When EIS alum Don Francis submitted a comprehensive $33 million prevention plan, suggesting blood testing and education at drug treatment and STD clinics, CDC director Jim Mason approved it and sent it to Washington. The plan was rejected by the Reagan administration in early February 1985.

In March, when blood donors were first screened using the new tests, Ward began a study in cooperation with the Atlanta Red Cross to see whether the tests worked. He proved that those with high reactivity on the initial ELISA test were more likely to be positive on subsequent tests and that virtually everyone found to be positive by Western blot did indeed have identifiable AIDS risk factors. The tests did not work, however, for those who had been infected shortly prior to blood donation. After accumulating eight such cases, Ward concluded that there was a six-week period between initial infection and when the production of HIV antibodies would show up on a test. That made it important that donor self-deferral should continue.

On October 2, 1985, movie star Rock Hudson died of AIDS, marking a sea change in the public and political attitude toward the disease. The money spigot finally turned on. EIS alum Jeff Harris was appointed head of the barely extant AIDS program at the U.S. Agency for International Development the next year and built the division into an effective partner with EIS alum Jonathan Mann's Global AIDS Program at the World Health Organization. In 1987 President Ronald Reagan finally acknowledged AIDS, calling it "public enemy number one" six years after the epidemic commenced.

An estimated twelve thousand people had been infected by transfusions administered before the HIV blood test was available. The transfusion data provided precise infection dates, Ward realized, allowing him to estimate the incubation period. "We conclude that most recipients of HIV-infected blood become seropositive," he wrote. "AIDS develops in about half these recipients within seven years." In time, it would become clear that the average incubation period for AIDS was ten years.

Examining Ward's figures in 1986, EIS alum Walt Williams, an African American, noticed that blacks and Hispanics were overrepresented. He and EIS alum Martha Rogers in the AIDS unit collaborated on a study. "Most people continue to think of AIDS as a disease of homosexual white males," they wrote. "However, AIDS cases are occurring three times more frequently among black and Hispanic men than among white men." And the difference was even greater for minority women.

A larger proportion of black and Hispanic men were bisexual, and more minority men and women were intravenous drug users, sharing nonsterile needles. Women prostituting themselves to feed their drug habits spread AIDS heterosexually, and they passed the disease to their babies in the womb.

Williams and Rogers urged that much of the $50 million allocated to AIDS prevention in 1987 should be targeted at minority populations at risk. To avoid mother-to-child transmission, they suggested the support of more family planning and drug abuse clinics and the distribution of free sterile needles. Only military recruits could be forced to take AIDS blood tests, but people attending STD clinics should be urged to submit to voluntary testing. Few of these suggestions were implemented, and the rapid spread of AIDS among blacks and Hispanics continued.

In 1987 Don Francis published a comprehensive article in the *Journal of the American Medical Association*. "Virtually all future infections can, at least theoretically, be prevented," he wrote, since the disease could only be transmitted through blood or semen. "Individuals should be able to modify their behaviors to protect themselves from infection." All they needed was "information, motivation, and skills." He suggested voluntary, confidential blood testing for high-risk groups, contact tracing, counseling, and gay bathhouse closure. His article caused hardly a ripple.

A Scathing Skit

In their April 1986 skit, EIS officers let loose with their frustrations over how AIDS was being treated, mocking CDC director Jim Mason. "Oh, but dear," the actor portraying Mason said to his wife, "I get so worried and embarrassed when I talk about AIDS. I just can't say those words." The EIS skits have always used black humor to release tension over the difficult life-and-death issues EIS officers deal with. That sort of sophomoric irreverence is a part of their culture just as much as their efforts to save lives.

Gay EIS officer Juan Rodriguez sang about how to rise within the CDC bureaucracy by playing up to the boss, but the song (a takeoff on "Dance: Ten; Looks: Three" with its "tits and ass" refrain from *A Chorus Line*) had an underlying sexual innuendo. "Kiss his ass, butter up his derriere. Get real close to it, make the most of it." A few years later Rodriguez would die of AIDS.

16
UNEXPECTED CONNECTIONS

DURING THE REAGAN years, EIS officers encountered novel challenges in addition to AIDS. In 1983 pediatrician Ed Lammer, in the Birth Defects Branch, conducted investigations of sudden infant death syndrome (SIDS), including a case-control study of a SIDS cluster among the Oglala Sioux on the Pine Ridge Indian Reservation in South Dakota, where eleven babies had died inexplicably in little over a year. Most deaths had occurred during the winter. Lammer found that many mothers of SIDS infants were anemic and had gotten pregnant shortly after giving birth to another child. While he didn't isolate the cause of the syndrome, at least he dispelled rumors that the deaths were due to vaccinations or contaminated water.

Soon after the South Dakota investigation, Lammer visited Dalton, Georgia, where a young mother had lost three children to SIDS. The woman's great-grandmother told the EIS officer that there had been twelve SIDS deaths over six generations in the maternal line, suggesting a possible genetic component to the syndrome. The mother, a heavy smoker, had first become pregnant at eighteen, and by twenty-two she had conceived five times, miscarrying twice.

Lammer wrote that genetic factors might predispose an infant to SIDS, "given the added insults from maternal and other environmental risk factors." Still, he cautioned, "the etiology of the great majority of

SIDS cases continues to elude researchers." That remains true, though placing babies on their backs to sleep appears to help. Recent research indicates, as Lammer suggested in his report, that SIDS babies may have an abnormal breathing control mechanism in their brains.

His next investigation involved a clearer etiology. In September 1982 pharmaceutical giant Hoffmann-La Roche had begun to market Accutane, its brand name for vitamin A derivative isotretinoin, a miraculous acne cure. By July 1983 four pregnant women who had taken Accutane had borne babies with severe birth defects. Hoffmann-La Roche revised the package to warn women of the potential risks, but cases continued to occur, as each month an additional ten thousand women of childbearing age began taking the acne medication.

In July 1984 Lammer studied all 154 Accutane-exposed pregnancies that had been identified since the product's release. Of those, 95 women had chosen to abort and an additional 18 babies had died in the womb or were stillborn. Of the remaining 41 live births, 18 had major congenital malformations, and half of them soon died. The evidence against Accutane was overwhelming.

Although Lammer published his report in the *New England Journal of Medicine,* the FDA continued to permit dermatologists to write prescriptions for the acne medication. After the Accutane patent expired in 2002, generic isotretinoin became widely available on the Internet from countries where a prescription is not required.

Working Both Sides of the Cuyahoga River

In the spring of 1984 Cleveland pediatric hematologist Peter Coccia called Bruce Evatt, the EIS alum who headed the CDC effort to track AIDS in hemophiliacs, to report that ten of his young black patients with sickle cell anemia and a white patient with a hereditary blood disorder had developed acute aplastic crises within the preceding five weeks. An "aplastic crisis" means that something is preventing new red blood cells from being formed, producing severe anemia and dehydration in sickle cell patients. Such crises are rare, yet here was a cluster. Two of Coccia's patients were brothers. Could an infectious agent be involved?

On May 1 Evatt sent EIS officer Terry Chorba to Cleveland. In an article about aplastic crises, Chorba found that a Haitian researcher had associated parvovirus B19 with the condition in 1981, and that in 1983 a British doctor had found the same virus in children with fifth disease. Life-threatening aplastic anemia primarily affected black children with sickle cell anemia. Fifth disease, so-called because it was the fifth kind of rash identified after measles and three others, was officially named erythema infectiosum. When it affected white children, it briefly caused a bright red rash that gave it yet another nickname, "slapped cheek syndrome."

Chorba, who joined Ohio-based EIS officer Jon Sudman, asked Coccia if he knew of any fifth disease cases, and Coccia referred him to hematologist Betty Kruzinsky at Metropolitan General Hospital on the city's west side. Cleveland was neatly divided and segregated by the Cuyahoga River. To the east lived African Americans. On the west side were mostly middle-class whites, whose children were having an outbreak of bright red cheek rashes.

Chorba and Sudman, with help from two CDC Public Health Advisors, drew blood from patients and their families on both sides of the river. Chorba returned to Atlanta with 840 blood samples. The blood from the black aplastic crisis patients was teeming with parvovirus B19, while the white fifth disease patients' samples had antibodies to B19, though by the time they developed a rash, the virus itself had disappeared.

Chorba's paper on the concurrent outbreaks proved that parvovirus B19 caused both aplastic crises and fifth disease. The virus also produced a rash in black children that wasn't visible on their cheeks. B19 is highly contagious. People infected as children are immune for life, but others who had not been infected could develop serious problems. Chorba's EIS classmate Janet Kinney later found that pregnant women with fifth disease might have spontaneous abortions or fetal wastages.

An Exhausting Disease

Daniel Peterson, a doctor in Incline Village, Nevada, called the EIS on August 8, 1985. Since January he and his partner, Paul Cheney, had seen at least one hundred patients with an illness characterized by malaise, fatigue, sore throat, tender lymph nodes, and enlarged spleens. Although the symptoms sounded like infectious mononucleosis, the patients tested negative to the diagnostic heterophile antibody test.

In January 1985 virologist Stephen Straus had published an article in the *Annals of Internal Medicine* signaling a possible new disease: "Persisting Illness and Fatigue in Adults with Evidence of Epstein-Barr Virus Infection." After reading the article, Peterson and Cheney sent their patients' blood to a California lab, where all tested positive for EBV antibodies.

The syndrome itself was not new. In a 1959 article reviewing twenty-three worldwide outbreaks, EIS officer D.A. Henderson had described the "protean symptomatology, including fatigue, headache, alternations in emotional status, aching muscular pain, paresis [weakness] and paresthesias [tingling, numbness]." He noted that "females have been more frequently and severely afflicted" and that "the nature of these diseases has suggested to most a viral etiology." At that time, however, no virus could be found.

Peterson called again in September; he was continuing to see new cases. On September 18 EIS officer Gary Holmes flew to Nevada and began to interview patients who had been overwhelmingly tired for at least a month. From the thirty-one who fit those criteria, he eliminated those with diagnosed ailments such as congestive heart failure, thyroid diseases, cirrhosis, Crohn's disease, anemia, or persistent bacterial infections.

Of the remaining fifteen, thirteen were women, most with histories of overachievement as long-distance runners, business executives, or supermoms. Now they could barely drag themselves out of bed. While he set up a case-control study, Holmes asked the California lab to retest the patients' blood samples, and he sent sera back to the CDC and an independent lab at Georgetown University. The findings were inconsistent. Even the California lab couldn't replicate its earlier results. It also turned out that almost everyone had EBV antibodies. The results for the controls were almost indistinguishable from the cases. Since there was no compelling evidence that the disease was caused by EBV, Holmes and a group of consultants suggested calling it chronic fatigue syndrome.

For his five-plus-year career at the CDC, Holmes was the chronic fatigue expert, growing increasingly frustrated. Congress passed legislation forcing the CDC to set up surveillance for the ailment. "But how do you do that for a disease with no diagnosis?" Holmes asked. "Frankly, that's why I left the CDC. I was tired of dealing with chronic fatigue syndrome." Yet doctors kept referring chronic fatigue patients to him. He concluded that most of them suffered from severe depression and treated them with some success with antidepressants. By 1990 an estimated 1 million people had been diagnosed with chronic fatigue syndrome. No virus or other infectious agent has yet been identified as its cause.*

Serendipity at BU

On January 15, 1985, a young Venezuelan woman matriculated at Boston University, then came down with a fever and rash. The BU infirmary sent her to the university hospital, but her measles remained undiagnosed, since most physicians didn't look for it in adults. As a consequence, measles spread quickly to a hundred students.

Near the end of February EIS officer Bob Chen arrived to investigate. Meanwhile, measles had also broken out at Ohio State University and Principia College, a Christian Science school in Illinois. For the unimmunized students at Principia, the epidemic was worse, with three dying from respiratory complications. But why were supposedly vaccinated college students in the other schools coming down with the disease?

Chen suspected that childhood measles vaccinations might not confer lifelong immunity. The only way to find out was to test blood

---

*In October 2009 researcher Judy Mikovits published an article in *Science* claiming that xenotropic murine leukemia virus (XMRV), a retrovirus, had been found in two-thirds of her study's chronic fatigue patients, versus 3.7 percent of healthy controls. CDC expert William Reeves faulted the publication for failing to explain how CFS cases or controls were selected or classified. He noted the importance of others verifying the reported findings but doubted that XMRV would turn out to be the unique causative agent for CFS.

from students *before* they contracted measles. Chen called the Boston Red Cross. Why yes, just two weeks before the epidemic, they had conducted a blood drive at BU. By serendipity, Chen was able to test pre-exposure blood for eight students who had come down with measles and compare the results with seventy-one donors who remained well.

Seven of the eight students who became ill did have measles antibodies, but with pre-exposure titers (amounts) of 120 or less. Those who remained well had higher titers. He also found that students with intermediate titer levels didn't come down with classic measles, but they did have mild fevers, aches, or headaches. Four years later, in large part because of Chen's investigation, a two-dose measles policy was endorsed.

Mumps and Slumps

Because of its expense and the mild nature of the disease, the mumps vaccine, licensed in 1967, was not recommended for universal use until 1977, creating a cohort of unvaccinated young adults. On August 18, 1987, at the Chicago Mercantile Exchange, the faces of two young men began to swell and their salivary glands ached. Two months later, as aggressive traders screamed in the pits, days before the market crash of October 19, 1987, they sprayed saliva, creating ideal conditions for the spread of the virus. By October 25, when EIS officer Karen Kaplan arrived, 116 employees at three futures exchanges had contracted the disease, which can cause miscarriages in women or (rarely) sterility in men.

The news was kept out of the papers until after an emergency vaccination campaign and the end of the outbreak. As with measles, two doses of mumps vaccine eventually became the standard recommendation.

Toxic Spills

Toxic spills proliferated in the mid-1980s. By far the worst occurred on December 3, 1984, in Bhopal, India, when a Union Carbide pesticide plant released 40 tons of methyl isocyanate gas that immediately killed three thousand people and ultimately caused the deaths of an estimated sixteen thousand. The Indian government refused to allow a CDC investigative team led by EIS alum Jeff Koplan into Bhopal. With tact and diplomacy, they finally got to spend a few days at the accident site but could make only limited recommendations.

In the United States, on August 11, 1985, a West Virginia Union Carbide pesticide plant released a plume of twenty-three different chemicals into the air. EIS officer Ruth Etzel rushed to the scene. No one died, but 135 people sought hospital care. Most residents had not heard the warning siren. Even had there been an effective warning, no one knew what to do.

"Chemical releases such as [this] are not uncommon," Etzel wrote. From 1980 to 1985, more than 420 million pounds of chemicals had been released in U.S. industrial spills, killing 139 people and causing 4,768 injuries. She recommended that industrial plants be located away from densely populated areas, that hazardous chemicals be stored in small amounts, that backup and safety systems be checked frequently, and that better evacuation plans and warning methods be developed.

Pesticide in Sierra Leone

In June 1986 Etzel and EIS officer Don Forthal flew to Sierra Leone to investigate a cluster of sudden deaths. On May 20, in the village of Kenema, twenty-seven people had become dizzy and weak, vomited, and then developed tremors, frothed at the mouth, and lost consciousness. Five children and two adults died. Suspecting that their bread was contaminated, the villagers threw it out. Six ducks who ate the crumbs dropped dead. The next day a similar outbreak occurred in another neighboring village, and again on June 1 in Kenema. A total of fourteen people died.

Etzel and Forthal traced the bread to a local baker and then to a flour mill in Freetown, the capital. No toxin could be found. Finally the EIS officers located the driver and truck that had delivered the load of flour. The truck's metal floor was still contaminated with the toxic pesticide parathion, which had apparently been carried in the same load with the flour. Etzel suggested that parathion be banned in countries without sufficient regulations. Yet even in the United

States, agricultural workers were sometimes poisoned when applying the pesticide.*

Vitamin E Shots

An Ohio hospital notified the CDC in March 1984 that three premature babies had yellow skin, bloated stomachs, low platelet counts, enlarged livers, and kidney failure. Two had died. Despite extensive testing, no infectious cause could be found. Then a Tennessee hospital alerted the CDC to a similar outbreak in its neonatal intensive care unit. Three of the eight premature babies had died. Walter Williams, a recent EIS graduate, was dispatched on April 3.

At the Tennessee hospital, Williams pored over the premature babies' charts, working eighteen-hour days until he finally found what he was looking for. All of the sick infants had received a new intravenous vitamin E preparation called E-Ferol. Born with low vitamin E levels, preemies had traditionally received supplements by intramuscular injection. E-Ferol, licensed in December 1983, allowed easier administration through an IV tube. Williams notified EIS officer Bob Gaynes, who was still working the Ohio cases, in which he soon found an association with E-Ferol. A few days later a third hospital called the CDC from Spokane, Washington, to say that four premature babies had died there. They, too, had been given E-Ferol.

A national recall halted the epidemic. The FDA had approved E-Ferol without testing because its constituents were similar to other harmless products. "The pharmaceutical industry and federal regulatory agencies should give special consideration to evaluating the safety of new medications that will be used to treat infants," Williams and Gaynes wrote in their paper on the outbreak.

Hard to Wear the White Hat

In March 1985 EIS officers Sue Binder and Wendy Kaye went to rural Montana to evaluate arsenic exposure in the area surrounding a

---

*In the United States, more than one hundred people died of parathion poisoning before the pesticide was finally banned there in 1999.

copper smelter operated until 1980 by the Anaconda Copper Mining Company.* A century of smelting operations had left the soil rich in heavy metals. Arsenic, considered a carcinogen, was of primary concern. Because young children were more likely to ingest dirt, Binder and Kaye tested the urine of two- to six-year-olds. The kids in the main mill town had arsenic levels around 14 micrograms per liter, compared to the 11 micrograms in control children of a nonmill town. But the ten children in the tiny community of Mill Creek, adjacent to and downwind of the smelter, had elevated counts of 66 micrograms per liter.

As a result of the study, EPA officials relocated ten Mill Creek families to Butte. "The people loved Mill Creek," Binder recalled. "They owned their own land, hunted, grew vegetables. They were poor but making it." She felt that relocation was correct from a public health perspective. "But sometimes it's really hard to wear the white hat."

Sudden Death in Brazil

Just after Christmas 1984 EIS officer David Fleming arrived in Brazil, in the rural town of Promissão, where ten children had died in the previous two months. The victims' symptoms had been similar to the effects of meningococcal meningitis, a relatively common disease in Brazil, but no *Neisseria meningitidis* bacteria were found in the blood or cerebrospinal fluid of the victims. Many lived on the outskirts of town near the sugarcane fields, so Fleming suspected a pesticide. The sudden onset and quick death made that scenario likely. Or maybe these were cases of hemorrhagic dengue fever, carried by mosquitoes. Yet laboratories found no evidence for either hypothesis. Fleming watched helplessly as children died of internal bleeding that turned them purple. All he could do was name the disease Brazilian purpuric fever.

Fleming learned of identical cases that had occurred earlier in 1984 in seven other towns. Of the thirty-eight total cases, twenty-seven had died, for a 71 percent mortality rate. Fleming realized that he needed

---

*There are approximately 500,000 abandoned mine sites in the United States, and 50 billion tons of mine waste pollute 2 million acres.

help. EIS officer Seth Berkley, who spoke Portuguese, flew to Brazil in late January 1985.

Fleming and Berkley conducted a case-control study, based on interviews with the children's parents. The only thing that stood out was that more case children had recently suffered from purulent conjunctivitis, or pinkeye, caused by the common *Haemophilus aegyptius* bacterium. Months later, from a skin scraping of one of the dead children, the CDC lab identified *H. aegyptius* with an unusual DNA segment called a 25-megadalton plasmid, but that didn't prove anything, and the specimen had been collected in nonsterile conditions.

In December 1985 two cases were reported, followed by two more in January. All four children died. On February 9, 1986, Berkley again flew to Brazil. Soon after he arrived, eight more cases occurred in the town of São José do Rio Preto. Six died. Berkley rushed to the scene, but arrived too late to collect blood specimens. He conducted another case-control study, once again showing that the affected children had been recovering from routine conjunctivitis.

Before he returned to Atlanta, he urged better surveillance and specimen collection. Shortly after he left, Brazilian purpuric fever struck again in the town of Serrana. In this case, children were identified in time to collect blood specimens and to be treated with intravenous antibiotics. Even so, five out of eleven cases died. Berkley flew back to Brazil with EIS officer Lee Harrison. The blood specimens yielded *H. aegyptius* with the same unique plasmid profile. A mutant strain of the usually mild bacterium had turned it into a killer.

Harrison continued to monitor the disease for several years, but the cases dwindled and then vanished as mysteriously as they had appeared, demonstrating that nature sometimes produces mutations that have no staying power because they provide no evolutionary advantage.

An Import from Mecca

On August 9, 1987, EIS officer Patrick Moore got a call from a New Jersey public health official about a case of meningococcal meningitis in a pilgrim who had just flown back from the annual hajj in Mecca. A similar call came from New York the next day. Moore and Lee Harrison rushed to JFK Airport to meet the next flight from Saudi Arabia.

The bacterium *Neisseria meningitidis,* which causes meningococcal meningitis, usually lives harmlessly in the throat, but the polysaccharide capsules of some types facilitate their invasion of the bloodstream and cerebrospinal fluid. For unknown reasons, North Americans do not normally have epidemics of Group A, the most lethal type. Yet Group A sweeps through sub-Saharan Africa every few years, killing children with horrific swiftness. Those who survive can lose hands or feet when intravascular blood clots prevent sufficient flow to the extremities.

Moore and Harrison set up a medical gauntlet on the airport tarmac, taking throat swabs from all who had been to Mecca or Medina, giving them antibiotics, and asking them to fill out questionnaires. They did the same thing for the next three nonstop flights from Saudi Arabia. Of the 550 passengers, 36 were carrying Group A *N. meningitidis.* Seven had begun to develop early symptoms of severe headache and neck rigidity. Two other U.S. pilgrims had died of the disease in Saudi Arabia.

Moore and Harrison were able to treat only a quarter of the U.S. citizens returning from the hajj, but fortunately there were no more cases after the nine they identified. EIS officer Ben Schwartz flew to Saudi Arabia to investigate and concluded that over ten thousand hajj pilgrims had contracted the disease. Many carried it back to sub-Saharan Africa, where a huge epidemic took place in 1988 and 1989.

In 1988 Moore flew to Chad to help with a massive vaccination campaign. "We stopped meningitis cold in that country, with 95 percent coverage," Moore recalled. He also looked into a 1968 hypothesis of EIS officers Marc LaForce and Lowell Young, who had posited that flu might predispose people to invasive Group B meningococcal disease.* In Chad, Moore found that meningitis patients were twenty-three times more likely to have had an upper respiratory virus before its onset than matched controls.

---

*See pages 89–90.

Parasites Are Us

The WHO malaria eradication program was dead by the 1980s, as the effort was clearly failing and had never even begun in Africa. In July 1982, when reports reached the CDC that drug-resistant strains of the protozoan parasite had jumped from Asia to East Africa, EIS officer Ira Schwartz flew to Zanzibar, the island off the mainland coast of Tanzania. Half of the malarial children failed to clear the *Plasmodium falciparum* parasite after a dose of chloroquine, the popular, inexpensive treatment, and in vitro testing showed that two-thirds of the isolates were drug-resistant.

"Over the decade," Schwartz said, "we watched drug-resistant malaria spread inexorably from east to west across Africa." Alternative malaria drugs such as mefloquine and doxycycline were more expensive with worse side effects. Malaria continued to kill more than a million Africans a year.

In 1986 malaria reached California, though not the resistant African strain. In August a fifty-eight-year-old resident of San Diego County with a high fever and diarrhea was admitted to the hospital, where *Plasmodium vivax* was found in his blood. Chloroquine worked just fine, and he quickly recovered. But where had he gotten the parasite? He had not traveled to any malarial countries. EIS officer Bernard Nahlen joined California-based EIS officer Yvonne Maldonado to investigate.

The victim lived across the street from a marsh, near which hundreds of illegal Mexican migrant workers camped. Nahlen and Maldonado interviewed 319 migrants, took blood smears, and treated cases with chloroquine. In June, they learned, five migrants, who had probably brought the parasite with them from Mexico, had come down with malaria. Three weeks later twenty more migrants contracted the disease, transmitted by the local *Anopheles freeborni* mosquitoes that bred in the marsh.

If one of those mosquitoes had not bitten the local white resident, it is possible that the epidemic — the largest U.S. cluster in thirty-two years — would have gone unrecognized.

Punching Holes in the Brain

EIS officer Rob Janssen, a neurologist, read articles on Creutzfeldt-Jakob disease (CJD) as he flew on January 15, 1987, to New Haven, Connecticut, to examine a twenty-eight-year-old woman at the Yale University Medical Center. In mid-November 1986 she had begun to stumble. Within two weeks she needed assistance with walking. In early January she began to jerk spasmodically and then became demented. By the time Janssen arrived, she could not communicate. A brain biopsy revealed characteristic CJD spongiform encephalopathy — her brain had holes like the ones in Swiss cheese.

The invariably fatal brain disease affects one in a million people, almost all of them elderly. Cases of CJD in young people had been caused by corneal transplants and human growth hormones from diseased patients. Janssen found that this young woman had had an operation on April 23, 1985, to remove a benign tumor. Some of the protective brain covering, called dura mater, had also been removed and was replaced with a patch of Lyodura, dura mater harvested from cadavers and sold by a German company.

The company did not keep detailed records on the bodies from which it harvested dura mater, and it mixed dura from multiple donors in a single lot. It subjected the product to irradiation, but that killed only bacteria and viruses. CJD is caused by bizarre proteins called prions that do not contain DNA or RNA. After May 1, 1987, the company stopped comingling cadaveric dura mater and added sodium hydroxide disinfection. But the Lyodura already used by that date would cause nearly two hundred additional cases of fatal CJD over the ensuing years, particularly in Japan, where the product had been widely utilized.

Behave Yourself

As horrifying as CJD was, the primary human killers in developed countries stemmed from behaviors such as smoking, drinking, violence, poor eating habits, lack of exercise, and reckless driving. When EIS alum Jim Marks took over the Nutrition Division in 1982, he discovered that two Public Health Advisors were working on a Behavioral Risk Factor Survey (BRFS), in which state health officers called randomly selected households to ask about behaviors such as alcohol intake, smoking, and seat belt use. Marks supported and expanded the program.

When the first complete data set was finished in 1983, EIS officer Kirsten Bradstock found that one out of five adults had reported consuming five or more drinks on a single occasion during the past month. "Young males ages 18–24 reported the highest prevalence of binge drinking (51.9 percent)," she wrote. While they comprised only 15 percent of the population, these young men accounted for nearly half of all fatal single-vehicle accidents involving alcohol.* More men also reported driving after drinking too much.

Bradstock looked at the correlation between drinking and other risk factors. A third of all respondents smoked, and heavy smokers were four times more likely to be chronic drinkers. Over half of the people contacted didn't wear seat belts. High stress levels correlated with drinking. "Interventions that aim at first identifying the primary causes and then reducing identified patterns of poor health practices may prove more effective than those that target a single behavior," she concluded. But the BRFS data couldn't identify primary causes, and no one knew what preventive measures worked best.

Jim Marks realized that, instead of a onetime behavioral snapshot, the BRFS should be administered regularly, allowing epidemiologists to track the impact of prevention programs and new legislation. The BRFS thus became an annual survey.

In October 1983 the Rhode Island state epidemiologist, EIS alum Richard Keenlyside, asked for help analyzing data sets in preparation for presenting an injury-control program to the governor. EIS officer Leslie Boss took on the job, finding that injuries were the leading cause of years of potential life lost before age sixty-five. Motor vehicle crashes topped the list, followed by suicides, falls, homicides, fires, poisonings, and drownings.

---

*At CDC, *accident* soon became a forbidden word, since it implied that pure chance was responsible. Instead, EIS officers speak of preventable injuries.

Boss found that 20 percent of the vehicle-related deaths involved pedestrians. Fewer than one in ten car crashes resulted in injury or death, compared to 90 percent of motorcycle crashes. While women were more likely to attempt suicide, men were more successful in killing themselves. African Americans were four times more likely to be murder victims. Most falls occurred among the elderly in their own homes. Fires and smoke inhalation killed more blacks and Hispanics, probably due to overcrowding, poor housing conditions, and lack of smoke detectors. Over a third of the fires were associated with smoking.

Suicide Missions

Of all those causes, suicide was the most disturbing and inexplicable public health problem. In 1983 EIS officer Jim Mercy wrote, "Between 1970 and 1980, 49,496 of our nation's youth age 15 to 24 committed suicide." Over the decade, the suicide rate in this age group had increased 40 percent.

In Plano, Texas, a Dallas suburb, eight teenagers committed suicide in a little over a year (1983 to 1984). In Clear Lake, Texas, a Houston suburb, four teens killed themselves within an eight-day period in October 1984. Rumors of teen suicide pacts flew in both cities. EIS officer Lucy Davidson and EIS alum Mark Rosenberg, the chief of the Violence Epidemiology Branch, investigated.

Davidson combined the two clusters into a single case-control study of fourteen adolescent suicides, eleven of whom were male. She and Rosenberg chose three controls for each suicide of the same grade, gender, and school. Their questionnaire asked about exposure to suicide and interpersonal violence, physical and emotional health, personality, behavior patterns, and life events. They conducted "psychological autopsies" of the cases, asking parents, friends, and teachers for information.

The study found little evidence for the contagion hypothesis. All the suicides had taken place prior to the airing of four made-for-television movies about suicide in 1984 and 1985. Although some suicide victims were best friends, others did not know one another. Cases and controls were equally exposed to extensive local media coverage after the initial suicides.

Some patterns emerged from the case-control study. Those who had killed themselves were perceived as being generally unhappy and easily hurt or offended. Many had recently broken up with a boyfriend or girlfriend. Several had criminal records. Cases were more likely to have previously damaged themselves physically, such as pounding a wall with a fist, and were more likely to be violent toward others. They had moved more frequently than controls. Many were cared for by stepparents or grandparents. Some cases had talked, dreamed, or written about death or suicide. More cases had been close to someone who had died violently (though not necessarily from suicide).

Seven of the cases had shot themselves, all with guns kept in unlocked storage. Five others had used carbon monoxide from auto exhaust, and two had hanged themselves.

On February 11, 1986, a sixteen-year-old boy shot himself in Spencer, Massachusetts. Counselors learned that eight other high school students—six girls and two boys—had recently attempted suicide. Administrators invited external counselors into the school; they offered individual and group therapy. Yet over the next two months, nine more students (mostly girls) attempted suicide. None succeeded.

In October the head of the local counseling center invited EIS officer Patrick O'Carroll to assess what had happened. "There was a group of four to six individuals," he reported, "who seemed particularly fascinated by suicide." They were close friends, primarily dating others within the clique. An excluded girl who wanted desperately to join finally gained acceptance by making repeated suicide attempts. O'Carroll also found that many of the suicide attempters had recently moved to the area. Half of their families were "severely disrupted." Some parents were alcoholics. Others had sexually or physically abused their children. O'Carroll concluded that it was counterproductive to bring counselors into the school, where they inadvertently abetted attention seekers.

The next spring tragedy struck in Bergenfield, New Jersey. On

March 11, 1987, two sisters drove into a garage with their boyfriends. The boys had been drinking and all four teens had snorted cocaine. They closed the garage door, left the motor running, and were found dead. Shortly thereafter, a teenage boy and girl broke into the same garage and were found unconscious in their car by alert police at 4 A.M. They barely survived.

Two days later O'Carroll arrived and discovered that three of the four who had committed suicide had dropped out of school. The older male had a history of alcohol abuse, and both boys had scars on their wrists. Both had been friends of an eighteen-year-old who had fallen off a cliff six months earlier, and one had witnessed it. O'Carroll also learned that two young local men had been hit by trains in the past few months, and another had drowned, apparently by intent. Yet when he examined the overall suicide rate for the county, it was actually lower than the national average.

In November O'Carroll attended a meeting of key responders to nine recent suicide clusters in as many different states. He subsequently wrote the CDC's recommendations for communities with suicide clusters. Among those recommendations: appoint one agency to coordinate the response; "avoid glorification of the suicide victims and minimize sensationalism"; partner with the local media if possible; set up an ongoing surveillance system to identify suicide attempts; ask teachers and students to spot those at high risk; and provide appropriate counseling.

O'Carroll knew that teen suicide clusters accounted for only 5 percent of all adolescent suicides, at most. What about all the others? "We wanted to interview dead people," he recalled. With colleagues, O'Carroll arrived at an ingenious solution. Through emergency room surveillance, they could identify near-fatal suicide attempts that people had survived only through flukes. A few years later in Houston, the CDC team found 153 victims of nearly lethal suicide attempts between the ages of thirteen and thirty-four and interviewed them within a week of their hospitalization, comparing them with neighborhood controls.

The results were surprising. Having a suicidal relative, friend, or acquaintance apparently was not a contributory factor. Exposure to accounts of suicidal behavior in the media actually *lowered* the risk of suicide. Those who had made serious attempts to kill themselves tended to be depressed, to be alcoholics, to have moved in the previous year, or to have ended a relationship recently. Unlike the white suburban teens of the suicide clusters, these suicidal people were more likely to be African American or Hispanic and to have a lower household income. The study showed that the majority of suicidal people weren't copying anyone. They were just miserable and saw no reason to go on living.

Bang, You're Dead

Gun control issues were among the most controversial areas into which EIS officers ventured. In January 1987 Patrick O'Carroll and Jim Mercy seized an opportunity after Detroit passed a city ordinance mandating jail time for anyone carrying a gun in a vehicle or in public. Detroit had the nation's highest homicide rate, and two-thirds of the murders were committed with firearms. "Some kids got into schoolyard arguments that ended with *Shut up. Bang, you're dead*," O'Carroll recalled.

O'Carroll and Mercy designed a study to measure the impact of the new law. They found that the rate of gun violence continued to increase, but more slowly than it had before. When it became apparent that the new law was not being enforced, however, the rate escalated again.

Homicide was the eleventh leading cause of death in the United States, and it was the primary cause of death for black males fifteen to thirty-four. Over half of all murders were committed with handguns. Yet there was little available epidemiological evidence to support gun control legislation. "Due to the clear public health implications of this question, we must carefully test the hypothesis that handgun accessibility increases the risk of homicide," O'Carroll and Mercy concluded.

Eat Right, Stop Smoking and Drinking, and Get Off Your Butt

By the mid-1980s evidence was mounting that even nonsmokers were at risk of cancer and heart disease from breathing cigarette smoke. At the April 1986 conference, Michigan-based EIS officer Rob Anda reported on a statewide survey of smokers who were asked whether their doctors had advised them to quit. Less than half had been admonished, even when they had a history of high blood pressure, diabetes, obesity, or oral contraceptive use. "Although a physician's advice to quit smoking may have limited efficacy," Anda noted, "most smokers do see a physician at least once a year." If all doctors had told their patients to quit smoking, and even 5 percent heeded the advice, Anda figured that sixty-five thousand Michigan residents would have given up cigarettes in one year alone.

A growing body of evidence showed that babies of women who smoked were more likely to be stillborn or have low birth weights, while their mothers had more pregnancy complications. EIS officers David Williamson and Juliette Kendrick found that 21 percent of pregnant women still smoked — less than the 30 percent of nonpregnant women, but still alarmingly high. They found that unmarried pregnant white women were 40 percent more likely to smoke than their nonpregnant counterparts.

Still, behavioral norms were changing. The Behavioral Risk Factor Surveillance System (BRFSS) had shown that a third of the U.S. population smoked in 1983. By 1987 smoking was restricted in all New York State workplaces. Seat belt use also increased dramatically during the 1980s, in large measure because of new legislation. EIS officers both tracked these trends and helped them on their way.

Williamson and Kirsten Bradstock used BRFSS data to link alcohol consumption and obesity, showing that women on diets were more likely to engage in binge drinking. They hypothesized that women who were overweight and did not diet might be substituting food for alcohol as a way to cope with stress.

In 1988 Anda, Williamson, and EIS alum Pat Remington looked at data from the National Health and Nutrition Examination Survey

(NHANES), begun in the early 1970s and repeated every few years. They used an NHANES follow-up study of the 1980s to see how many people who admitted heavy alcohol use in the first study had died of fatal injuries. Those who had reported taking five or more drinks per occasion were nearly twice as likely to have died of injuries (mostly from car crashes or suicides) than more moderate drinkers, while those who said they had imbibed nine or more alcoholic beverages were 3.3 times more likely to have had fatal injuries. As with smokers, Anda suggested that physicians urge heavy drinkers to cut back.

A Faltering Founder and a Frustrated Chief

By 1987, when Alexander Langmuir turned seventy-seven, he had become increasingly critical of the CDC. He disparaged case-control studies and the use of computers. He incorrectly asserted that AIDS cases would soon peak and dwindle. The previous year Langmuir had written that the EIS, having "outlived its usefulness," should be abolished and subsumed within different divisions of the CDC.

During his tenure as EIS chief, Carl Tyler never doubted the continued relevance of the program. To seed other government agencies, he placed EIS officers at the FDA and NIH, and he welcomed a U.S. Department of Agriculture veterinarian as an EIS officer. Under Tyler, core EIS requirements, such as making a conference presentation and writing an *MMWR* article, were put in place. He also instituted "EIS rounds," during which officers could give constructive feedback.

By 1986 EIS officers received portable computers to take into the field. Tyler brought EIS alum Andy Dean back to the CDC, where Dean developed a computerized program called Epi Info that would allow EIS officers and other epidemiologists to enter data and calculate odds ratios, relative risks, and more sophisticated approaches such as multiple regression analysis to assess the impact and interaction of different factors.

Tyler encouraged the growth of the Global EIS Program, which started Field Epidemiology Training Programs in different countries. When pharmaceutical executive Charles Mérieux offered to fund

an EIS-like course for budding French epidemiologists, Tyler sent
EIS alums to teach the course for several years and recruited several
French EIS officers to come to Atlanta.*

During the Tyler years, the EIS classes became increasingly diverse. There were more foreign-born officers, women, minorities,
and nonphysicians. More officers entered in their thirties or even for-
ties, having already earned advanced degrees in public health or other
fields.

Despite these achievements, however, Tyler was frustrated. With
the CDC reorganization, most EIS officers were no longer directly
under his wing at the Epidemiology Program Office but were instead
assigned to centers and programs throughout the organization. Tyler's attempts to intervene in situations where he felt officers were
not receiving adequate supervision were rebuffed. His suggestion to
make Epi-Aid reports public rather than confidential was ignored. He
and CDC director Jim Mason clashed over budget-cutting exercises.
In January 1987 Tyler assigned himself to a monthlong sabbatical in
Oklahoma as an ersatz EIS officer, returning to Atlanta reenergized.
Impressed with action at the state level, he extrapolated figures from
field officers to estimate that state health departments were investigating some three thousand epidemics annually, far more than the eighty
or ninety yearly Epi-Aids conducted by CDC-based EIS officers.

Yet, suffering from undiagnosed sleep apnea, Tyler became increasingly irritable. Tensions built within the Epidemiology Program
Office.

---

*French EIS officer Alain Moren, who had served with Médecins Sans Frontières (Doctors
Without Borders), facilitated the 1986 Mérieux-sponsored course. He went on to cofound
(along with twelve other EIS alums) the European Programme for Intervention Epidemiology Training (EPIET), based largely on the EIS program.

17
EMERGING INFECTIONS

In the summer of 1988 CDC director Jim Mason reassigned Carl Tyler, and in August 1989 EIS alum Steve Thacker took over as director of the Epidemiology Program Office (EPO). That same year Bill Roper (who had once been accepted into the EIS but hadn't ended up serving there) replaced Mason as head of the CDC.

Thacker continued the trend toward diversification. In 1990 an equal number of women and men entered the Epidemic Intelligence Service, and nearly a fifth were members of racial/ethnic minority groups. Ten officers came from foreign countries.

In 1991 Thacker appointed EIS veteran Ward Cates as director of the EPO Training Division. Cates then hired EIS alum Polly Marchbanks, a nurse with a Ph.D. in epidemiology, as the EIS chief to run the program under the supervision of Cates and Thacker.

During all the job changes, EIS officers continued to battle diseases. Since 1981, when listeriosis was traced to coleslaw in Nova Scotia,* other outbreaks had been associated with milk and cheese, but no one knew the origin of sporadic listeriosis cases. Of the 1,850 annual U.S. cases, most were isolated, and about a quarter of the victims died. During their two EIS years, Anne Schuchat and Bob Pin-

---

*See pages 205–206.

ner studied these cases in collaboration with health officers in four states. Schuchat conducted hundreds of telephone interviews, speaking to each victim (or a surviving relative), along with two controls, about food consumption and other matters. In December 1988 an Oklahoma woman was hospitalized with listeriosis. In her refrigerator were Plantation brand turkey franks that yielded the same bacterial strain. So did two unopened Plantation packages from the local store.*

Until this proven instance, the food industry had maintained that *Listeria* bacteria in meat did not cause disease. In early May the USDA instituted a zero-tolerance policy for *Listeria* in ready-to-eat meats. Schuchat's case-control study also implicated meat from deli counters, undercooked chicken, and soft cheeses.

She also studied Group B streptococcal disease, which had emerged in the 1970s as the leading cause of childbirth infection and death in the United States. One in three women harbored the bacteria in the vagina without any symptoms. Research had shown that if such women were treated with antibiotics after the onset of labor but before delivery, their babies did not acquire the infection. Yet hospitals did not routinely test women for Group B strep. Schuchat's subsequent research led to testing and treatment of women giving birth that has reduced infant Group B strep by 70 percent and has prevented some forty-five thousand infections since 1990.

The Womyn's Malady

On August 17, 1988, EIS officer Lisa Lee flew to Michigan. The thirteenth annual Womyn's Music Festival had attracted seven thousand women, mostly lesbians, from forty-eight states and several foreign countries. From August 10 to 14, they had camped in rural central Michigan, listening to music and celebrating life in the absence of men (thus "womyn's"). Recent EIS grad Steve Ostroff accompanied

---

*EIS officer Jay Wenger was dispatched to the Plantation Foods plant in Waco, Texas, where he found that the same forklifts were used to move raw turkey hot dogs and the cooked product, allowing cross-contamination.

Lee, but as a man he was not allowed onto the festival grounds. Soon after the festival ended, thousands of attendees became extremely ill. Lee found that just before the festival, some of the staff contracted diarrhea caused by *Shigella sonnei,* so they took extra precautions, placing buckets of bleach solution outside toilets and in the kitchen for handwashing. Nonetheless, the *Shigella* bacterium, which requires only a small infectious dose, sickened more than three thousand festivalgoers.

The EIS officer interviewed staff members and ill Michigan attendees. She also mailed out a questionnaire to a sample of two thousand other women who had attended the festival. The resulting case-control study implicated the tofu salad served on the last day. It had been prepared by fifty women who had diced several hundred pounds of uncooked tofu, then mixed it by hand with chopped vegetables. The salad was served for both lunch and dinner.

Lee concluded that the bleach solution for handwashing had lost its potency. Many women reported that they had not washed their hands after using the toilet, in part because the handwashing solution looked filthy. Bacteria were efficiently transmitted by the hand-mixed tofu salad. At future events, Lee suggested installing piped water for handwashing, as well as reducing the number of cooks and choosing recipes that required minimum handling of uncooked items.

Following the outbreak, Lisa Lee, a Chinese American, flew to Beijing to present her findings at an international epidemiology conference. Her Chinese colleagues were impressed that Americans ate tofu, contaminated or not. There were plans to start an EIS-like Field Epidemiology Training Program in China, but two weeks later, on June 4, 1989, the Tiananmen Square massacre occurred, and plans were scrapped for another ten years.

The Chinese Connection

That was unfortunate, because the Chinese not only had public health problems but exported them to other countries. On the morning of February 13, 1989, three students at Mississippi State University reported to the student health service with nausea, vomiting, cramps, and diarrhea. When the doctor there learned that all had eaten omelets at the student cafeteria, he called the cafeteria manager and asked him to close the omelet line. Then another student with similar symptoms appeared. For lunch, he had eaten a hamburger with mushrooms. The doctor asked the cafeteria to stop serving mushrooms and alerted the state health department.

EIS officers Katherine Hendricks and William Levine identified a total of twenty-two sick students, nine of whom had been hospitalized. The EIS officers' case-control study implicated canned mushrooms traced to a Memphis warehouse. Their labels indicated that they came from the People's Republic of China. A lab identified staphylococcal enterotoxin in the mushrooms.

Two months later there were two outbreaks in pizza joints in McKeesport and Philipsburg, Pennsylvania. Canned mushrooms imported from China were again implicated by EIS officers David Dennis and Youngsook Cho, and the FDA banned importation. A further FDA investigation in China revealed widespread environmental contamination with enterotoxin-producing staphylococci in several mushroom-canning factories. These were the first known instances of a contaminated food product from China causing an epidemic of these proportions in the United States, but there would be more deadly products coming out of China in years to come.

Quicksilver Paint

In the summer of 1989 a four-year-old Michigan boy had been hospitalized with acrodynia, a rare type of childhood mercury poisoning. The boy's illness became apparent ten days after the interior of his family's home was painted. Because of the August heat, the family kept the windows closed and the air conditioner running.

EIS officer Mary Agocs found that the homeowners had used latex paint made by the Mercury Paint Company. About a third of the latex paint then produced in the United States contained phenylmercuric acetate to prevent the growth of bacteria and mildew. The Detroit firm's paint contained three times the Environmental Protection Agency's recommended mercury limit.

Agocs conducted a study of nineteen families in the Detroit suburbs who had recently used the same brand of paint, finding high mercury concentrations in their urine. She calculated that the paint would continue to emit mercury for at least another eight years.

No one knew the impact of low levels of mercury in humans, but Agocs feared that even minute amounts of mercury, like lead, might produce subtle nerve problems without noticeable symptoms. The CDC recommended that the EPA stop the use of mercury in latex paint, and the following year the EPA instituted the ban.

A Foggy Outlook

On November 7, 1989, EIS officer Charles Hoge went to Bogalusa, Louisiana (population sixteen thousand), to investigate an epidemic of acute pneumonia. Hoge and Louisiana-based EIS officer Frank Mahoney identified the infectious agent as *Legionella pneumophila,* but the source of the infection wasn't clear. New cases kept occurring, with the most susceptible dying.

Most prior outbreaks of Legionnaires' disease* had been traced to cooling towers or other aerosol-producing apparatuses. A paper mill located in the city center featured twenty cooling towers as well as four paper machines that emitted aerosolized water along Main Street. The officers collected water from the cooling towers. Many samples yielded *Legionella* bacteria, but not the strain identified in patients.

Using thirty-one confirmed victims of a possible eighty as official cases, Hoge and Mahoney chose age-matched controls who were also patients of the admitting doctors. Cases were no more likely than controls to have visited the paper mill or other cooling tower locations. However, many cases had shopped at a Winn-Dixie grocery store on the opposite side of town.

A follow-up questionnaire indicated that cases were more likely to have shopped in the Winn-Dixie for over thirty minutes and to have bought vegetables near an ultrasonic misting machine that sprayed the produce to keep it fresh. The water in the machine's reservoir held

*See page 179.

the same strain of *Legionella* that had killed fourteen people. When the machine was removed, the epidemic stopped.

These ultrasonic machines, known as "foggers," constituted about 10 percent of those used in supermarkets nationwide. The more common sprayers came on only intermittently and hosed the vegetables with larger drops. In contrast, the foggers ran continuously, producing water particles small enough to be inhaled deep into the lung's bronchioles.

When their blood was tested, the Winn-Dixie employees showed elevated antibodies to *Legionella*, though none of them had been ill, just as no one who worked in the lobby of the Bellevue-Stratford had caught the disease in 1976. Healthy younger people were less susceptible than the elderly and those with underlying health problems.

Hoge and Mahoney's investigation led to the national removal of such foggers from supermarkets. The EIS officers cautioned that ultrasonic home humidifiers might also cause problems if not washed frequently. Legionnaires' disease nonetheless remained a huge problem, putting at least eleven thousand people in U.S. hospitals every year.

An Alternative Cure That Killed

In October 1989 normally athletic thirty-nine-year-old Bonnie Bishop could barely walk into her doctor's office in Santa Fe, New Mexico. A blood test revealed an extremely high level of eosinophils, white blood cells produced by the immune system to fight disease. Her doctor, suspecting cancer, referred her to William Blevins, an oncologist. She became so weak and bloated with fluids that she had to be hospitalized. An operation drained more than a gallon of fluid from her body, but there were no tumors, and exploratory biopsies revealed no leukemia.

Blevins asked Bishop's mother to bring him the contents of her daughter's medicine cabinet, which held, among other things, a food supplement containing L-tryptophan. Sold over-the-counter without a prescription, during the 1980s L-tryptophan had become an increasingly popular alternative remedy for sleep disorders, premenstrual syndrome, and depression.

Within a few days Blevins learned of two other New Mexico women with similar symptoms and eosinophil counts. Each had been taking L-tryptophan. On October 30 Blevins notified the New Mexico Health Department and Gerald Gleich, a noted authority on eosinophils, at the Mayo Clinic in Minnesota. Gleich, in turn, called EIS alum Ed Kilbourne at the CDC.*

On November 7 *Albuquerque Journal* reporter Tamar Stieber published an article about the three New Mexico cases. Ailing women in New Mexico who read the article and had taken L-tryptophan contacted the state health department. State epidemiologist Millicent Eidson, an EIS alum, called the CDC for help. On Thursday, November 9, EIS officer Rossanne Philen flew to New Mexico. That same day Kilbourne notified all state health departments of the possible L-tryptophan problem.

Philen and others combed through thousands of medical reports at nine New Mexico laboratories, looking for high eosinophil counts. They found twelve cases, then located twenty-four controls in their neighborhoods. By Sunday night they found that every case patient had taken L-tryptophan but that only two controls had taken it.

Investigators were working in parallel in Minnesota, where EIS officer Ed Belongia was assigned. "We have to jump on this," said state epidemiologist Mike Osterholm. "It's a public health emergency. We have to know if the association is real." By chance, state pathologists were meeting on Saturday, November 11. Belongia and Osterholm went to the meeting, explained the newly identified syndrome, and asked for cases, then called Minnesota rheumatologists.

By that afternoon they had found twelve cases. Calling similar phone numbers to locate age-matched controls, they and their colleagues conducted a case-control survey. By noon on Sunday, the results showed that all of the cases had taken L-tryptophan and none of the controls had.

Osterholm called a press conference encouraging people to contact the health department if they were taking L-tryptophan. The

---

*EIS alum Ed Kilbourne was the son of virologist Ed Kilbourne Sr. See page 161.

FDA issued an advisory to "temporarily discontinue" use of the product. On November 16 a Minnesota case died. By that date, the CDC had learned of 243 potential cases of the newly named eosinophilia-myalgia syndrome (EMS), reported from thirty-five states and the District of Columbia. The following day the FDA requested a recall of all L-tryptophan products. Eventually, over 1,500 cases in the United States would be identified, with 37 deaths. As many as 60,000 EMS cases might have occurred worldwide.

The biggest question was whether concentrated L-tryptophan itself was lethal or if selected products were somehow contaminated. The Minnesota team mounted a cohort study of L-tryptophan users, comparing those who got sick with those who didn't. Belongia led the study, asking all L-tryptophan users who called the state health department to save their pill bottles. To avoid potential bias from such self-referrals, he also found other consumers through a laborious random-digit-dialing phone survey. Then he set about comparing the retail brands used by sick and well L-tryptophan users. Six Japanese manufacturers supplied powdered L-tryptophan to U.S. pill makers, but the brand names had to be traced back to specific lots made by particular companies.

By February 1990 Belongia and his colleagues had identified Showa Denko K.K. as the manufacturer of twenty-nine out of thirty L-tryptophan products associated with EMS cases (the single exception probably came originally from Showa Denko as well).

Osterholm and Belongia met with Showa Denko executives. The Japanese businessmen were cooperative and concerned, handing over documents that showed key manufacturing changes late in 1988, including an altered filtration process and a new strain of bacteria. The twenty-nine cases had all consumed products made after these changes. Although the Showa Denko powder was 99.6 percent pure, the minute contaminant was enough to cause the epidemic.

The mystery unraveled further when EIS officer Mary Kamb went to Spartanburg, South Carolina, where an inordinate number of severe EMS cases had been reported by February 1990. Most of them were patients of one psychiatrist who prescribed L-tryptophan for their depression and bipolar disorder. Kamb and EIS colleague Kees Nederlof found forty-seven definite cases and sixty-eight with milder symptoms among the patients in the practice. Showa Denko products were implicated, but beyond that, the EIS officers were able to examine the impact of daily dosage. Half of the patients who used more than 4,000 milligrams per day developed EMS (three died), while those on lower doses often had milder symptoms. There was a clear dose-response relationship.

The exact chemical contaminant that caused the epidemic has never been identified. Both the L-tryptophan and Spanish toxic oil culprits remain mysteries.* The symptoms and long-term effects are alike. No animals have been similarly sickened by the products, making it very difficult to conduct meaningful experiments.

"Most people assume that someone has looked at any product they can buy in the United States and that it has been determined to be safe," Belongia said. "But the lack of monitoring for alternative medicines and health food supplements puts the public at risk." The FDA has been banned from monitoring such products by the U.S. Congress, acting under pressure from interest groups.

Importing Ebola

On November 27, 1989, Tom Geisbert at the U.S. Army Medical Research Institute of Infectious Diseases (USAMRIID) in Fort Detrick, Maryland, stared in disbelief through his electron microscope.† There, in the cells of a monkey that had died in a holding facility in Reston, Virginia, swirled the unmistakable snakelike shape of a filovirus. Only two — Marburg and Ebola — were known to exist. Both were deadly hemorrhagic viruses that killed from 50 percent to 90 percent of the people they invaded.

The following day the Fort Detrick scientists tested the virus against human antibodies for Marburg and the two known types of

---

*See pages 204–205.

†USAMRIID is the stepchild of the Fort Detrick facility at the heart of the American biological warfare program until it was halted by Nixon in 1969. See page 97.

Ebola. It tested positive for Ebola Zaire, the most virulent strain. They called the CDC.

After Marburg had invaded humans in Marburg, Germany, through imported Ugandan green monkeys in 1967, all U.S. monkeys were quarantined for at least a month before being distributed to research labs. In October 1989 Hazleton Research Products had imported one hundred macaques from the Philippines to their quarantine facility in Reston. Recent EIS grad Steve Ostroff assembled a list of all humans who had potential contact with the Reston monkeys. He identified six people (mostly animal handlers) considered high risk.

Ostroff knew that Ebola transmission required close contact with blood. The caretakers at Reston had taken reasonable precautions with the monkeys, wearing protective gloves and masks. Yet on the morning of December 4, an animal handler named Keith felt sick and dizzy. As he worked, he felt worse and worse, then rushed outside and vomited in the parking lot. The extermination of the 450 remaining Reston monkeys was authorized immediately. The sick handler recovered quickly after a stay in isolated intensive care. He may have had a panic attack.

In the meantime, EIS alum Mark White, in the Philippines to establish an EIS clone (Field Epidemiology Training Program), visited the monkey holding facility from which the macaques had been shipped. None of the animal handlers had gotten sick, though 10 percent of the monkeys had died.

On Christmas Day, 1989, the twenty-one-day surveillance time — longer than any known Ebola incubation period — ended, and no humans had come down with the disease. Hazleton imported more macaques from the Philippines, housing them in the same Reston building. By mid-January they, too, began to die from Ebola. A month later an animal handler performing a necropsy on a dead monkey sliced open his thumb. He did not get sick, but he did develop antibodies to Ebola. So did three other Reston monkey handlers. This clearly was a new strain of Ebola that could infect people but did not make them sick.

In 1989 twenty-two thousand Philippine macaques had been

shipped to the United States. EIS officers discovered that the Reston Ebola strain (as it was named) had turned up in monkeys in Pennsylvania and Texas. When tested, other animal handlers, including those in the Philippines, had Ebola antibodies. "Hundreds of persons in multiple states were exposed before the threat was even recognized," Ostroff observed. He added that the monkey outbreak "illustrates our global vulnerability for rapid movement of highly pathogenic microbes."

Flesh-Eating Microbes

In January 1990 three people in Pima County, Arizona, died of a strain of Group A streptococcal infection. A new strain of the bacteria that normally causes sore throats, as well as scarlet and rheumatic fever, *Streptococcus pyogenes,* had been identified a few years earlier. Dubbed flesh-eating strep, it produces a toxin that attacks skin and muscle tissue. Unless it is treated aggressively early in the illness, it causes a form of toxic shock syndrome, killing many of its victims.

In March 1990 EIS officer Charles Hoge went to Pima County to investigate. The flesh-eating strep had attacked 12 people, but there were four different serotypes, and he could trace no contact between patients. He went through microbiology records at ten local hospitals, looking back to 1985. He found 128 cases with *S. pyogenes,* but only 6 suffered from toxic shock, with its characteristic peeling of skin from the feet and hands along with liver-kidney damage and low blood pressure. With a median age of fifteen, these patients were much younger than the others and, aside from the toxic shock, appeared to be healthy. All 6 cases had occurred since 1987, with a preponderance in Native Americans, though Hoge couldn't tell if it had to do with living conditions or genetics.* He called for ongoing studies of the disease.

As the EIS officer was writing his report, Jim Henson, the fifty-three-year-old creator of the beloved Muppets, thought he might be coming down with the flu. On May 13, 1990, he consulted his North

---

*Recent research has implicated genetic factors as contributors to strep toxic shock cases. Several vaccines against Group A strep are in various stages of development.

Carolina doctor, who recommended aspirin and rest. The next day Henson coughed up blood and had difficulty breathing. He entered a New York hospital on May 15. His organs failing from strep toxic shock, he died the next day. As the world mourned Henson's untimely death, flesh-eating strep dominated headlines.

Later that year Wisconsin-based EIS officer Jay Butler investigated a family cluster of Group A strep. In November the twenty-five-year-old son, a graduate student, came down with a sore throat. He had visited his parents briefly. Eleven days later his father developed a pustular infection on his right index finger, then his left hand. The lesions ruptured, draining yellow fluid. On December 12 the mother saw her gynecologist for a vaginal discharge. He gave her a suppository for suspected candidiasis. For the next four days she vomited, then developed diarrhea, fever, and chills. She was finally admitted to the hospital on December 18 with strep toxic shock syndrome. Fortunately, she recovered.

The CDC found twelve such family clusters that had occurred since 1988, in which four toxic shock victims died. During the same period, there had been five clusters of hospital-acquired invasive strep infections, and five nursing home outbreaks, with more deaths. Just why it caused sore throats in most children but could become flesh-eating strep in adults wasn't clear. "We live in a sea of bacteria, fungi and viruses," EIS alum Larry Altman reminded *New York Times* readers. "Why one individual can be overwhelmed by certain dangerous microbes . . . remains a puzzle."

Cat-Scratch Serendipity

In 1990 EIS officer Brad Perkins was working on another puzzle. Occasionally, a child scratched by a cat develops a solid lump at the site a week or two later. The child may have a slight fever, headache, chills, fatigue, and swollen lymph nodes. Usually, cat-scratch disease is mild, but sometimes it leads to encephalitis, convulsions, conjunctivitis, or pneumonia. Since its identification in 1889, no one had figured out what caused it, so in between outbreak investigations, Perkins pursued the mystery as a long-term project.

He worked at the same time on bacillary angiomatosis, a disease in AIDS patients that causes black skin lesions and can affect virtually every organ. "We applied a new DNA technology and identified a bacteria called *Bartonella henselae* as its cause," Perkins said. As controls for an experiment on the new bacteria, he chose some of his cat-scratch specimens. To his astonishment, they tested positive to *Bartonella*. It turned out that the AIDS patients had also been scratched by cats.

The next year Connecticut-based EIS officer Doug Hamilton investigated the cases of two elementary school boys who had seizures, then fell into comas for several days before recovering. Hamilton discovered that both boys had new kittens. Sure enough, the children tested positive for *Bartonella*.

With more than 27 million U.S. households owning felines, Perkins estimated that cat-scratch disease affects approximately twenty-two thousand people a year in that country alone.

"The Health Educators Told Us"

Cholera continued its inexorable spread during the drawn-out seventh world pandemic that had begun in 1961. In November 1990 cholera broke out in southern Malawi, where refugees from the civil war in neighboring Mozambique had fled. The largest camp, built to hold fifty thousand people, then had a refugee population of seventy-four thousand.

EIS officer David Swerdlow arrived at the camp alone with a laptop computer and a few lab supplies. In the sweltering heat, he set about answering two questions. *Why were so many people dying? How was cholera being spread?*

"I found that children were more likely to die," he said, "so I suggested setting up a tent just for children, with the best nursing care." He also identified an overreliance on intravenous tubes, often left in place for a week or more, which led to infections and septic shock. Even when they were offered lifesaving oral rehydration solution (ORS), sick refugees weren't getting enough, so Swerdlow assigned "ORS officers" whose only job was to tell people to drink, drink, drink.

But how were people getting cholera in the first place? Deep boreholes provided clean water, though not enough. Swerdlow asked how long refugees waited in line, how they transported the water. Did they wash their hands? *Yes, the health educators told us.* Where did they wash their hands? *In the water buckets.* You mean, the same container you drink from? *Yes, there is no other place to wash our hands.* It was a perfect way to transmit cholera. "Use of narrow mouthed water containers would probably decrease the likelihood of contamination," he wrote in his report.

After One Hundred Years of Solitude

On January 29, 1991, Rob Tauxe received a call from EIS alum Marjorie Pollack, who was directing Peru's fledgling Field Epidemiology Training Program (FETP). "We have a cholera outbreak here in Peru," she reported.

There had been no cholera in Latin America for nearly a century. On February 10 Tauxe and EIS officer Allen Ries flew to Piura, Peru, where EIS officer Duc Vugia later joined them. They discovered that the chlorine tanks delivered to the water treatment plant contained no chlorine, and they identified unboiled water and produce from street vendors as transmission agents.

After writing an *MMWR* article to alert the medical community to the arrival of cholera in Latin America, David Swerdlow caught a plane for Peru, along with EIS officer Eric Mintz. In Lima, Swerdlow and Mintz were escorted to the health department in a bulletproof car due to fears of Shining Path rebels.* With two Peruvian FETP trainees, they drove north to Trujillo, the country's third-largest city, where cholera had struck a third of the citizens. Their case-control study implicated water. The EIS officers then identified multiple problems with the water system of interconnected wells, with only sporadic chlorination. People dug holes to tap illegally into the water lines, reducing water pressure and allowing backflow contamination.

Because running water was available only an hour a day in poorer

---

*The EIS officers were later pulled over as suspected terrorists when the red Igloo coolers they carried for stool and water samples were mistaken for bombs.

neighborhoods, most families stored water in household containers, which held more fecal coliforms and vibrios than the pipes. As in Malawi, people's hands were contaminating the same water they dipped into for a drink. In their report, Swerdlow, Mintz, and the FETP trainees recommended improvements in the municipal water system as a long-term solution. In the meantime, people should boil or disinfect their water and store it in narrow-necked vessels.

Cholera moved swiftly inland from the coast. In May 1991 EIS officer Rob Quick joined five Peruvian FETP colleagues in Iquitos, a commercial hub at the headwaters of the Amazon, where a hundred new cholera cases a day were overwhelming the local hospital facilities.

"The hospital was doing a great job with limited resources," Quick recalled. He and his colleagues did a case-control study, which implicated untreated drinking water, unwashed fruits and vegetables, and leftover cooked rice. The fresh produce was probably polluted as water splashed into the shallow canoes carrying it to market. "Extreme poverty, lack of water treatment, and near-universal use of the river for cooking and drinking water, bathing, and raw sewage disposal offer ideal conditions for rapid dissemination of infection," he and his colleagues concluded in their report.

Though residents in the shantytown area where most cases lived knew that they should either boil or chlorinate their water, few did so. Boiling was expensive and time-consuming. Bleach was available but was used mostly for laundry. People said the bleach-treated water tasted bad and feared it might be toxic.

Quick found that most of those who died of cholera were coming from remote villages, so he enlisted naval speedboats to take his team upriver, where they documented a 13.5 percent case fatality rate in twelve villages. In most other areas of Peru the mortality rate was less than 1 percent. People waited until they were really sick before starting on the four-hour boat ride to Iquitos. Many died en route, while others were beyond help by the time they reached the hospital.

Quick pondered the situation. *We've been to the moon, we've got these cities where good sanitation and water are foregone conclusions. Yet here I am in a place where something as simple as water can kill you.* He decided to join the CDC Enterics Branch after his EIS service.

By the end of 1991 over 300,000 Peruvians had contracted cholera, and 3,000 had died. Within three years the bacteria spread throughout Latin America, infecting over a million people and killing 10,000 of them.

In February 1992 more than one hundred passengers on an airplane en route from Peru to Los Angeles contracted cholera from cold seafood salad. EIS officer Rich Besser was appalled to find that a cholera diagnosis had not been considered for seventeen people who sought treatment. None received proper oral rehydration, and one died.

Nevertheless, the United States and other countries with good sanitation systems had little to fear from rampant cholera. Elsewhere in the world, over a billion people depended on unsafe sources for drinking water. Cholera, *Shigella, Campylobacter,* rotavirus, and other microbes caused waterborne diarrhea that killed more than 2 million children annually.

Obviously, the long-term solution would be to fix the world's infrastructure so that everyone could turn a tap and drink safe water. To do that just in Latin America would cost $200 billion. In the meantime, Rob Tauxe considered the lessons learned in cholera investigations: Promote household use of a narrow-mouthed container with a spigot to prevent people from sticking their hands in the water. Teach people to put diluted bleach into the water. Simple and cheap.

In 1992 Eric Mintz noticed a five-gallon jug in a CDC janitor's closet that, when modified for a spigot, served the purpose. In November that same year in La Paz, Bolivia, on a shoestring budget, Rob Quick introduced the narrow-mouthed container and little bottles of bleach. Families quickly accepted the system. In a subsequent Bolivian study, Quick found that this simple solution resulted in a 44 percent reduction of diarrhea. This was the origin of CDC's Safe Water System, which has spread throughout the developing world and saved thousands of lives.

The Resurgence of TB

Emerging Infections, a study commissioned by the Institute of Medicine of the National Academies, was published in 1992. The authors noted that drugs and pesticides, while potent weapons, could "inadvertently contribute to the selection of certain mutations, adaptations, and migrations that enable pathogens to proliferate." Human technology, jet travel, population growth, and manipulation of the environment could have unforeseen consequences. Among the reemerging microbes they mentioned were cholera and tuberculosis (TB).

People become infected with TB by breathing *Mycobacterium tuberculosis,* though most people's immune systems combat the bacteria to prevent clinical illness. The infection can persist for years, however, and can become active at any time, especially if the immune system becomes impaired. The debilitating disease primarily affects the lungs, causing bloody coughs, fever, night sweats, fatigue, pallor, and weight loss; thus its early name, consumption.

With the arrival of antibiotics such as streptomycin in the 1940s, TB cases had steadily declined until the mid-1980s, when four factors — the AIDS epidemic, diminished TB control efforts, rising poverty and homelessness, and immigration from countries with high TB prevalence — contributed to their rise.

In October 1990 New York City EIS officer Tom Frieden got a call from Harlem Hospital's Karen Brudney: "Tom, I'm seeing a big increase in resistant TB, especially among AIDS patients and the homeless." Brudney had found that 89 percent of the Harlem TB patients were lost to follow-up (failing to return for medication, with no known address) or had died after they were discharged. Having failed to complete their course of antibiotic therapy, which was supposed to last at least six months, many were readmitted with active TB, only to be discharged and lost again. It was a perfect recipe for developing drug resistance.

The incidence of tuberculosis in New York City had more than doubled in the previous ten years. In consultation with EIS officer Sam Dooley of the TB unit in Atlanta, Frieden planned a major project — every New York City lab would send all positive TB cultures to him during April 1991 to be tested for drug susceptibility. The city-wide dragnet identified 518 patients with positive TB cultures, a third of whom had isolates that were resistant to one or more antibiotics. Nearly one in five patients had multidrug-resistant tuberculosis.

Frieden asked for EIS reinforcements. In two hospitals, officers Michele Pearson and John Jereb identified forty patients with mul-tiple-drug-resistant tuberculosis (MDR-TB), mostly AIDS victims who had been previously hospitalized with another MDR-TB patient. At one hospital, three of four health-care workers who had contracted tuberculosis died.

Although TB patients were supposed to be isolated, the bacteria could waft into the corridor when they coughed. Also, "patients on isolation often left their rooms," the EIS officers wrote. "Although re-quested to wear masks when out of their rooms, many reportedly re-moved their masks to talk or smoke." As stopgap measures, fans were placed in windows to blow air out of the rooms, and more stringent isolation was imposed.

In November 1991 a hospital in upstate New York reported that thirty-five health-care workers had positive TB skin test conver-sions after caring for patients who were inmates. That led EIS officers Sonia Richards and Sarah Valway to the nearby prison, where they traced MDR-TB to prisoners transferred from New York City jails. Seven HIV-positive inmates had died from resistant tuberculosis, as had a prison guard whose immune system was suppressed by cancer treatment.

In December an outbreak occurred in Elmhurst Hospital in Queens, which housed a unit for HIV-positive prisoners from the Rikers Island Correctional Facility. Of the seventeen MDR-TB pa-tients on the unit, fourteen had died. When EIS officer Victor Coro-nado visited the jail, he found infirmaries with no isolation capacity. In his report, he concluded, "Due to unanticipated release and incor-rect home addresses, many inmates with TB were reportedly lost to follow-up," thus further spreading the disease.

In January 1992 the CDC called a meeting of tuberculosis experts in New York. MDR-TB cases had been found in sixteen states, but 60 percent of them were in New York City. The New York City Health Department opened a TB hotline for doctors and allotted $8 million in federal, state, and local funds, in part for Public Health Advisors who would make sure that TB patients continued to get appropriate treatment after being discharged.

Patients with MDR-TB needed to continue therapy for eighteen months or longer, using a complicated combination of second-line medications with disagreeable side effects. Frieden championed directly observed therapy, in which health workers watched patients swallow their medicine every day.

Near the end of Frieden's second EIS year in May 1992, New York City health commissioner Peggy Hamburg appointed him director of the city's Bureau of Tuberculosis Control. "By December 31, 1992, we will have 500 TB patients on directly observed therapy," he announced to his 144-person staff.

With additional money and staff (topping $40 million and six hundred employees), they did. "Outreach workers traveled to patients' homes and workplaces," Frieden later wrote, "as well as to street corners, bridges, subway stations, park benches, and even 'crack dens' in abandoned buildings, to ensure that patients were appropriately treated."

In October 1992 Marci Layton, a new NYC EIS officer, helped investigate a hotel on the Upper West Side where the city rented rooms for 83 otherwise homeless AIDS patients. She found that 16 of the residents had tuberculosis, but only 8 were still on their TB therapy. Half had been "lost to medical follow-up." Since there were 1,725 AIDS patients in thirty-two single-room-occupancy city hotels, that meant some 850 might have MDR-TB. Directly observed therapy was begun for all such AIDS/TB residents.

A few hard-core patients (often those who were homeless and addicted to crack) repeatedly eluded treatment. In 1993 NYC health regulations were modified to allow forced detention of such patients until they were cured. The program provided effective treatment and served as a national model for detention as a last resort.

New TB cases had declined by 15 percent by the end of 1993. The rest of the country followed New York City's lead in aggressive TB treatment, but the problem was far worse internationally, especially in Africa, where AIDS was rampant. "The tuberculosis bacterium infects approximately 1.7 billion people," Frieden wrote, "causing about 8 million cases and . . . 3 million deaths annually worldwide." Frieden would move to India in 1996 to help expand effective tuberculosis diagnosis and treatment to millions of patients.

The Ethical Folic Acid Test

On June 24, 1991, Godfrey Oakley, EIS alum and head of the CDC Birth Defects Division, got a call from British researcher Nick Wald: "Godfrey, we're stopping our trial. It works." Wald had launched his double-blind controlled folic acid trial in 1983, enrolling women whose previous pregnancy had produced a child with a neural tube defect. "Folic acid prevented 72 percent of the NTDs!" Wald proclaimed.

Oakley compared the moment to the invention of the Salk polio vaccine. But the discovery left him with a dilemma: What should the CDC do about its long-planned Chinese trial? In May 1983, while in China at a conference on perinatal surveillance, Oakley had discovered that the number of Chinese children born with spina bifida and anencephaly was seven times higher than the United States. Data extracted from an Agent Orange study had found that mothers who took multivitamins early in their pregnancies had fewer babies with NTDs, and Oakley had suspected that folic acid was the crucial ingredient.* Because so many American women already took multivitamins, a randomized clinical trial in the United States would be nearly impossible. But in China, virtually no women took vitamins. He had successfully found funding and in 1988 work had finally begun on the study's design. But it would now be unethical to do a controlled trial, giving some women placebos instead of folic acid.

Oakley and his colleagues decided to do a clinical trial to prove the efficacy of folic acid among *all* women, whether or not they had

---

*See pages 201–202.

experienced an NTD pregnancy. In July 1991 EIS alum R. J. Berry moved to China to begin the program. With the CDC's help, the Chinese mounted a massive public health campaign to give folic acid to 150,000 women from 1993 to 1995.

In September 1992 the U.S. Public Health Service recommended that women of reproductive age take 400 micrograms of folic acid every day, estimating that this would cut the incidence of U.S. neural tube defects at least by half. In 1998 the FDA mandated fortification of U.S. cereal grain products, but only to the degree sufficient to ensure that the average woman would consume 100 micrograms of folic acid.

The results of the massive Chinese study, published in 1999, proved incontrovertibly that folic acid reduced the risk of NTDs, but most of the world's nations have not yet acted on that knowledge.

The Desperate Ones

After the U.S.-led coalition drove Iraqi troops out of Kuwait in the 1990–1991 Gulf War, the Kurds in northern Iraq rebelled. EIS officer Don Sharp joined a multinational team in October 1992 to assess the embattled Kurds' basic humanitarian needs. He found near-empty stockrooms, no surgical equipment, and marginal nutrition. Kurdish doctors reported cases of brucellosis, diarrhea, hepatitis, acute respiratory infections, intestinal parasites, measles, and typhoid. Pediatricians noted increased malnutrition in children. Physicians ranked fuel, food, and shelter as top priorities, followed by medicine and clean water.

Because of an internal embargo imposed by Saddam Hussein, Sharp urged that UNICEF move fuel, food, drugs, vaccines, and surgical supplies from Turkey into Iraqi Kurdistan — a delicate matter, since the Turks despised the Kurds. Thanks in part to Sharp's advocacy, much-needed aid and medical supplies did flow across the border.

In 1991, in nearby Somalia, the ouster of the president was followed by a civil war among feuding warlords that, in conjunction with a severe drought, produced a humanitarian disaster. In November

1992 EIS officers Lynn Quenemoen, Brad Gessner, and Tony Marfin flew into Mogadishu, the chaotic Somali capital, supposedly to assist WHO and the USAID Disaster Assistance Response Team (DART), but they mostly worked independently.

"Everything in Somalia ran on bribery and intimidation," Quenemoen recalled. Trucks swerved through the countryside with thirteen-year-olds perched atop them chewing hallucinogenic qat leaves and wielding AK-47s or rocket launchers. "Once, Brad and I were in a prop plane, about to land, when they started shooting at us, so the pilot had to pull up." On November 20 the EIS officers arrived in Baidoa, 150 miles west of Mogadishu. "Access to the whole town was not possible because it was not safe," they wrote in their report in the *Lancet*, "so we surveyed only people in displaced persons camps."

Nearly 40 percent of household occupants in the camps had died during the past seven and a half months, including three-quarters of the children under five, mostly from measles or diarrhea in conjunction with severe malnutrition. It was the highest mortality rate ever recorded in medical literature.

"There wasn't much grieving," Quenemoen recalled. "People were too famished and ill, lying in these little huts on death's doorstep." The EIS group reported back to Washington every day through the DART satellite phone. They left Somalia on December 6, 1992, three days before a multinational U.S.-led military intervention that restored a semblance of order and alleviated the famine. A series of EIS officers later cycled in to help. But when pictures of Somali rebels dragging dead U.S. soldiers through the streets hit American TV screens, politicians began to question the wisdom of such humanitarian military missions in Africa.

Gessner and Quenemoen concluded that well-intentioned aid often made matters worse. "Much of the food sent to Somalia was stolen," Gessner said, "then sold in Kenya to buy weapons that perpetuated the fighting." The donated food that did reach the population was distributed at large, crowded camps where communicable diseases were rampant. Warlords fought over the imported resources, driving off foreign aid workers.

By 1993 an estimated 41.5 million people worldwide were refugees, forced from their homes by violence. In July 1993 EIS officer Les Roberts, accompanied by EIS alum Brent Burkholder, went to Sarajevo, under siege by the Serbs in the wake of the breakup of Yugoslavia. Water treatment was a problem, with rates of hepatitis A and other waterborne diseases increasing. But Roberts estimated that 57 percent of all deaths in Sarajevo stemmed from violence.

He had heard "crazy rumors" that Serbian snipers were shooting children in the legs to lure adults into the street. Then he walked into a hospital ward filled with children whose legs had been shot. "I had nightmares for weeks afterwards," he said. "I had no capacity to process that level of evil."

In their report, Roberts and Burkholder urged that adequate vaccines and refrigeration capacity be provided to local *dom zdravljas* (health centers) before the winter, that feeding programs continue, and that undeterred access to central Bosnia be maintained. The most critical need was for diesel fuel. "Because of the fuel shortage," they wrote, "water pumps cannot function, health-care workers cannot travel to rural clinics, and some public health programs (e.g. garbage collection and vaccination campaigns) have been curtailed." They cabled a summary back to the U.S. State Department, and while changing planes in New York, Roberts heard President Bill Clinton on television saying that the highest priority in Bosnia was providing adequate diesel fuel.

In November 1993 Roberts flew with EIS officer Chuck Vitek to Armenia, where the ongoing war with Azerbaijan had cut off supplies of food and fuel. The EIS officers found that while city residents in the capital of Yerevan were near starvation, farmers in the countryside were growing plenty of food. Roberts and Vitek recommended purchasing produce from rural Armenians as a practical, cheap solution instead of the planned USAID food drop.

During the previous year civil war had erupted in Tajikistan between Islamic tribes and the communist government. Some sixty thousand Tajiks fled south to Afghanistan, then brought cholera back upon their return to their farm collectives. EIS officers John Murray and Paul Cieslak recommended the use of oral rehydration solution, chlorination, repaired pumps, and closed-mouth plastic jerry cans, though in the chaotic circumstances, their advice probably had limited impact.

Terrorism in NYC

Religious violence reached the United States on February 26, 1993, when a Ryder rental van exploded in the parking garage below Tower One of the World Trade Center in New York City. The conspirators were linked to the al-Qaeda terrorist organization. The blast killed six people and knocked out the electrical power to both towers, so that people in 198 elevators were trapped, and the public address system could not direct people to safety. The elevator shafts acted like chimneys, carrying smoke to the upper floors, where it escaped through heating and air-conditioning vents, then wafted into stairwells where thousands of fleeing employees jammed in long lines.

EIS officer Lynn Quenemoen uncovered these facts when he investigated the bombing in March 1993. Nearly a thousand occupants had suffered from smoke inhalation. He suggested more backup power sources, emergency lighting in the stairwells, smoke control, and fire drills for those working in high-rises, which saved some lives eight years later on 9/11, when terrorists flew airplanes into the World Trade Center buildings.

So Good It's Scary

On Saturday, January 16, 1993, EIS officer Beth Bell got a call from EIS alum Marcia Goldoft, her coworker at the Washington State Department of Health: "Beth, can you work tomorrow? This *E. coli* problem is looking worse than we thought." Earlier that week an unusual number of children had come down with bloody diarrhea, some on dialysis for hemolytic uremic syndrome (HUS).

On Sunday morning Goldoft went to Seattle Children's Hospital to interview the parents of the sick children. She and Bell used the children's best friends as controls for a case-control study. By that evening they had results from sixteen cases with matched controls.

Twelve of the cases had eaten Jack in the Box hamburgers, but none of the controls had. The following day Goldoft and Bell's boss, state epidemiologist John Kobayashi (another EIS graduate), called a press conference to announce that Jack in the Box hamburgers could be lethal, and that the company was withdrawing the implicated lots.

In Idaho, Nevada, and California, EIS officers Paul Cieslak and Abby Shefer investigated cases of bloody diarrhea and HUS, part of the same multistate outbreak caused by Jack in the Box hamburgers. A new method called pulsed-field gel electrophoresis (PFGE) used in laboratories provided a DNA fingerprint of an *E. coli* O157:H7 strain that matched all of the cases and bacteria found in the withdrawn hamburger patties.

More than seven hundred cases were eventually identified. Four children died, and many more suffered multiple organ damage and permanent paralysis. Ironically, the company's advertising slogan for its hamburgers at that time was "So good it's scary."

It was also scary that the outbreaks outside Washington State would have been missed completely were it not for publicity about the hamburger chain. In San Diego, California, six-year-old Lauren Beth Rudolph had eaten a Jack in the Box hamburger a week before Christmas. After suffering three heart attacks, she died in her mother's arms on December 28, 1992. Only in retrospect did anyone realize why she had died.

EIS officer Jessica Tuttle, with USDA veterinarian Tom Gomez (an EIS alum), conducted the trace-back investigation. The meat came from the United States, Canada, Australia, and New Zealand, up to five hundred carcasses mixed together in one hamburger lot. Tuttle and Gomez visited five U.S. slaughterhouses linked to the implicated meat and saw many obvious ways that fecal matter could contaminate the meat. "The meat traceback provided insight into the enormous complexity of the farm-to-table continuum for meat," Tuttle concluded. She suggested "zero tolerance of this [*E. coli*] organism in processed food."

By their prompt action, Bell and other EIS officers had prevented thousands of people from eating contaminated hamburgers. It was a watershed outbreak, providing a national wake-up call that would produce stricter agricultural regulations and better surveillance for foodborne illnesses.

The Brew That Made Milwaukee Infamous

On Monday, April 5, 1993, Kathy Blair, the epidemiologist for the Milwaukee Health Department, called the Wisconsin Department of Health Services in Madison about diarrheal illness reported in the Milwaukee media. EIS alum Jeff Davis, the Wisconsin state epidemiologist, advised her to submit stool isolates to labs and to collect specific data.

By the next afternoon Blair was frantic. The labs couldn't find anything in the stool samples, but she was inundated with calls from the public and the press. Most of the calls seemed to be coming from the southern part of the city, where several schools had closed. On Wednesday morning Davis, Bill Mac Kenzie, his Wisconsin EIS assignee, and two coworkers drove to Milwaukee to investigate.

Mac Kenzie and Davis suspected a waterborne outbreak, since the illness appeared to be citywide. They met with the Milwaukee mayor, health department, and water treatment officials and learned that the city drinking water was provided by two treatment plants, one mostly for the south side, the other for the north, though the system was interconnected, with substantial overlap in the central city. Both plants took their water from Lake Michigan through separate pipes extending a mile offshore.

The water department officials stated that recent water quality met EPA standards and included no coliforms (fecal contamination). The turbidity of the water from the southern Howard Street plant had been higher recently, but it was still within historical limits. The system used sufficient chlorine along with coagulants, sedimentation, and rapid sand filtration. Davis insisted on seeing plant turbidity data from the last ten years.

Later that afternoon Mac Kenzie was summoned by the city lab chief. As the EIS officer peered into a microscope, the lab man explained that he was looking at *Cryptosporidium* protozoa, and that another city lab had found them in seven other stool samples that same day. An alert physician who cared for HIV patients had ordered the out-of-the-ordinary tests.

First identified in humans in 1976, these protozoa came to prominence as opportunistic parasites in AIDS patients. The *Crypto* parasites did not require a mosquito vector or other host, since they could complete their entire life cycle within one host. They thrived in calves and could reach humans through contact with oocysts in cow manure.

Mac Kenzie knew that the parasite was resistant to chlorine. He told Mayor John Norquist and Davis about the *Cryptosporidium* and his suspicion that this outbreak was associated primarily with the Howard Street water treatment plant. The mayor immediately issued a boil-water advisory.

A survey of nursing homes, whose occupants did not travel around the city, showed that the elderly north-side residents had no *Crypto* parasites in their stools, while half of the south-side occupants tested positive — all except one south-side nursing home, where the water came from a well.

This was strong circumstantial evidence, but how to prove that the water from the south-side treatment plant had contained the protozoa? A week into the investigation, EIS alum David Addiss fielded a call from a south Milwaukee company that made ice sculptures. The company had two blocks of ice made on March 25 and April 9, the day the water plant had shut down. Might they be of some use? Tests revealed that the melted ice did indeed contain *Cryptosporidium*.

Snowmelt and spring rain had probably transported the *Cryptosporidium* that made it through the municipal water filters, and when the filters were backwashed to clean them, more protozoa had washed through. When a few people became ill, their watery stool had flushed into the treated sewage that flowed into the lake, where the counterclockwise flow delivered it to the southern intake pipe. This set up a cycle in which *Cryptosporidium* became more and more concentrated in the south Milwaukee drinking water.

Mac Kenzie and his colleagues estimated that more than 400,000

Milwaukee residents had contracted diarrhea from *Cryptosporidium*, making it the largest documented waterborne disease outbreak in U.S. history. The epidemic had a major public health impact. In the ensuing years, most municipal water systems improved their filtering systems, limited turbidity levels, and eliminated backwashing practices.

Navajo Flu

On May 9, 1993, Florena Woody, a twenty-one-year-old Navajo long-distance runner, died while struggling for breath. Five days later her fiancé, nineteen-year-old marathon runner Merrill Bahe, collapsed on his way to her funeral and died soon after. The couple had lived together in a trailer in Littlewater, New Mexico. Their autopsies revealed plasma-soaked lungs that weighed twice as much as normal. They had essentially drowned in their own fluids.

Within a week Woody's brother and his girlfriend, who had visited the deceased couple frequently, couldn't breathe. Both barely survived in intensive care units. By the end of the month, nineteen similar unexplained cases were found, twelve of whom died. Aside from the Littlewood cluster, the others didn't know one another. They lived in far-flung rural isolation across the Navajo nation of 175,000 people spread over 17 million acres in New Mexico, Arizona, Utah, and Colorado, known as the Four Corners area.

On Saturday, May 29, EIS officers Jeff Duchin and Ron Moolenaar and recent EIS grad Jay Butler joined a brainstorming meeting of some forty doctors and public health officials in Albuquerque. Could it be pneumonic plague, leptospirosis, inhalational anthrax, pulmonary tularemia, legionellosis, rare viruses, toxins? Or an influenza strain similar to the 1918 variety that had killed healthy young people?

Tests on autopsy samples for all known bacteria were negative. EIS alum Jim Cheek, who worked for the Indian Health Service, had thought it might be phosphine, used to kill prairie dogs, but his search of the abandoned Woody-Bahe trailer found nothing but scavenging mice. The national media ran stories about the so-called Navajo flu, fostering racism and paranoia. Waitresses serving Navajos wore rubber gloves.

Duchin studied medical charts, finding that the disease began with fever, muscle aches, headache, cough, and nausea, then produced shortness of breath, high white blood cell counts, and bilateral lung infiltrates. Within eight days of the first symptoms, most victims were dead. Moolenaar sent autopsy specimens to the CDC labs and helped to plan a case-control study to be run by Arizona-based EIS officer Paul Zeitz.

EIS officer Ben Muneta, the grandson of a famed Navajo medicine man, worked for the local Indian Health Service. Tribal elders told him that similar deaths had occurred in 1918 and 1933, when harsh winters were followed by excessive spring rains that made the desert bloom, as it had in the spring of 1993. The elders linked the deaths to mice, which descended from the mountains in droves in such years, feasting on the large pine nut harvest.

Back in Atlanta, CDC labs tested the samples Moolenaar had sent. C.J. Peters, the head of viral Special Pathogens, oversaw testing against rare viral strains, and by June 4 he had a match: hantavirus.* Asian hantaviruses caused internal bleeding and shut down the kidneys, whereas the Four Corners epidemic flooded the lungs. This was a new strain.

Asian hantaviruses were carried by rodents, so attention turned to Four Corners mice. Using the recently developed technology of polymerase chain reaction (PCR), which allowed the amplification of tiny bits of genetic code, the CDC lab identified the viral fingerprint and found it in deer mice (*Peromyscus maniculatus*) that had been trapped in victims' homes. The rodents carried the virus in their urine. When people stirred up urine-soaked dust and breathed the aerosolized virus, they contracted what was now named hantavirus pulmonary syndrome (HPS).†

Deer mice thrive throughout the United States, with the exception of the Southeast. Cases soon cropped up outside the Four Corners

---

*See page 4.

†Jim Cheek realized how lucky he had been not to contract the disease as he rummaged without protection around Florena Woody's trailer.

region. By the end of 1995, 124 hantavirus cases had been confirmed in twenty-four states.

As a freshman EIS officer in 1978, Rick Goodman had investigated the case of a young Idaho father who suddenly had trouble breathing and died inexplicably with fluid-filled lungs. In 1993 it dawned on him that the Idaho victim might have died from pulmonary hantavirus. The hospital still had the paraffin tissue block from his autopsy, and the CDC labs were able to isolate hantavirus from it. Twelve other retrospective cases were also identified. Viruses are traditionally named for a place where they are found (Marburg, Lassa, Ebola). The CDC suggested naming this one Four Corners virus, but the Navajo community objected. Perhaps Muerto Canyon virus, after an arroyo near Florena Woody's trailer? When the Navajo protested again, the CDC virologists gave up and called it the Sin Nombre virus (SNV) — "virus without a name" — now its official moniker.

Farewells to Uncle Lyle and Alexander the Great

The year 1993 marked transitions for three public health leaders. CDC director Bill Roper was replaced by David Satcher, the first African American leader of the agency, and the Epidemic Intelligence Service saw the departure of two men.

After twenty-seven years of sending more than five hundred EIS officers out on state assignments, Lyle Conrad refocused his attention during his final two years at the CDC on revamping epidemiology in the former Soviet republics, where 200 million people needed help. He continued to assist with recruitment of state EIS officers, but mostly, after forays to Moscow and Siberia, he trained Russians who came to the CDC for instruction.

Conrad had worked in twenty-nine countries during the course of his public health career, but his greatest pride was the "care and feeding" of state-based EIS officers. "Lyle Conrad was consistently hard on his bosses and gently supportive of anyone he supervised," Bill Mac Kenzie observed. "Lyle is always the champion of the underdog."

On November 22, 1993, Alexander Langmuir died of kidney cancer at the age of eighty-three. His forceful presence and perfectionism had set high standards for scientific rigor, clear writing, and diligence in the field. He had introduced the concept of surveillance in public health and led the EIS into new areas such as family planning, chronic diseases, environmental health, birth defects, toxic hazards, occupational health, drug addiction, famines, disasters, and international health.

Although Langmuir had briefly considered that the EIS might have outlived its usefulness, by the time of his death he clearly regarded it as his greatest legacy. In November 1993, as Langmuir lay near death, EIS alum Steve Schoenbaum paid a call, commenting on a nearby photograph taken that spring featuring Langmuir, in black tie, surrounded by six deans of schools of public health, all EIS alums. "What a wonderful field," Langmuir said. "We should drink a toast to epidemiology!" They located a bottle of champagne, popped the cork, and Langmuir managed a sip. He died a week later.

In his final days, Langmuir's daughters demonstrated a new tenderness toward their father. "He let me be close to him and do things for him for the first time," said Susan. She knew that her father was an atheist who did not believe in an afterlife, but she now told him to consider that he was going to history, where he would join those he loved and admired, such as his uncle Irving, his wife Leona, Eleanor Roosevelt, Abraham Lincoln, "and the *other* Alexander the Great."

18
ROUGH SLEDDING

In 1994, DUE TO government cutbacks, the CDC had to drop four hundred positions, which would eliminate the incoming EIS class. To circumvent this disaster, the new recruits were designated EIS "fellows" who were neither official CDC employees nor officers in the Commissioned Corps of the U.S. Public Health Service. The Epidemiology Program Office found money in the tight budget for the program. At the same time, the CDC Foundation, a private nongovernmental organization, was created to supplement the CDC budget, independent of political influence.

Hell on Earth

On April 6, 1994, an airplane carrying the presidents of Rwanda and Burundi was shot down, sparking the Rwandan genocide, in which an estimated 750,000 minority Tutsis were slaughtered by members of the Hutu tribe. Spooked by the recent failed humanitarian military mission in Somalia, neither the UN nor the Clinton administration would intervene.

In mid-May EIS officer Les Roberts was asked to assess the Rwandan situation for the World Health Organization (WHO). Roberts ventured into areas controlled by the Rwandan Patriotic Front, the Tutsi rebels under the command of Paul Kagame. He saw the remains of the genocidal carnage committed by the Hutu extremists, but he also learned of retaliatory massacres committed by the invading Tutsi army. He found the countryside nearly deserted — an eerie emptiness in what had been the most densely populated country in Africa.

The remnants of the Hutu army, along with terrified Hutu families, fled into neighboring Zaire, Tanzania, and Burundi on July 14. The majority of the refugees, some 800,000, poured into Goma, Zaire, dispersing to three camps hastily set up on the outskirts of town.

On the afternoon of July 19, Roberts arrived in Goma on a UN supply helicopter. He made his way to the Mugunga camp, where French doctors with Médecins du Monde were trying to treat more than a thousand cholera victims. The doctors had run out of oral rehydration salts, and there were few IV drips available. A third of the dehydrated refugees were dead by day's end. One woman's full-time job was to pluck surviving babies from their deceased mothers and take them to orphanages. Roberts thought, *This is the worst spot on earth.*

Goma sat on impenetrable solidified lava, so cholera-laden excrement flowed into nearby Lake Kivu, where desperate refugees scooped buckets of polluted drinking water. Roberts wanted to enlist refugees to put chlorine into the water, but his WHO supervisor insisted that he maintain mortality statistics instead.

As the disaster in Goma unfolded, President Clinton authorized aid to the refugees, and charitable organizations from around the world rushed to help. On July 30, 1994, EIS officers Scott Dowell and Brad Woodruff landed in Goma, and in the next few days more EIS officers arrived. Dowell and Woodruff focused on the twenty-one camps for ten thousand "unaccompanied children," who were either orphans or separated from their families.

"Every morning we would see a little pile of what looked like firewood stacked outside the camp entrances," Dowell said. They were bodies of children who had died overnight. The well-intentioned health volunteers for AmeriCares and most other NGOs knew little about appropriate cholera treatment.

By early August there were sufficient supplies of oral rehydration salts and intravenous solutions, but, as Dowell wrote later, "staff responsible for oral rehydration rarely understood that there was a specific quantity of fluid to be given over a specific period of time." One misguided charity had sent Gatorade, which caregivers gave to the dying children, only making them worse. Another center administered intravenous dextrose, which contained no essential sodium and was harmful. Yet another facility had no access to water.

Dowell and Woodruff provided on-the-spot training in the use of oral rehydration and set up a surveillance system to monitor deaths and conduct nutritional surveys. "We'd enter a room packed with children, the floor covered with stool and vomit," Dowell recalled. "Of forty kids, ten would be severely dehydrated and two or three dead." By the time they made it around the room to treat the fortieth patient, another child would have died. In one camp the toll for infants under a year of age reached 800 deaths per 100,000 in a single day, over three hundred times higher than the rate before the crisis.

Additional EIS officers arrived, seeking to save lives, even as their own were threatened. They watched helplessly as people accused of theft or of being Tutsis were stoned to death or beheaded with machetes. David Swerdlow and EIS officer Alfredo Vergara focused on refugee nutrition. EIS officer Orin Levine, the son of an EIS alum, took charge of a meningitis vaccine initiative, while Don Sharp administered measles immunization.

In August, after cholera had run through the entire population, the diarrhea flow turned bloody due to *Shigella* bacteria. The CDC people found that the officially sanctioned nalidixic acid treatment as well as donated tetracycline and the antibiotic Bactrim were useless because of resistant *Shigella*, but that ciprofloxacin, available from the U.S. military, was effective.

Every night the EIS officers discussed a profound ethical dilemma. Many of those they cared for were *genocidaires*. Were the camps just facilitating their continued reign of terror? There was no easy answer.*

"The immediate, medical cause of most deaths was diarrheal dis-

---

*In November 1996 the Goma camps were broken up. Approximately 100,000 Hutus who fled were killed by the Rwandan Patriotic Front.

ease," the EIS officers and other authors wrote in a summary paper, "but the underlying causes were the historical, ethnic, demographic, socioeconomic, and political factors that led to the collapse of Rwandan society and to this mass population migration.... The world was simply not prepared for an emergency of this magnitude." As a result of their critique, standards for NGO training and response to such disasters were strengthened.

By the end of August almost fifty thousand refugees had died, but the cholera/shigellosis epidemic was over, and the mortality rate had decreased dramatically. The first wave of EIS officers headed home.

The Return of Ebola

Scott Dowell flew back to Zaire in May 1995. Ebola had erupted in the first major epidemic since the 1970s. Because epidemiologists had arrived as prior human outbreaks were ending, they hadn't been able to study ongoing transmission.* This epidemic in the town of Kikwit (population 200,000) was still raging. Dowell came into Kikwit a few days after the arrival of three CDC men from viral Special Pathogens. Investigators from other nations were also converging on the town.

Ebola had been amplified primarily in a hospital setting, and by the time the international team arrived, the Kikwit General Hospital had been abandoned except for a few patients and health-care workers in the last stages of the hemorrhagic disease. "The first day or two, we cleaned up the hospital so it could be reopened and divided up tasks," Dowell recalled.

Wearing protective garb and air filters that covered his nose and mouth, he helped with patient care. The tropical heat was unbearable. "I squashed around in the puddles of sweat filling my boots," he said. "My hands were shaking, trying to draw blood without poking myself. My goggles fogged up, and when I wiped them, I thought, *Oh my god, I just touched the skin on my face with the glove.*"

Dowell interviewed surviving family members and contacts with the help of a translator. His study revealed that Ebola spread only dur-

---

*See pages 170–175.

ing the terminal stages in which patients were bleeding out. In Zaire, hospitalized patients were usually cared for by family members, who often slept with them. At funerals, family members tenderly washed and kissed the body, allowing further transmission.

EIS alum Ali Khan conducted standard trace-back epidemiology to identify the index patient. He concluded that Gaspard Menga, a forty-two-year-old farmer and charcoal maker, had been the first case when he became ill on January 6. Khan could track subsequent transmission from contacts with Menga. Assuming that the farmer had caught the virus from an animal or insect near his charcoal pit in the rain forest, investigators trapped and studied thousands of animals. None harbored the virus.

After the hospital was sterilized and barrier nursing practices with gloves and masks enforced, only one more Ebola case was contracted there, but the virus continued to spread slowly in the community. EIS officer Peter Kilmarx took on the job of surveillance, directing a team of local medical students, tracking down rumors, and centralizing the data. "Cases were frequently hidden because of stigmatization and the perception that transportation to the hospital was a death sentence," Kilmarx wrote. "There were two reports of people from Kikwit being killed in other villages because of fear of contagion."

When Kilmarx and Dowell left Zaire in mid-June 1995, the epidemic was nearly under control. The last Ebola patient died in Kikwit on July 16, 1995. Of the 315 identified cases, 81 percent were fatal, and a quarter of the dead were health-care workers.

Contaminated Ice Cream

In October 1994 Minnesota-based EIS officer Tom Hennessy investigated a major epidemic of *Salmonella enteritidis*.* In a case-control study, he and his colleagues found that eleven of the fifteen cases had eaten Schwan's ice cream, versus only two controls. Even though the laboratory had not yet been able to culture bacteria from the ice

---

*See pages 226–227.

cream,* state epidemiologist Mike Osterholm announced the results, and the company closed its plant and recalled its products nationwide.

Hennessy thought that ice cream, with eggs as an ingredient, seemed a logical culprit. But Schwan's ice cream contained no eggs. Tanker-trailer trucks hauled the pasteurized premix to the Marshall, Minnesota, plant, which Hennessy found pristine. He discovered, however, that truck drivers were "back-hauling" liquid raw eggs on their return trip, and they were not cleaning their tankers sufficiently to prevent cross-contamination. An estimated 224,000 people throughout the continental United States had gotten diarrhea from eating Schwan's ice cream. This was the largest common-source outbreak of salmonellosis ever recognized in the United States.

Dragnets for Microbes

Despite the huge number of Schwan's victims, fewer than three hundred cases were actually reported to the CDC. The epidemiologists arrived at the larger estimate by extrapolating attack ratios to the number of total customers. In fact, most diarrhea is never reported. During his final year as an EIS officer, Fred Angulo focused on this problem.

Angulo and EIS alum David Swerdlow proposed FoodNet, an active surveillance system in which clinical laboratories in five states would be contacted regularly to determine what they found in stool samples, looking for rates of *Salmonella, Shigella, Campylobacter, E. coli* O157:H7, and *Listeria,* among others. It was launched in January 1996 and later expanded to ten states, with subsequent efforts to pin down which foods carried which microbes.

At the same time, the CDC launched PulseNet, a national molecular subtyping network in which regional labs were trained in pulsed-field gel electrophoresis, the method of DNA fingerprinting that had

---

*The lab eventually found *Salmonella* in the ice cream, but locating it was difficult because the bacteria hid inside fat cells.

been pivotal in the 1993 Jack in the Box *E. coli* O157:H7 investigation.* Now laboratory technicians and epidemiologists could work collaboratively to identify and track down epidemics.

Angulo also worked on a national study of *Salmonella* resistance. He learned of Scott Holmberg's pioneering 1983 investigation that had linked animal feed to human disease† and became convinced that indiscriminately administering antimicrobials to animals was foolhardy. No one kept track of such feed supplements, though the administered drugs amounted to an estimated 29 million pounds annually.

In 1995 the FDA authorized the use of fluoroquinolones (i.e., Cipro) in chickens and turkeys, to promote growth and prevent disease. In response, Angulo created the National Antimicrobial Resistance Monitoring System (NARMS) for Enteric Bacteria. Launched in 1996, it documented an alarming increase in fluoroquinolone resistance in the ensuing years. The FDA finally reversed its approval of the drug for poultry, but limiting antibiotic use in U.S. food animals remained a challenge. Angulo would oversee FoodNet and NARMS at the CDC for many years.

Lives and Dollars Up in Smoke

In 1994 EIS officer Mike Siegel, assigned to the CDC Office on Smoking and Health, conducted a cost-benefit analysis of tobacco in the state of Georgia. "For a long time, most Southern states had ignored this health issue," Siegel said, "because of the powerful tobacco industry lobby."

In the previous full year, Georgia farmers had grown 96.3 million pounds of tobacco and sold it for $159 million. Revenue from sales of cigarettes, cigars, and chewing tobacco amounted to $1.203 billion, with another $176 million flowing in from state tobacco taxes. Tobacco provided jobs, directly or indirectly, for 35,860 people who earned $1.230 billion. Thus, the annual economic benefit of the nicotine-laden plant came to $2.768 billion.

---

*See pages 280–282.
†See pages 219–220.

Annually in Georgia there were 10,650 smoking-attributable deaths from cancer, heart disease, respiratory failure, and fetal/infant fatality. That translated to 177,424 years of potential life lost due to premature smoking deaths. Siegel estimated the state's direct and indirect smoking-related medical costs at $2.9 billion per year, while smoking had caused 91.4 million work-loss and bed-disability days in Georgia in 1993, amounting to $6 billion in lost productivity. Thus tobacco cost about $8.9 billion per year. Siegel presented his findings to the Coalition for a Healthy and Responsible Georgia (CHARGe), which pushed for and eventually got smoke-free restaurant legislation in the state.

He also studied the impact of brand-specific cigarette advertising on youth smoking, demonstrating that the three most heavily advertised brands — Marlboro, Camel, and Newport — were also the most popular among the 3 million adolescent smokers in the United States. The rate of teenage smoking began to rise in 1988, the year that the Joe Camel campaign launched nationally. Camel's market share among teens rose by 5.2 percent from 1989 to 1993, as advertising spent on the brand increased from $27 million to $43 million annually.

Siegel testified as an expert witness in seven tobacco cases, leading in part to the massive 1998 nationwide tobacco master settlement agreement in which the industry agreed to pay $206 billion and sponsor antismoking ads. As a result, a pack of cigarettes cost forty cents more, and youth smoking rates began to drop.

Gulf War Syndrome

Since the end of the Persian Gulf War in early 1991, a growing number of the 700,000 U.S. veterans had complained of a wide range of health problems that came to be known as Gulf War syndrome. In May 1994 *Esquire* published an article claiming that thirty-seven out of fifty-five babies born to Mississippi National Guard veterans who had served in the Gulf were "not normal." EIS officer Alan Penman investigated and found that three babies in the National Guard units were born with severe defects, while two had minor problems. The rates fell within the expected range.

In December 1994 EIS officer Rita Washko went to Lebanon, Pennsylvania, where members of a local Air National Guard unit were reportedly suffering from irritable bowel syndrome, joint pains, aching muscles, and memory problems. Katherine Leisure, a local infectious disease doctor, had diagnosed most of them, concluding that they had contracted an illness from sand fly bites in the desert. That sounded somewhat plausible, since a total of thirty-two Gulf War veterans did come down with leishmaniasis, a disease caused by a parasitic protozoa carried by sand flies.

Though sympathetic to the suffering veterans,* Washko concluded that Gulf War syndrome was not a bona fide physical ailment. The fifty-nine veterans whom she and her colleagues interviewed and examined had no consistent constellation of symptoms. Asked to name their most bothersome symptom, 27 percent listed fatigue and 14 percent diarrhea. Washko concluded that they were probably depressed or had post-traumatic stress disorder. "Many participants related a complex of symptoms which has imposed restrictions on their daily activities," she reported. Still, she thought that they had been "influenced by suggestions from the media."

Gulf War syndrome resembled chronic fatigue syndrome, whose sufferers quickly joined ranks with the veterans. Legislators would throw more than $115 million into studies of the amorphous ailment by 1998, with more money to follow.

EIS alum Phil Landrigan, an environmental epidemiologist, was appointed to Bill Clinton's Presidential Advisory Committee on Gulf War Veterans' Illnesses, which took two years to reach the same conclusion as Rita Washko. EIS alum Bob Haley disagreed. He studied twenty-three Houston veterans and concluded that they suffered from low-level pesticide and chemical weapons aerosols, but Landrigan and many others criticized the studies, which relied on unverifiable self-reported exposures. Gulf War syndrome remains a disputed phenomenon today.

---

*Washko's father and his six brothers had served in World War II, where one was killed. She herself had been in the Army Reserves for ten years.

Homegrown Terror

On the morning of April 19, 1995, a decorated Gulf War veteran named Timothy McVeigh (who didn't claim to suffer from Gulf War syndrome but who was clearly troubled) parked a rented Ryder truck in front of the Alfred P. Murrah Federal Building in Oklahoma City, lit the fuse to the five thousand pounds of ammonium nitrate fertilizer and fuel inside, and walked away. A total of 168 people were killed by the resulting blast. EIS officer Roberta Duhaime, a veterinarian on leave from the U.S. Department of Agriculture,* was running late for a 9 A.M. meeting to discuss a study with fellow USDA employees at the Murrah Building. Seven of her friends and coworkers were killed.

Atlanta EIS officers Ann Dellinger, Patrick Kachur, and Gail Stennies rushed to help Duhaime assess the damage, focusing on injuries sustained by rescue workers. This bombing came only two years after that of the World Trade Center. "We must now more seriously prepare for domestic acts of terrorism," the EIS officers concluded.

Taking the Heat

A muggy tropical air mass settled over Chicago on Wednesday, July 12, 1995, sending temperatures to 103 degrees Fahrenheit, then to a record 106 the following day, which felt like 126 degrees due to the high humidity. As the scorching temperatures stretched over the weekend, emergency rooms overflowed. Mayor Richard M. Daley's administration belatedly declared a state of emergency and rushed to provide food, water, and transportation to air-conditioned centers, but over seven hundred residents died during the weeklong heat wave.

EIS officers Jan Semenza and Joel Selanikio flew to Chicago on July 20. They documented 1,072 more hospital admissions than the average for comparable weeks, mostly due to dehydration, heatstroke, and heat exhaustion. Many affected people had underlying health problems.

Semenza and Selanikio assembled and trained an eighty-person

---

*The USDA and Department of Defense each sponsored one or two employees as EIS officers.

staff to conduct a case-control study, finding that isolated, poor elderly men without air-conditioning were the predominant victims.
Older women apparently maintained more support systems. A disproportionate number of victims were alcoholics living in run-down
single-room-occupancy hotels on the top floor, under black roofs
that hastened snowmelt in winter but absorbed brutal heat in the
summer.

EIS officer Ed Kilbourne had documented similar patterns in a
1980 heat wave in Kansas City and St. Louis, where he discovered that
fans simply blew more hot air and did not help. As sociologist Eric
Klinenberg observed in his book *Heat Wave: A Social Autopsy of Disaster in Chicago,* the real culprit was not nature but a dysfunctional social system that neglected those who were poor, old, sick, and alone.

The Republican Revolution and Gun Control

With the restoration of the EIS budget, the "fellowship" program was
terminated, and new officers could once again join the Commissioned
Corps, with its twenty-year retirement option. When EIS chief Polly
Marchbanks decided to return to research, EIS alum Joanna Buffington took over as administrator of the EIS program.

In November 1994 conservative Republicans had won both houses
of the U.S. Congress, which spelled trouble for the CDC National
Center for Injury Prevention and Control, where EIS alums Mark
Rosenberg and Jim Mercy continued to study the impact of firearms.*
They recruited Etienne Krug, a thirty-four-year-old Belgian, as their
EIS officer for the incoming class of 1995.

"I grew up in Europe," Krug said, "where firearms are not available
at all. They are considered very unsafe to have in your home." So he
decided to compare the rate of firearms deaths in the United States
with other developed countries. The results showed children under
the age of fifteen were twelve times more likely to be killed with a gun
in the United States, compared to the other countries' combined average rates. Krug's study also pointed out that while the overall annual

---

*See pages 216, 253.

death rate for children in the United States had declined substantially since 1950, the child homicide rate had tripled.

When the *MMWR* published his findings in February 1997, Krug was interviewed on international TV and radio, resulting in an anonymous death threat. The Republican Congress had just passed a bill eliminating the $2.6 million Division of Violence Prevention budget for firearms research and ordering the CDC never to advocate gun control. Thus, when pressed by reporters about whether tougher laws should be passed, Krug answered, "That is up to legislators to determine based on the data." The congressional ban on CDC gun control advocacy remains in place.

In the textbook *Violence in American Schools,* published in 1998, Rosenberg and Mercy cited a survey in which 7.9 percent of students nationwide said that they had carried a gun in the past month, noting that there had been 105 documented school-associated violent deaths in a recent two-year period — averaging more than one killing per school week.

On April 20, 1999, at Colorado's Columbine High School, two disturbed students, armed with two pump-action shotguns, a semiautomatic rifle, and a semiautomatic handgun, killed twelve fellow students and a teacher and wounded twenty-three others before committing suicide. Despite huge media attention and discussions of gun control, no meaningful legislation ensued.

Five months later Mark Rosenberg, who had become a lightning rod for criticism by the National Rifle Association and gun lobbyists, was removed as director of the National Center for Injury Prevention and Control, shortly after an Institute of Medicine study concluded that "institutional rivalries and resentments" were impeding collaboration on injury prevention.

"Mark was a visionary with respect to injury and violence prevention whose persistence helped move this field forward immensely," Jim Mercy observed. The CDC would continue to conduct limited firearm-related research but with a slashed budget and a focus on less controversial aspects such as proper gun storage (an important issue, but only part of the problem).

Death in Haiti

In November 1995 an infant died in the Port-au-Prince University General Hospital, and by May 1996 thirty-two children were dead. Before dying, the children had suffered from severe vomiting, pancreatitis, respiratory failure, facial paralysis, liver damage, and kidney failure. EIS alum Neal Halsey, a Johns Hopkins professor studying mother-to-child HIV transmission in Haiti, learned of the cases and alerted the CDC.

Without an official request from the Haitian government, the CDC could not send a team. Officials were angry at the CDC for stigmatizing Haitians during the early AIDS days* and so instead asked the Pan American Health Organization (PAHO) for help. PAHO finally summoned the CDC, and EIS officer Kate O'Brien flew to Haiti late on Friday, June 14, 1996, immediately going to the Port-au-Prince hospital.

All of the children had had some kind of preliminary illness, usually with a fever. O'Brien concluded that a toxic substance, perhaps in a children's medication, was probably the culprit, since the illness didn't appear to be infectious.

A doctor gave O'Brien eight bottles of medications that two hospitalized children had been taking. Six were unlabeled, but two were Afebril and Valodon, liquid acetaminophen preparations, both made by Pharval, Haiti's major pharmaceutical company. She sent the bottles to the CDC labs in Atlanta.

The University General Hospital kept no admission or discharge records. Nonetheless, O'Brien learned of enough cases to begin a case-control study, using children hospitalized with fever but no urinary retention (a symptom of the kidney-failure cases) as controls. With fresh cases arriving at the hospital every day, O'Brien identified sixty-three cases with known medications, of whom fifty-five had taken either Afebril or Valodon, all from three consecutive lot numbers, compared to only five controls with exposure to the Pharval drugs.

---

*See pages 211–212.

Six days into the investigation, EIS officer Joel Selanikio arrived in Haiti to help. The next day O'Brien learned that the CDC labs had found that both Afebril and Valodon samples contained about 15 percent diethylene glycol (DEG). Similar to antifreeze, DEG had become notorious in the United States in 1937, when its use in a medication killed more than a hundred people. DEG's illegal use had killed children in South Africa, India, Nigeria, and Bangladesh.

O'Brien and Selanikio stayed up all night, conferring with the Haitian minister of health, the American ambassador, and one of the members of the Boulos family who owned Pharval. On Saturday morning the minister announced that no one should take Afebril or Valodon, the police removed products from store shelves, and a broad media campaign was launched, including bullhorns in the streets.

The following week, seven more children were admitted to the hospital, but all had taken the drugs prior to the public warning. After that, there were only three more victims. Of the 109 identified cases, 88 children died, most of them younger than five.

In collaboration with David Pulham, an FDA investigator, Selanikio began the trace-back investigation. Pharval had purchased drums of DEG-contaminated glycerin from a Haitian distributor, who had bought it through a German chemical broker, which had bought the glycerine from Vos, a Dutch company.

FDA investigator Ann deMarco took up the trail in Europe, finding that the contaminated glycerin had been purchased from Sinochem International, a Chinese trader. After much stonewalling, Sinochem revealed that the Tianhong Fine Chemicals Factory had produced the glycerin, but by the time an FDA representative got to the plant, it was no longer making the product and denied any wrongdoing.

"China is turning into one of the major bulk pharmaceutical producers in the world," wrote FDA deputy commissioner Mary Pendergast in 1997. "Unless they have an open, transparent and predictable system, it is going to be rough sledding in the years ahead."*

---

*In ensuing years, many other contaminated products exported from China would sicken or kill people and pets, including DEG-contaminated glycerin consumed in Panama in 2006 and 2007.

Hitchhiking Microbes

On June 13, 1996, FoodNet surveillance picked up six *E. coli* O157:H7 infections in Connecticut, where EIS officer Betsy Hilborn was stationed. Seven more cases were identified in Illinois. The *E. coli* all had the same molecular fingerprint.

Hilborn subsequently found twenty-one cases in Connecticut. Her case-control study singled out mesclun, a mix of salad greens such as arugula and radicchio. She alerted EIS officer Jonathan Mermin, who was conducting the Illinois investigation. He reinterviewed patients and came to the same conclusion. Hilborn and Mermin's trace-back investigation led them to Fancy Cutt Farms in Hollister, California.

Hilborn and Mermin went to the Fancy Cutt fields, where they identified multiple possible sources of contamination. Beef cattle grazed near the lettuce, and roaming free-range chickens could have spread the cow manure to the fields. But the most likely culprit was the primary wash tank for the greens, where unchlorinated well water was recirculated and inadequately filtered. When the well water was replaced three times a day, the outbreak stopped.

It's the Strawberries!?

In late May 1996 a Canadian company physician in Calgary, Alberta, called the CDC about an unusual cluster of *Cyclospora* infections among company employees who had attended a meeting at an athletic club in Houston, Texas. The CDC notified the Texas Department of Health, which had no EIS assignee and conducted an initial investigation on its own. The Texas officials found additional cases among people who had eaten at the same club as well as at a Houston restaurant.

The *Cyclospora* parasite causes watery diarrhea that can last for six weeks and sometimes recurs, though it is treatable with Bactrim (sulfamethoxazole trimethoprim). It doesn't usually kill, but the abdominal pain can be excruciating. Little was known about the spherical protozoa other than it seemed to afflict people primarily in the tropics in springtime. No one knew whether it had an animal or insect reservoir as part of its life cycle.

Texas investigators concluded from food-consumption interviews that California-grown strawberries had been contaminated with the parasite and issued a public warning. The California Strawberry Commission objected and pointed out that there were no cyclosporiasis cases in California or anywhere else in the western United States. Strawberry sales plummeted anyway.

Throughout June other *Cyclospora* outbreaks popped up in Florida, South Carolina, Illinois, Ohio, Pennsylvania, Connecticut, Massachusetts, New Jersey, and New York, and many sufferers had indeed eaten strawberries. On July 1 *Time* magazine ran a story headlined THE STRAWBERRY SICKNESS.

By that time, however, EIS officer Michael Beach, finally invited to Texas to help with the investigation, was beginning to doubt that strawberries were to blame. About half of the guests who attended a May 30 party in Dallas had somehow ingested *Cyclospora*. Honeydew melon shells filled with raspberries and a cluster of strawberries had been on the table. Raspberries and blackberries were scattered over other dishes. While strawberries had been served for several weeks by the kitchen where the party was held, fresh raspberries and blackberries had arrived only two days before the party.

"Although raspberries cannot be definitively implicated as the vehicle of transmission," Beach concluded, they were probably the source of the parasite. Because strawberries and raspberries were often served together, the California produce might have been falsely implicated.

The raspberries at the party had been grown in Guatemala. During her June 1996 investigation, Florida-based EIS officer Dolly Katz became increasingly suspicious of raspberries. The previous year Florida had had forty-eight cases of cyclosporiasis. The investigation by EIS officer Emily Koumans had been inconclusive, though she had suggested that Guatemalan raspberries might be involved. With 180 cases in 1996, Katz had a better chance to prove the connection.

While 65 percent of the victims remembered eating raspberries, 87 percent recalled strawberry consumption. Yet over half of the controls had also eaten strawberries, while only 7 percent had consumed raspberries, thus implicating the Guatemalan raspberries seven times more than strawberries. Katz suspected that because raspberries were not as memorable as the bigger strawberries, the victims underreported their consumption.

The Florida cohort study of nine *Cyclospora* clusters — mostly in people dining at home — clinched it. Fresh raspberries were the only food served at all nine dinners. On July 3 the state of Florida issued a consumer warning against raspberry consumption.

EIS alum Barbara Herwaldt, based at the CDC Division of Parasitic Diseases, coordinated other studies around the country that also implicated raspberries, which explained why a disproportionate number of patients were wealthy adults who ate the expensive, more perishable fruit. In the spring and early summer of 1996, there were nearly fifteen hundred cases of confirmed cyclosporiasis in the United States and Canada. In mid-July EIS officers Marta Ackers and Victor Cáceres visited several Guatemalan farms, but they could prove nothing.

The initial misidentification of strawberries cost the California growers more than $20 million in lost sales. The next spring over a thousand documented cases of cyclosporiasis in the United States and Canada were traced to Guatemalan raspberries. The United States banned raspberries from Guatemala for the 1998 season, while Canada allowed the importations. Toronto berry eaters contracted more cases of cyclosporiasis. Had EIS officers not raised the alarm about Guatemalan raspberries, more U.S. cases would likely have occurred. Nonetheless, further *Cyclospora* outbreaks occurred anyway, traced by EIS officers to Peruvian mesclun and Mexican basil.

Health-Conscious Sprout Eaters

From February through early June 1997, *Salmonella* cases in Missouri and Kansas with the same molecular fingerprint kept occurring. From their initial interviews, EIS officers Kate Glynn* and Tadesse Wuhib

---

*A month later Glynn investigated a hamburger-related *E. coli* O157:H7 outbreak identified by PulseNet in Colorado. Her study contributed to FDA approval, in December 1997, of irradiation of meat products to kill bacteria.

suspected that alfalfa sprouts might be involved. The lab results confirmed that sprouts from a local grower contained *Salmonella*.

The EIS officers could find no fault with the operation, concluding that the seeds arrived already laden with the bacteria. The warm, misty sprouting environment then provided perfect growing conditions for the microbes. Crunchy seed sprouts, consumed by many health-conscious young women, sometimes turned out to be hazardous, causing a series of outbreaks around the world in the late 1990s.

A month later EIS officers Thomas Breuer and Roger Shapiro were called to Michigan to investigate an outbreak of *E. coli* O157:H7. Again, alfalfa sprouts were the carriers. Soon similar cases were identified in Virginia. Although a different sprouter was implicated in each state, they had all received seeds from the same distributor. The seeds were traced back to four Idaho farms where deer — frequent visitors — may have deposited *E. coli* O157 in their droppings.

It was difficult to find the source of contamination for sprout cases, since seeds were grown primarily for animal feed and mixed from a wide number of farms, sometimes sitting for years in storage. Soaking the seeds in a chlorine solution before sprouting was not entirely effective. While washing produce before eating made sense, *E. coli* O157 was cultured from the inner tissues of sprouts, indicating that bacteria became internalized during the growing process. "Raw sprouts are inherently dangerous," concluded Shapiro. "They are the only food I stopped eating as a result of my EIS experience."

The U.S. food supply, repeatedly touted as the safest in the world, was clearly not always so safe. International commerce, modern mass marketing, and demand for fresh produce at all times of year created opportunities for hitchhiking microbes.

19
APPROACHING A NEW MILLENNIUM

IN FEBRUARY 1997 EIS officers Yvan Hutin and Joel Williams, with EIS alum Ali Khan, traveled to the village of Akungula in Zaire, where a prolonged outbreak of monkeypox had occurred. After the eradication of wild smallpox in 1977, public health officials feared that monkeypox, a close relative, though not as lethal, might evolve to take its place. Surveillance of the disease from 1981 to 1986 indicated that it did not spread as easily as smallpox from person to person. Yet the outbreak that had begun in 1996 affected dozens of people in what appeared to be prolonged chains of transmission.

The investigation took place in the midst of a civil war. In the capital, Kinshasa, the CDC team shared a hotel with Serbian mercenaries before being flown on a forty-year-old prop airplane to a Catholic mission, and then driving over terrible roads to Akungula.

For a week Hutin interviewed people in twelve villages, while Williams collected sixteen species of animals, dissecting and bleeding them to check later for monkeypox virus. After six days in the villages, the satellite phone brought alarming news — rebel forces were approaching fast, pushing the retreating Zairian troops before them. The team had to leave immediately, since both sides were reputed to murder with impunity. The wild ride with daredevil drivers to the Catholic mission was terrifying.

When Hutin, Williams, and Khan finally got into the airplane, panicked locals tried to board. A security guard shot into the air, and the EIS officers dropped to the floor as the plane took off. Then, during a severe hailstorm, the plane went into a sharp nosedive. Williams prayed for his life, while Hutin started a quick farewell note to his wife and children, but the pilot somehow pulled up in time.

When the CDC labs tested Williams's samples, they found that African squirrels and Gambian rats, a Congolese delicacy, carried monkeypox virus. Hutin's interview data documented eighty-eight clinical cases of monkeypox during the past year. In one household, eight consecutive cases had occurred, apparently confirming prolonged chains of person-to-person transmission. "I hate to be accused of pushing the alarmist button," said one scientist, "but for practical purposes, smallpox is back."

Fortunately, Hutin eventually concluded that monkeypox was not capable of sustained transmission. It was likely that new cases kept occurring due to contact with squirrels and Gambian rats. Also, some of the cases were probably chicken pox, which was also common in the Akungula area.

The Zairian civil war had begun in the east, near Goma, where refugee camps once more were set up. On April 1, 1997, EIS officer Arthur Marx arrived to help UNICEF and the UN High Commissioner for Refugees assess health needs in the north Kivu area. Shortly after he arrived, cholera broke out among 90,000 Rwandan refugees in three temporary camps between the cities of Kisangani and Ubundu. Humanitarian workers were not allowed to stay overnight and had to commute six hours each way from Kisangani. Each night scores of unattended patients died of dehydration. Marx counted 1,500 deaths before the evening of April 20, when armed militias attacked, driving everyone out. Only 37,000 refugees were eventually repatriated to Rwanda. Most of the others probably died.

Marx made it back to Goma but had to be evacuated on May 10 for his own safety. A week later rebel forces took Kinshasa. Laurent Kabila changed the country's name from Zaire to the Democratic Republic of the Congo, and the country descended into years of blood-drenched conflict.

The Spoils of War

On April 25, 1997, EIS officer Deborah Levy and her supervisor in the CDC Division of Parasitic Diseases, EIS alum Anne Moore, flew into southern Sudan, another war-torn area, to study an epidemic of African trypanosomiasis, or sleeping sickness. Once infected with the parasite *Trypanosoma brucei gambiense* by the bite of an infected tsetse fly, a victim develops fever, headaches, and joint pains, and the lymph nodes swell into balloons. In the second phase, as the parasite invades the brain, victims often sleep during the day but cannot rest at night. Untreated, the disease leads to coma and death.

International Medical Corps (IMC) representatives had found that 23 percent of those they screened in the town of Ezo were infected. Levy and Moore designed a random cluster survey, beginning with outlying villages. They had managed to interview and collect blood from two hundred people in five villages when on May 10, their vehicles were seized at gunpoint by rebel soldiers. Levy and Moore were evacuated, flown out on a small plane that dashed in from Kenya despite a Sudanese threat to shoot it down.

Their randomized survey, completed by the IMC staff they had trained, showed that nearly 20 percent of the population in fifteen villages had the parasite in their blood, suggesting some five thousand cases in Tambura County. Unless treated, they were doomed to die.

"The reemergence of trypanosomiasis as a major public health threat is occurring because disease control activities have been sharply reduced or curtailed for a decade or longer," Levy and Moore wrote, "as a consequence of war, civil strife, and economic crisis." They noted that the parasitic disease in the Democratic Republic of the Congo was challenging AIDS as the leading cause of death. "Furthermore, the presence of war [in both countries] may have contributed to the transmission of sleeping sickness by promoting behaviors which have increased man-tsetse fly contact," as villagers hid in the bush from air raids, forced army recruitment, or tribal strife.

The CDC survey led indirectly to a $2 million grant from the Office of U.S. Foreign Disaster Assistance. Drug maker Aventis resumed production of eflornithine, a modern treatment with few side effects, and donated it to save lives. West African trypanosomiasis cases subsequently dropped dramatically.

An Anthropologist Listens

EIS officer Holly Ann Williams, a pediatric nurse with a doctorate in anthropology, arrived in May 1997 in Zambia, an African country not at war but suffering from malaria. She documented that most malaria was resistant to chloroquine, the inexpensive first-line drug. Health officials had not shifted to sulfadoxine-pyrimethamine (SP), the second-line drug, fearful that parents would not accept it, since it did not reduce fever, as did chloroquine. Williams held informal focus group discussions with parents and found that they knew perfectly well that SP worked better and were grateful that she was there to make sure their children were getting the proper dosage.

In August Williams went to eleven refugee camps in western Tanzania. Refugees from Rwanda, Burundi, and the Democratic Republic of the Congo had all found their way to the Kigoma region near the shores of Lake Victoria. She discovered that drug-resistant malaria was indeed a problem, but over half the fever cases diagnosed as malaria didn't yield positive blood smears. Antimalarial drugs were being inappropriately administered, enhancing drug resistance. Williams recommended distribution of more insecticide-treated bednets and a scientific study to determine the extent of drug-resistant malaria.

One day she heard children arguing over something outside her bamboo hut. "They were fighting over a toy," Williams recalled. "It was a dead bird." It was a poignant moment for her. "I thought, *Maybe, just maybe, if these drugs work, these kids will have a slightly better chance of making it to age eight.*"

This Is How It Begins

In May 1997 a three-year-old boy died of influenza in Hong Kong. In August the strain was determined to be H5N1. No human had ever caught flu with this hemagglutinin protein, which had previously afflicted only poultry. Indeed an H5N1 epidemic in Hong Kong's rural New Territories in March 1997 had killed thousands of chickens on three farms.

In the CDC Influenza Branch, EIS alum Keiji Fukuda got the call about the boy with the bird flu. *This is how it begins,* he thought — the onset of the next flu pandemic. He and EIS officer Catherine Dentinger arrived in Hong Kong on August 20. While the boy had had no contact with the sick chickens in the New Territories, they discovered that pet chicks and ducklings at his day-care center had died shortly before he became ill. Fukuda, Dentinger, and others collected blood samples from about two thousand possible contacts, finding antibodies to H5N1 in nine people, including one of the child's doctors and a classmate, as well as five poultry workers in the New Territories. None had become ill. After two and a half weeks, the CDC team flew home. Relieved, Fukuda thought it might have been an anomaly.

Then in late November 1997 the Hong Kong lab identified another H5N1 sample from a two-year-old boy who had been hospitalized briefly but recovered. Fukuda headed for Hong Kong again, this time with second-year EIS officer Carolyn Bridges. By the time they arrived on Saturday, December 6, two more H5N1 cases had been identified — a thirteen-year-old girl struggling on a respirator, and a fifty-four-year-old man who had died that day. Within a few days EIS officers Tony Mounts and Seymour Williams arrived with two other staff.

Over the next three weeks there were fourteen more cases and two deaths. Avian flu was identified in 10 percent of chickens in the live markets inside Hong Kong. But people weren't supposed to catch flu directly from chickens. In theory, the flu virus had to mutate within another intermediary such as a pig.

The biggest concern was whether human-to-human transmission was taking place. "The population density of Hong Kong is amazing," Bridges observed. "If this flu could easily jump from human to human, it would just explode." In the worst-case scenario, a person might simultaneously contract H5N1 and H3N2, the common human virus, and the adaptable microbes would trade genes, with a resulting strain that could spread simply and quickly. With the regular flu season due to begin in February, such a viral reassortment was a real possibility.

Looking for evidence of human-to-human spread, Bridges interviewed and helped draw blood from close contacts of cases and from health-care workers exposed to H5N1 patients. Williams studied cohorts of a day-care case, while Mounts looked for risk factors in a case-control study.

On December 28, 1997, the eighteenth victim, a thirty-four-year-old woman, was hospitalized, and the Chinese authorities decided to kill all of the birds in chicken farms, wholesale markets, and live-bird stalls in Hong Kong. It took three days to slaughter 1.6 million birds. In the ensuing weeks, no new cases occurred, though two more women in intensive care died. Thus, six out of eighteen hospitalized patients died, yielding a 33 percent mortality rate.

Poultry workers objected to the slaughter, pointing out that they themselves weren't getting sick. Bridges drew blood from the workers, finding that 10 percent of them had antibodies to H5N1. Her other studies found that 6 of 51 household contacts and one person on a tour bus with a victim tested positive, as did 8 of 217 exposed health-care workers. She concluded that the bird flu had indeed been transmitted from person to person, but that it required extremely close contact. Mounts' case-control study showed that the primary risk factor for contracting H5N1 was recent exposure to live poultry — not exposure to someone else with the infection.

Pounding on Polio

With major funding from Rotary International, the World Health Organization had pursued polio eradication since 1988, thanks in large part to leadership from EIS alum Bill Foege. For every person paralyzed by polio, there are two hundred infected people without symptoms who can pass on the disease to others. Yet the Pan American Health Organization (PAHO) had eliminated polio in Latin America by 1991 by sponsoring repeated National Immunization Days, in conjunction with mopping-up operations in any areas with a subsequent outbreak. PAHO had even arranged "days of tranquility" during civil wars in El Salvador and Peru in which *pax polio* was declared long enough for children to be immunized.

Even though the last wild polio outbreak in the United States had occurred in 1979,* some ten people contracted polio every year from the live attenuated vaccine itself, usually the first dose. For years, public health authorities had debated whether to switch back to the killed Salk vaccine (now much improved), which required an injection but was completely safe. The main resistance came from those who feared that if the United States switched to the more expensive inactivated vaccine (IPV), it would doom the worldwide eradication effort. The much more costly killed vaccine would require medical professionals to give the injections, whereas anyone could administer the oral vaccine with minimal training.

In June 1996 the Advisory Committee on Immunization Practices finally voted to begin a gradual shift. Beginning in 1997 children received two doses of IPV, followed by two administrations of OPV. Still, there were a few cases of OPV-associated polio, and three years later the United States switched entirely to the inactivated vaccine.

As an EIS officer (1995–1997), Linda Quick had helped set up some international polio surveillance and worried over paralysis caused by the oral vaccine in the United States. After graduation, she remained with the CDC Polio Eradication Branch. The change in U.S. policy did not adversely affect the polio eradication effort, but constant travel to monitor progress was exhausting Quick. In the fall of 1998 she and others hatched an idea for an army of public health recruits to help with polio surveillance. New CDC director Jeff Koplan, who had helped eradicate smallpox in Bangladesh as an EIS officer,[†] enthusiastically backed the plan to send EIS officers (and other volunteers) overseas for three-month tours to conduct polio surveillance.

---

*See pages 194–195.
† See pages 155–156.

Quick stayed in Atlanta, sending out the first wave of officers in January 1999 for the Stop Transmission of Polio (STOP) program to Nepal, Bangladesh, Yemen, and Nigeria.

In Nigeria, EIS officers Tracee Treadwell and Tim Thomas found that many newly paralyzed people sought treatment from witch doctors, who believed that polio was caused by evil spirits. Nonetheless, these traditional healers recognized that the vaccine was reducing the number of cases. Treadwell and Thomas told them, "We have a spirit in this bottle."

As with smallpox, one of the most challenging areas for polio eradication was India. In May 2000 EIS officer Gwen Hammer joined the STOP program in Bihar and discovered that a major hospital there was distributing nonpotent polio vaccine. On each vial, a telltale dot turned black if the cold chain had been broken — i.e., if the vaccine had been unrefrigerated and lost its potency. She taught health workers to look for the black dot and spoke about her discovery and solution at community meetings.

The EIS officers who took on polio went to some of the most desolate places on earth. By the end of 2000 polio eradication appeared to be an attainable reality. Only ten countries still had active, endemic polio cases, with 719 paralytic polio cases worldwide during the year, a 99 percent reduction since the eradication program had begun in 1988. The last wild type 2 poliovirus was isolated in October 1999, and only India, Pakistan, Somalia, and Nigeria still harbored type 3.

A Triathlon to Remember

EIS alum Doug Hamilton took over as EIS chief in the spring of 1998, renaming the position EIS director. Hamilton's first major challenge occurred in July. Two patients in a Madison, Wisconsin, hospital suffered from high fevers, achy muscles, red eyes, diarrhea, and jaundice, one with a failing kidney. An alert doctor discovered that both had recently competed in a local triathlon as well as a similar June event in Springfield, Illinois. He notified the Wisconsin Department of Health, which learned of a third hospitalized athlete in Illinois. The Wisconsin epidemiologist called the CDC and sent specimens from the patients, one of which tested positive for leptospirosis.

Hamilton sent EIS officers Juliette Morgan and Mike Bruce to Madison on Friday, July 17. There they learned that there were more ailing athletes in Illinois, and since the average incubation period for leptospirosis is two weeks, the Illinois event, the sixteenth annual Iron Horse Triathlon, held on June 21, was more logically implicated. Morgan and Bruce rented a car and drove through the night to Springfield.

Leptospira, large spiral-shaped bacteria known as spirochetes, commonly afflict animals. Human illness results from contact with the urine of an infected animal. Thus, the second venue for the triathlon, Lake Springfield, fed by a 265-square-mile watershed, was the likely source of the disease.

The EIS officers learned that 876 people from forty-four states and seven countries had competed in the event, so the CDC put out an international media notice. Local officials issued a health advisory against swimming in the lake, and EIS officer Adam Karpati arrived to look for illness in local residents.

Meanwhile, more than seventy new EIS officers in Atlanta stayed in the evening after their training course, calling triathlon participants and finding that 13 percent had been ill, some critically. No one died, but many were misdiagnosed and subjected to unnecessary spinal taps. Two had their gallbladders removed.

The cohort study revealed that people whose swim time exceeded forty-two minutes, and those who recalled swallowing more than one mouthful of lake water, were more likely to contract leptospirosis. Karpati found a few cases in local residents, but no animal reservoir was ever discovered.

Death by Design?

In the fall of 1997 Oregon passed the Death with Dignity Act, which allowed physicians to prescribe lethal doses of barbiturates to terminally ill patients who chose to take them. The law required those who wanted to die to express their wishes orally and in writing, then wait fifteen days and reaffirm their decisions. Two physicians had to agree that the patients were unlikely to live longer than six months. The doctors had to refer them for counseling if they were depressed and to discuss all feasible alternatives, such as hospice or palliative care. Doctors could prescribe but not administer the fatal medicine. Legislators also ordered the Oregon Health Division to collect data on all such physician-assisted suicides.

Arthur Eugene Chin (known as Gene), the state EIS officer, tracked the fifteen people who took advantage of the new law to end their lives in 1998. He decided not to intrude on the patients or their family members. Instead, he interviewed the doctors who had prescribed the lethal medication, seeking information about the patients' medical history and attitude. For each case, he sought three matched controls who had died within thirty days of the patient's death, then interviewed the doctor who had signed the death certificate, asking the same questions.

Neither cases nor controls were concerned about financial issues. Only two of the cases (13 percent) worried that they were a burden on family, friends, or caregivers, whereas 35 percent of the controls did. Only one case patient expressed concern about inadequate pain control, compared to 35 percent of the controls. The real difference was that 80 percent of the people who chose to end their own lives were concerned about loss of autonomy due to their illness versus 40 percent of the controls. Cases were also more concerned about loss of control of bodily functions. "Many physicians reported that their patients had been decisive and independent throughout their lives," Chin wrote, and they had "a long-standing belief about the importance of controlling the manner in which they died."

More cases than controls were single or divorced, leading some critics to conclude that they chose death because of social isolation, but it may be that they were simply more independent. Many of the doctors who prescribed lethal medication told Chin how difficult it had been. "It was an excruciating thing to do," said one. "It made me rethink life's priorities."*

The Bat Connection

In March 1999 EIS officers Tony Mounts, Paul Kitsutani, and Mike Bunning departed for Malaysia to investigate a newly discovered virus. Beginning in the fall of 1998, some young pigs in the city of Ipoh, 145 miles northwest of the capital of Kuala Lumpur, began to twitch, cough, bite at their bars, and lose their footing. Their urine turned bloody. Many adult swine without symptoms suddenly collapsed and died. Then thirty-one pig farmers developed fevers, becoming lethargic and disoriented. Five fell into a coma and died.

One desperate Ipoh farmer advertised on the Internet, selling sick swine on the cheap to farms fifty miles south of Kuala Lumpur, where more than two hundred farmers contracted the disease.[†] When CDC labs analyzed spinal fluid from patients, they found something similar to Hendra virus, which had been identified in 1994 in Australia, where it killed thirteen horses and their trainer. The pig variant was named Nipah virus, after a village where the fire-sale pigs had been sent, and was designated a biosafety level 4 pathogen, equivalent to Ebola.

"People left their farms, their pigs, everything they owned. Whole villages just fled," recalled Bunning. The outbreak was finally brought under control at the end of May 1999, by which time a million pigs had been sacrificed and 108 out of 280 identified human cases had died. The EIS case-control study indicated that direct contact with sick pigs was a primary risk factor.

The related Hendra virus had been traced to fruit bats, so Bunning suspected that Malaysian bats might serve as the reservoir for Nipah

---

*In the first ten years of the Oregon Death with Dignity Act, 341 patients chose to end their lives. Most were white, well-educated people with terminal cancer whose primary concern was loss of autonomy.

[†]Mike Bunning learned of the Internet pig sale from a farm widow who had lost her husband, son, and granddaughter to the disease after purchasing sick pigs. Risking ostracism in the Chinese community, she talked to the EIS officer, begging him: "Never let this happen again."

virus as well. He helped to capture a variety of them, including the giant fruit bats known as flying foxes. Sure enough, Nipah antibodies were eventually found in the flying foxes. A dead bat or its feces might have fallen into a feedlot, or bats may have dropped contaminated, partially eaten fruit into pigpens.

In April 1999 EIS officer Paul Arguin flew to Singapore to investigate Nipah virus in slaughterhouse workers who had been infected by imported Malaysian swine.* His case-control study found that people who unloaded the pigs and chased them into the abattoir were infected as the terrified pigs lost bladder function. Their urine contained the virus.

In the ensuing years, Nipah virus jumped to Bangladesh and neighboring parts of India, often killing 75 percent or more of its victims. Bunning thought the actual mortality in Malaysia may have been near that figure, since many Chinese laborers who died were buried secretly to avoid the slaughter of their pigs. "If Nipah had been communicable between humans," Bunning observed, "the world as we know it today would be different."

A Deadly Combination

Multiple-drug-resistant tuberculosis (MDR-TB)[†] had grown into a disastrous problem in many countries by the end of the decade. EIS officer Kayla Laserson jetted around the world doing battle with the disease. In March 1998 she found inadequate treatment and no formal surveillance in the small port town of Buenaventura, Colombia. She suggested strict directly observed treatment (DOT) with first-line drugs. For those who already had multiply resistant TB, she recommended DOT with second-line drug regimens.

Second-line drugs were expensive and could produce severe adverse side effects, for which she advised "careful monitoring." Activist clinicians such as Paul Farmer had been pushing the World Health

---

*Arguin had spent the previous summer hunting bats in the Philippines, proving that they carried *Lyssavirus,* a type of rabies that kills virtually 100 percent of its untreated victims. Bats had also been found to harbor antibodies to the dreaded Marburg and Ebola viruses.
†See pages 273–276.

Organization to expand treatment for those with MDR-TB and to negotiate with pharmaceutical companies for lower-priced second-line drugs, and a month after Laserson's Colombian investigation, WHO changed its policy to a DOT-plus program to include those additional drugs to treat MDR.

In the former Soviet Union, the situation grew desperate. At the April 1999 EIS conference, Laserson presented a Late Breaker report, "The Sky Is Falling," in which she warned of the growing TB problem in Russian prisons and marginalized populations.*

As a new century loomed, MDR-TB appeared to be a particularly frightening problem in conjunction with HIV infection. With AIDS destroying the immune system, latent tuberculosis became active and lethal. Adding multiple-drug resistance to the equation usually resulted in a quick death. The problem continues today.

A Troubled Vaccine

In the spring of 1999 Tim Naimi and ten other EIS field officers had to determine if a new oral rotavirus vaccine was causing intussusception, a rare condition in which a portion of an infant's small intestine is blocked, sliding inside itself like a collapsible telescope. The new vaccine, called RotaShield, had been approved by the FDA the previous fall, and in November 1998 babies began to receive the recommended doses at two, four, and six months of age.

In prelicensure studies, five cases of intussusception had occurred among 10,054 vaccine recipients and 1 case in 4,633 controls — not a significant difference, but enough to make Wyeth Lederle list the condition as a potential adverse reaction. By June 17, 1999, 12 cases of intussusception had been reported through the Vaccine Adverse Event Reporting System (VAERS), passive surveillance that relied on people contacting the manufacturer, FDA, or CDC.

Twelve cases were fewer than the number expected by chance alone, but most of the babies had developed the condition within a

---

*Late Breaker presentations at annual April EIS conferences are added at the last minute.

week of receiving the first dose of the vaccine. On June 22, 1999, EIS officers around the country were tasked with searching hospital records to identify all cases of intussusception that had occurred since November 1, 1998, then finding four controls for each case—babies born in the same hospital at the same time. EIS officer Lynn Zanardi, assigned to the National Immunization Program, took overall charge.

In Minnesota, Naimi and colleagues quickly found eighteen infants with intussusception, five of whom had been given RotaShield. Four of the five vaccinated children required surgery, versus only five of the thirteen unvaccinated cases. All five had come down with the condition within two weeks of receiving the injection. The Minnesota data convinced the Advisory Committee on Immunization Practices (ACIP) to recommend that the FDA suspend the rotavirus vaccination program on July 16, 1999, until the results of the combined case-control study being conducted by EIS officers were known.

By October, EIS officers had found 429 cases, of which 74 (17.2 percent) had received the vaccine. A disproportionate number had come down with the condition within a week of getting the first dose. It appeared that the RotaShield vaccine caused intussusception in about 1 in 10,000 vaccinated infants, which would result in about 360 excess cases per year if all U.S. babies were vaccinated.

On October 22, 1999, ACIP called a permanent halt to the vaccination program and the vaccine was withdrawn, although it was not a clear-cut decision. Severe diarrhea in the United States caused by rotavirus in children younger than five accounted for an estimated fifty thousand hospitalizations and twenty to forty deaths per year. Those deaths had to be weighed against a bowel obstruction that might require surgery but rarely killed.

EIS alum Roger Glass was devastated. He had studied rotavirus for twenty years and helped work on a vaccine.* The decision to withdraw RotaShield in the United States meant that it would never be approved for use in the developing world, where rotavirus annually

---

*See pages 224–225.

killed an estimated 600,000 children under five. The risk of intussusception was trivial in comparison to the lives that would be saved, but
no one dared promote a product for African or Asian infants that was
deemed unfit for American babies. Years would be lost while alternative rotavirus vaccines were developed.

Reading This May Save Your Ass

EIS officer Gwen Hammer arrived at the STD Prevention and Control Division of the San Francisco Department of Public Health in August 1999 in the middle of a syphilis outbreak among gay men. With an
effective drug cocktail to combat AIDS on the market, HIV infection
was no longer an automatic death sentence, and a new generation of
gay men soon forgot the lessons of the past. With the help of the new
drug Viagra, men could engage in marathon sex sessions that left their
penises and rectums raw and easily infected. Hammer and EIS alum
Jeffrey Klausner, director of the STD prevention and control services
at San Francisco's public health department, took out a full-page ad in
a local gay paper about the syphilis outbreak, calling it "A Time-Bomb
We Can Defuse!"

Some gay activists refused to believe that there was an outbreak.
Nor did they believe that HIV caused AIDS, proclaiming that the
drug cocktails were useless and toxic. "Who is this secret agent Hammer?" asked their spokesman, and why was she engaged in a "relent-
less crusade to demonize gay male sex"?

Hammer persisted despite death threats, then left for three months
of polio eradication efforts in India. When she returned the following summer, a shigellosis outbreak had erupted in the gay community. In response, Hammer passed out a flyer at gay events headlined
READING THIS MAY SAVE YOUR ASS. "Shigella is transmitted by
fecal-oral contact — simply put: SHIT!" she had written for the flyer,
adding that the illness caused stomach cramps, bloody diarrhea, and
fever. "Avoid mouth-ass contact."

Hammer conducted a telephone survey with men who had contracted shigellosis that revealed half had had oral-anal contact. The
San Francisco health department offered free *Shigella* screenings, is-

sued press releases, sent out thousands of notices to community agencies and providers, and set up a website. Within a few months the epidemic numbers dwindled.

Death of the Constant Gardeners

On Monday, August 23, 1999, EIS alum Marci Layton, the chief epidemiologist for the New York City Department of Health, got a call from Deborah Asnis, a doctor at Flushing Hospital Medical Center in Queens. Asnis had two puzzling patients, men of sixty and seventy-five, who both had lost the use of their arms and legs, had high fevers and excess white blood cells in their spinal fluid, and seemed confused. Layton urged Asnis to send blood and spinal fluid samples to the state lab in Albany for testing.

On Friday afternoon Asnis called again. She now had two more cases, an eighty-year-old man and an eighty-seven-year-old woman. A neurologist overheard Asnis's call and said that he was treating another encephalitic patient in a nearby hospital.

On Saturday Layton and Annie Fine, who had stayed at the NYC health department after finishing her EIS stint there in 1998, drove to Flushing Hospital to see the patients, three of whom were now on respirators. The only thing they had in common was living within the same two-square-mile area of northern Queens. While Layton and Fine were at the hospital, a feverish, combative, hallucinatory fifty-seven-year-old man was admitted from the same neighborhood. By the end of the weekend they had identified eight such patients in Queens hospitals.

Layton called the CDC on Sunday to ask for help. EIS officer Kristy Murray, assigned to bioterrorism, flew up on Tuesday, by which time more cases had appeared. The next day she visited hospitals to review charts and interview patients.

Layton summoned Denis Nash, a freshman EIS officer in the New York City AIDS unit. On Wednesday, September 1, Nash toured patients' homes, traveling in a health department van with an exterminator, animal-disease expert, and entomologist. When they arrived at the eighty-year-old man's home, they met his wife and family, who were about to leave for the hospital to say their final farewells — he was to be disconnected from his respirator.

His wife showed them around. In the backyard was a lush flower/vegetable garden, with five-gallon plastic buckets to collect rainwater during the summer drought. She explained that her husband had come out here to smoke in the early mornings. The entomologist identified *Culex pipiens* larval cases floating on the surface: mosquitoes. The EIS officer continued his tour, accumulating evidence of prime mosquito habitat — here a birdbath, there thick grass. They subsequently discovered that most of the victims had been avid gardeners.

The next day the eighty-seven-year-old woman died, and the day after that, New York and CDC lab tests were positive for St. Louis encephalitis (SLE) viral antibodies in blood and spinal fluid. At last, an answer, though a puzzling one, since SLE was not known to cause paralysis. Kristy Murray remained skeptical, since many tests were equivocal, and one of the patients she had examined tested negative for SLE. Nonetheless, Mayor Rudolph Giuliani held a press conference. Helicopters began spraying pesticide in Queens.

For the next few weeks cases spread to the Bronx and then to Brooklyn. Other EIS officers arrived to help. An encephalitis hotline was overwhelmed with 130,000 calls. Banner headlines in New York papers cried KILLER BUG and LET US SPRAY! Mayor Giuliani expanded the pesticide campaign to the entire city, which turned out to be a good idea, as another case patient showed up in Manhattan.

Some hotline callers asked about all the dead crows around the city. Could they have anything to do with this? At the Bronx Zoo, veterinary pathologist Tracey McNamara also noticed the dead crows. Then the zoo's flamingo, cormorant, pheasant, and bald eagle died. She sent specimens to the National Veterinary Services Laboratories in Iowa, which isolated a virus that the CDC lab at Fort Collins, Colorado, analyzed. It was West Nile virus, a close relative of SLE.

West Nile virus had never before appeared in the Western Hemisphere. First identified in the West Nile district of Uganda in 1937, it had caused its first major epidemic in Israel in 1953. The strain that was killing New York City people and birds turned out to be nearly identical to one found in an Israeli goose in 1998. Had a mosquito flown into an airplane in Tel Aviv and disembarked eight hours later at JFK Airport? Or had the virus been imported by an infected bird or person?

With the first hard frosts of November, the epidemic was over, at least for the time being. Of the sixty-two confirmed cases, seven died. In October EIS officers had gone door-to-door in Queens asking families to give blood samples. Three percent harbored antibodies to West Nile virus. A conservative estimate was that at least 8,200 residents had contracted the disease, but that most were asymptomatic.

For the elderly, however, the long-term impact could be severe. Many survivors still complained of serious symptoms a year and a half later. A third of those surveyed needed assistance with the chores of daily living.

The birdborne virus moved throughout the continental United States over the next few years, sickening thousands of people and killing hundreds. "The 1999 West Nile virus disease outbreak again proves," wrote the EIS officers, "that with the growing volume of international travel and commerce, exotic pathogens can move between continents with increasing ease."

Deadly Agents or Powder Puffs?

In the wake of the 1995 deaths in the Tokyo subways from the deadly chemical sarin, fears of terrorism of all kinds mounted in the United States. On October 30, 1998, EIS officer Marshall Lyon got a call from a worker at a Planned Parenthood clinic in Knoxville, Tennessee, which had received a letter that said, "You've just been exposed to anthrax. You will die within 24 hours." Over the next hour he got calls about identical letters sent to clinics in Louisville, Kentucky, and Indianapolis, Indiana. Lyon tried to calm the callers, telling them that if there was nothing in the envelope but the letter, anthrax exposure seemed unlikely.

All the centers had also called 911, bringing police, firefighters, emergency medical services, the FBI, and hazardous materials (hazmat) units to the clinics. By the time Lyon flew to Indianapolis on Monday to assess the situation, it was clear that the letters were hoaxes. Yet when another Indianapolis clinic received a similar letter that day, the scenario repeated itself. Then in Los Angeles on December 17, 1998, two anthrax letters were mailed to city offices, followed within the next week by phone warnings to a private business and a large federal building, from which fifteen hundred employees were evacuated. Lyon flew out. "It kind of boggled my mind," he recalled. "There was no assessment of the threat credibility." Lyon tried to preach some common sense. "You have to temper your response," he said, "or you will go broke."

Over the next few months, dozens of hoax letters, many containing talcum powder or white flour, arrived at schools, courthouses, media outlets, abortion clinics, and an IRS office.

On Christmas Day 1998 EIS alum Scott Lillibridge met with four colleagues to form the new Bioterrorism Preparedness and Response Program. "CDC didn't even have an anthrax lab," he recalled. He rectified that while helping to upgrade state laboratories and supporting plans for a pharmaceutical stockpile to deploy in an emergency. He also helped to recruit Kristy Murray from the 1999 class as the bioterror EIS officer.

Two books on biowarfare were published in 1999. In the last chapter of *The Biology of Doom,* Ed Regis noted that fifteen countries, including Iraq, Iran, and North Korea, were purportedly pursuing the development of biological weapons. In *Biohazard,* Russian defector Ken Alibek offered an insider's look at Biopreparat, the disbanded Soviet program that had weaponized smallpox and produced 1,800 tons of anthrax annually. No one knew where those biological weapons had gone.

In October 1999 the FBI issued a warning about terrorism linked to the turn of the century. The same month, *Hot Zone* author Richard Preston published an article in the *New Yorker,* speculating that the recent West Nile virus outbreak might have been the work of a terrorist. Preston quoted an Iraqi defector who said that Iraqi dictator Saddam Hussein had boasted that his labs could produce a West Nile virus "capable of destroying 97 percent of all life in an urban environment."

Kristy Murray had already concluded that the West Nile epidemic in New York City was not premeditated and she knew that a 97 percent mortality rate was absurd. With near hysteria in the air over the Y2K bug that would supposedly wipe out computers as dates turned on January 1, 2000, Murray got a call from Pennsylvania health authorities. The trucker who had delivered the ball to Times Square for the New Year's Eve celebration had just died of a rapidly fatal pneumonia, and so had his wife. Murray had nightmare visions of the giant glittering ball slowly descending at midnight, spraying deadly fumes over thousands of celebrants. But she learned, to her relief, that the trucker had carried a *wall*, not a *ball*—someone had misheard the word and panicked. The trucker and his wife were already unhealthy and morbidly obese. The twentieth century went out with a routine bang, not a fatal hiss.

20
FULL CIRCLE

THE MORNING OF SEPTEMBER 11, 2001, EIS officer Michael Phillips, assigned to the New York City Department of Health, was home sick with a bad cold, in the apartment he shared with his fiancée Sudha Renny, who worked with him. Living only a block southwest of the World Trade Center, Phillips heard an explosion, saw the smoking North Tower, then witnessed the second airplane hit the South Tower.

Renny had stopped at a bookstore in the basement of the World Trade Center that morning. She heard a *boom*, but she didn't think much of it and walked belowground to exit some distance from the towers. Only when she noticed papers floating down and people running past her did she look up and see what had happened. She called her fiancé: "Go to the river promenade. You walk north, I'll walk south along the railing."

In the chaos of fleeing crowds, they found each other. "We stood and stared up at those buildings, just dumbfounded," Phillips recalled. "We could see people jumping to their deaths from the upper stories." Then the towers collapsed.

They walked back to the health department on Worth Street, where EIS alum Marci Layton, the city's chief epidemiologist and assistant health commissioner, had activated the department's Emergency Operations Center and was dividing up tasks, ranging from monitoring rescue worker safety to rodent control in abandoned restaurants. She also set up an ad hoc clinic to care for dozens of dazed survivors who sought care. Layton asked Phillips to contact five local hospitals, where he found that there were few severe injuries. "Most of the people in the towers either got out intact or they died," he said.

In Atlanta, shortly before noon, CDC director Jeff Koplan ordered the evacuation of the building after learning that another airplane might be heading to devastate the Centers for Disease Control, perhaps hoping to release lab pathogens resting in a freezer.* Fortunately, the rumored attack proved to be a false alarm.

That day antibiotics from the CDC's new national pharmaceutical stockpile were flown to New York City on a small charter jet, with EIS officers Dan Budnitz and Sandra Berrios-Torres and EIS alum Tracee Treadwell on board. They joined the staff at the NYC Department of Health building on Worth Street, where they studied hundreds of charts, entering data on patients and planning what to do next. Around 2 A.M., they discussed the possibility of bioterrorism. Could the airplanes have been carrying microbes aerosolized on impact? Might there be a follow-up attack with a biological agent? The EIS had begun fifty years ago due to fears of bioterrorism, and now it was coming full circle.

"Have You Seen My Daddy?"

On Friday morning thirty EIS officers flew up to New York City on a retrofitted Australian Air Force C-130. Aside from military aircraft, they were on the only airplane in U.S. airspace. Four state-based EIS officers drove to join them. The officers dispersed to fifteen hospital emergency rooms in the greater metropolitan area, monitoring new patients and searching for evidence of bioterrorism, although they told no one, not wanting to foment panic. Working alternate twelve-hour shifts, they provided continuous syndromic surveillance. Af-

---

*Even though his wife was in labor, Scott Lillibridge stayed behind in the CDC building to make sure that all biosafety labs were guarded.

ter three days, fourteen more EIS officers were sent up, allowing for eight-hour shifts.

Everywhere they went, the officers saw homemade missing-persons posters on walls, in subways, outside hospital entrances. EIS officer Marc Traeger wept as he looked at a picture with childish scrawl: *Have you seen my Daddy?* In addition to their emergency room surveillance duties, many EIS officers, including McKenzie Andre, volunteered to help fit rescue workers at Ground Zero with respirators, though dedicated workers often spurned the protection.* "There were six people working in a basement in a nearby building who didn't want to come out, so I went in and fitted them with a flashlight," Andre said. "They were working forty-eight and seventy-two hours straight — they wouldn't stop. I was never more proud to be from New York."

Brad Winterton and four other EIS officers volunteered to remain when, after two weeks of uneventful surveillance in emergency rooms, the others returned to their regular posts on Friday, September 28. "Our mere presence had a tremendous calming effect on the city generally," he said.

A Death in Florida

On Wednesday afternoon, October 3, the Florida state laboratory called the CDC about a likely anthrax case. A disoriented, feverish sixty-three-year-old man named Bob Stevens had entered a Boca Raton hospital early on Tuesday, and then had a seizure. His spinal fluid had just tested positive for *Bacillus anthracis*. Specimens would arrive at the CDC the next morning.

The next day the CDC lab confirmed the diagnosis. Stevens, a photo editor at the tabloid the *Sun*, was suffering from inhalational anthrax, a rare, deadly disease. There had been only eighteen such cases in the United States during the twentieth century, and the last had occurred twenty-five years before.†

---

*In conjunction with the CDC, the New York City Department of Health conducted a long-term study of health problems in Ground Zero rescue workers, led by EIS alum Polly Thomas.

†See pages 27–28.

Anthrax spores can lie dormant in soil for decades until a grazing animal consumes them. In the moist warmth of the intestines, the bacteria activate and kill unless treated in time. Most human cases stem from close contact with infected animals when spores enter the body through a small cut and cause cutaneous anthrax, which is rarely fatal if treated. If inhaled, however, the spores kill 85 percent of those whose lungs are infected, though, based on Philip Brachman's decades-old studies of mill workers, it was believed that it took thousands of spores to cause a case.

On October 4 a CDC team, led by EIS alum Brad Perkins and including five EIS officers, flew to Boca Raton. There they joined Florida-based EIS officer Marc Traeger.

Since Bob Stevens had just returned from a trip to North Carolina, another team of EIS officers went there to retrace his path and search for other victims. Coming so soon after the 9/11 terrorist attacks, the unusual inhalational anthrax case caused understandable concern, but the CDC investigators thought it unlikely to be bioterrorism. Why would terrorists pick on one obscure photo editor at an insignificant tabloid?

On Friday morning teams of federal, state, and local public health officials fanned out in search of clues, taking air samples at the pier Stevens had last fished from, swabbing animal products at the Indian grocery and Chinese import store where he had shopped. Accompanied by FBI agents, Perkins took samples from the victim's home and office at American Media, Inc. (AMI), a tabloid empire that published the *National Enquirer, Sun,* and others. EIS officers set up surveillance of local patients in intensive care units. None had anthrax.

EIS officer Jim Sejvar drove to Miami, where a seventy-three-year-old AMI employee, Ernesto "Ernie" Blanco, was hospitalized with pneumonia. He had picked up and distributed the AMI mail. Despite massive doses of intravenous Ciprofloxacin (commonly Cipro), an antibiotic effective against many infections, he was having trouble breathing and required oxygen. Still, he didn't seem to be as ill as an inhalational anthrax victim was supposed to be. Sejvar took a nasal swab just in case.

In North Carolina, EIS officer Peter Dull went to Stevens's daughter's apartment, where the photo editor had slept, and to the Irish pub where he had eaten. Officers visited hospitals in western North Carolina and in the Charlotte area, looking for possible anthrax cases. Others retraced the victim's hike at Chimney Rock State Park in the western North Carolina mountains.

At 4 P.M. on Friday, Bob Stevens died. In the wake of the 9/11 attacks, the Bush administration tried to control and centralize communication, so CDC director Jeff Koplan was effectively muzzled, while HHS secretary Tommy Thompson, who knew little about medicine, gave a press conference. He asserted that Stevens may have contracted anthrax by drinking from a North Carolina stream. "We cringed when we heard Thompson's comments," Traeger said. No one could get inhalational anthrax from contaminated water.

On Saturday CDC's Sherif Zaki arrived in Florida to perform the autopsy on Stevens, then returned to Atlanta along with all the environmental and clinical samples collected thus far. At 6:25 P.M. on Sunday, October 7, Perkins and the Florida CDC team were eating dinner at a cheap Italian restaurant. "We were feeling pretty good," recalls Josh Jones. "We had worked hard and had found nothing of real concern." Then Perkins got a call from Zaki on his cell phone. The samples from Stevens's AMI computer keyboard and mail slot tested positive for anthrax. So did Ernie Blanco's nasal swab. *Bioterrorism*, Perkins thought. *It had to be an intentional exposure, probably from a letter.*

All AMI employees were called and told to report to the health department instead of work on Monday morning. In meetings that lasted until 3 A.M., the EIS officers helped to plan antibiotic distribution the following day, wrote press releases, and recommended a hotline for public inquiries. The next day several EIS reenforcements flew down.

FBI agents shut down the AMI office building. The CDC health team had to beg permission to enter and had to fight to make sure specimens were properly collected and labeled. The FBI agents at first refused to fly samples to Atlanta for testing, finally agreeing to send the specimens on a charter plane if an EIS officer accompanied them.

The CDC labs found that samples were positive for anthrax in the mail-sorting room, the text library, a basement ventilation filter, and the mail van that Blanco had driven. Subsequent sampling found anthrax on all three floors of the building. Over a thousand employees or building visitors received antibiotics and submitted to nasal swabs. Only thirty-six-year-old Stephanie Dailey, who helped distribute mail, had a positive nose swab, though she had no symptoms.* Dailey recalled opening a letter that produced a small puff like baby powder on September 25. She had thrown it out, wiped off her desk, and washed her hands.

Another employee recalled seeing Bob Stevens closely examining a letter with white powder as he held it over his keyboard on September 19. It appeared that there had been at least two anthrax letters, though neither was ever found.

Since anthrax spores were found in Blanco's van, the EIS officers decided to follow the mail trail backward, sampling as they went. They would then test and treat postal carriers who might be at greatest risk. They would begin swabbing the main Boca Raton post office on the evening of Friday, October 12. "We wanted to sample at night to be discreet and not make a big deal of it," EIS officer Josh Jones recalled. But on the morning of October 12, as Jones put it, "all hell broke loose."

Giving Anthrax the Finger in New York

The phone woke Marci Layton around 3 A.M. on Friday, October 12. The biopsy results on thirty-eight-year-old Erin O'Connor, assistant to NBC news anchor Tom Brokaw, were positive for anthrax. O'Connor, who had been treated with antibiotics for a rash on her chest, had alerted authorities after hearing about the Florida cases.

---

*The presence of anthrax spores in nasal passages is not necessarily dangerous, as long as the spores have not invaded the lungs or bloodstream.

Maybe she had the disease. After all, she had opened a threatening letter.

By the end of the day, three other media-related cases had been reported to Layton from ABC, CBS, and the *New York Post*. Claire Fletcher, twenty-seven, who worked for Dan Rather, had developed ugly facial lesions. Thirty-year-old Johanna Huden, an editorial assistant at the *New York Post*, had a black sore on the middle finger of her right hand, which had required surgery.

The other case was the seven-month-old baby of a producer at ABC's *World News Tonight* whose mother had taken him to work for a couple of hours. He developed a sore on his arm and nearly died of kidney failure, though blood transfusions, antibiotics, and intensive care saved his life. Over the next few days a total of seven media-related New York City cutaneous anthrax cases were identified.

Only two anthrax letters were found, addressed to Brokaw and the editor of the *New York Post*. Both tested positive for anthrax, were postmarked on September 18 in Trenton, New Jersey, and contained the same message in handwritten block letters: 09-11-01. THIS IS NEXT. TAKE PENACILIN NOW. DEATH TO AMERICA. DEATH TO ISRAEL. ALLAH IS GREAT.

The EIS officers conducting surveillance for bioterrorism in the city's emergency rooms reported to the NBC offices at Rockefeller Center, where they were each paired with a mental health counselor. For the next three days they handed out Cipro, took nose swabs (all negative), and tried to allay employee fears. As a member of the Armed Forces Medical Intelligence Center, recent EIS grad Mike Bunning was dispatched to test the thousands of suspicious powder specimens that concerned citizens sent. Public health laboratories across the country were overwhelmed with suspect powder samples.

In the midst of the unfounded fears, there was one truly frightening detail: The letter to the *New York Post*, which had given cutaneous anthrax to three people, was still taped shut when it was found. Unopened, it had still somehow leaked spores.

What Next? Where Next? Who Next?

On Monday morning, October 15, an intern in Senator Tom Daschle's office in the Hart Senate Office Building in Washington, D.C., opened a letter sealed with tape on all sides that released a puff of fine white powder. He placed the letter on the floor and called security. Daschle himself wasn't in the building, but thirteen of his staff were in the room at the time and were immediately put on Cipro. It wasn't until forty-five minutes later that someone thought to shut down the building's ventilation system. The letter's contents tested positive for anthrax, and it appeared to be of a finer consistency than the variety sent to New York — more easily airborne.

By the end of the day the entire building was shut down, as was mail delivery throughout the Capitol. Over the next three days EIS officer Scott Harper and his colleagues gave antibiotics to more than two thousand people who had been in the building. Twenty-eight nasal swabs tested positive, though no one contracted anthrax.

The Daschle letter featured the now-familiar handwritten capital letters, beginning with: YOU CAN NOT STOP US. WE HAVE THIS ANTHRAX. YOU DIE NOW. It had been postmarked in Trenton, New Jersey, on October 9, which meant that, like the New York media letters, it had traveled through a large postal distribution center in Hamilton, New Jersey.

After hearing about the New York cases, two New Jersey doctors had notified the state health office of possible cutaneous anthrax in Teresa Heller, a postal carrier, and Patrick O'Donnell, who worked in the Hamilton distribution center. On October 18 Heller's wound biopsy tested positive for anthrax. With two likely cases of cutaneous anthrax in mail handlers, a CDC team led by EIS alum Beth Bell flew up to New Jersey that afternoon, accompanied by EIS officers Jennita Reefhuis and Michelle McConnell. By the time they arrived, the Hamilton facility, which processed approximately 2 million pieces of mail per day, had been closed.

Reefhuis was assigned to study the distribution process. Not allowed inside the Hamilton plant, she toured similar facilities with postal inspector David Bowers. She watched as letters whizzed through high-speed sorting machines. "I could see how much dust was created just from regular letters," she said. "I realized that this was another potential route of exposure." Compressed air hoses were used periodically to blow dust out of the machines.

On October 19 another Hamilton postal worker was diagnosed with cutaneous anthrax. Reefhuis and Bowers understood how the two victims who worked in the giant distribution center might have been infected, but they puzzled over the case of Teresa Heller, the mail carrier in West Trenton. Then Bowers realized that letters intended for West Trenton had gone through the sorting machines right after the New York–bound anthrax letters. Could this be a case of cross-contamination?

The next day Leroy "Rich" Richmond was diagnosed with inhalational anthrax. Richmond worked at the Brentwood mail distribution center in Washington, D.C., through which the letter to Tom Daschle had gone. Brentwood was shut down the next day, but it was too late for Richmond's coworkers, Thomas "Mo" Morris and Joe Curseen, who died of inhalational anthrax over the next two days. A fourth Brentwood worker barely survived the disease, as did Richmond. David Hose, a fifth inhalational anthrax victim-survivor, sorted mail at a State Department annex.

The lessons learned from natural outbreaks didn't necessarily apply to refined anthrax. Apparently a victim did not have to inhale thousands of spores to become infected.* Anthrax could and did leak out of sealed envelopes. All anthrax powder was not equal — the variety sent to Daschle could leak more easily through sealed envelopes and remain longer in the air.

In New Jersey, a bookkeeper at a Trenton firm contracted cutaneous anthrax, apparently from cross-contaminated mail. In Florida, six post offices had tested positive for anthrax spores, though there were no cases in postal workers there. Some 85 million pieces of mail

---

*In his later years, Alexander Langmuir enjoyed pointing out that the number of organisms necessary for an infectious dose was always *one* — in the right place in the right conditions.

had gone through the Hamilton and Brentwood distribution centers since the first anthrax letters were stamped on September 18. How many had been cross-contaminated?

In response to the inhalational anthrax deaths among postal workers, the CDC dispatched a team of eighty people into the District of Columbia to conduct surveillance for new cases, collect environmental samples, enter data, and answer questions.

EIS officer Puneet Dewan was able to trace the path of the Daschle letter among the 59 million pieces of mail that had gone through the Brentwood center during the potential exposure period. Dewan concluded that those at greatest risk worked near sorting machine number 17 and in the governmental mail "riffling" area, where employees thumbed quickly through stacks of letters to make sure of their proper destinations.

All of the Brentwood anthrax victims were African Americans, like the vast majority of those who worked at the facility. Many of them felt that the CDC had acted in a blatantly racist manner, giving special treatment and antibiotics to the wealthy white politicians and shutting down the Hart Building while allowing the Brentwood facility, with its black workers, to continue to spread the anthrax that had killed two of their coworkers. In reality, the disease detectives just hadn't realized that the letters would leak.

EIS officers Jim Hayslett and Kevin Winthrop were given the unenviable task of meeting with angry, confused postal employees to answer their questions. Hayslett tried to defuse the tense meetings with his relaxed, easygoing manner. "Just keep asking questions until you get a comfort level," he would say.

Winthrop, equally sympathetic, sometimes felt that the ground was shifting beneath his feet, as the advice from Atlanta kept changing. Expensive Cipro had severe side effects. So when the anthrax strain was found to be susceptible to doxycycline, which caused fewer adverse reactions, CDC recommended the cheaper drug. "We ain't no guinea pigs!" a black worker complained, assuming that they were getting an inferior drug.

As Hayslett led one of the meetings, a black worker jumped up on a sorting table and yelled, "You fucked the Indians and you're gonna fuck us!" He then began chanting, "Tuskegee! Tuskegee!" in reference to the notorious Alabama syphilis experiments.* Hayslett calmly waited, and eventually other workers told the protester to sit down. "We want to hear what the man has to say."[†]

Wham! Another Wave

Kathy Nguyen, a sixty-one-year-old Vietnamese immigrant, was diagnosed with inhalational anthrax on October 28. She died three days later. Nguyen had lived a quiet, solitary life in her Bronx apartment, taking the subway to her stockroom job at the Manhattan Eye, Ear and Throat Hospital, where she did not handle mail. EIS officer McKenzie Andre joined EIS alum Steve Ostroff in the investigation, retracing Nguyen's steps for the last two weeks of her life. They authorized quiet tests of subway stations on Nguyen's route, all of which were negative. No one ever figured out how she had contracted the disease.

It seemed as though the anthrax cases would never end. "It was like getting slammed by an ocean wave," CDC director Jeff Koplan said. "*Wham!* You just have to keep moving and dive right in."

On November 16 an unopened anthrax letter addressed to Senator Patrick Leahy was found in mail that had been quarantined after the arrival of the Daschle letter. It, too, had been postmarked in Trenton on October 9.

Three days after the Leahy letter surfaced, Ottilie Lundgren, a ninety-four-year-old widow who lived alone in rural Oxford, Connecticut, was diagnosed with inhalational anthrax. She died two days later. The investigation team found anthrax spores at the regional post office that processed her mail. Working with postal inspectors, EIS officer Kevin Griffith found that a letter to a nearby Connecticut address had zipped through the Hamilton, New Jersey, sorting machine

---

*See page 122.
[†]Hayslett and Winthrop also met with about 150 deaf postal service workers, commonly employed in the clattering tumult of the mechanized mail system. At the end of the presentation, one worker signed that this was one of the few times when they had their questions answered.

twenty seconds after the Leahy anthrax letter. In the middle of the night, Griffith woke the house occupants where the letter had been sent. They found the suspect letter, which did indeed test positive for anthrax, though they were not infected.

Aftermath and Fallout

Ottilie Lundgren was the last anthrax victim of the 2001 bioterror spree. A total of twenty-two people had been infected, half of them with inhalational anthrax, and five inhalational victims had died. Of the 146 then-current EIS officers, 136 helped with at least one part of the investigation. Nearly a third of them went out twice, and some were redeployed four or five times.

Prompt investigation and prophylaxis undoubtedly prevented other anthrax infections and deaths. Health authorities had no way of knowing how many letters had been sent out to what locations, or whom they would infect. "What shook me," EIS officer Kevin Winthrop said, "is how one individual could drop a few letters in a mailbox and nearly shut down a country."

As a result of the anthrax investigation, blowers were no longer used to clean sorting machines, letters were irradiated, and other safety measures put in place. There was some good news, too. Untreated, the case fatality rate for inhalational anthrax from the letters approached 50 percent — less than the expected 85 percent rate — but when promptly treated, all but a few patients survived.

EIS alum Larry Altman, the *New York Times* science reporter, complained of the "distressing lapses in communication with the public" during the anthrax investigation, as did alum Philip Brachman. "You won't ever prevent hysteria," Brachman said, "but you feed hysteria by not releasing information." In future bioterror events, he advised that "a single and well-informed source" should be the spokesperson.

CDC director Jeff Koplan probably should have been allowed to be that person, but at the onset of the anthrax scare, he was forbidden to make public statements. HHS Secretary Tommy Thompson made his life miserable by insisting on personal updates several times a day. "The tone was not supportive," Koplan recalled. "There was harping criticism and undermining of our efforts." Koplan resigned in February 2002, soon replaced by Julie Gerberding.

The FBI and most other experts concluded that the perpetrator was probably a U.S. citizen, perhaps an unhinged scientist with the expertise to produce finely milled anthrax spores. The "Allah is great" message was probably a smoke screen.*

In the wake of the anthrax letters, the Bush administration and Congress threw billions of dollars into bioterror preparedness, much of it going to the CDC and to state health departments. HHS secretary Tommy Thompson called for an EIS officer in every state, but some states had weaker public health infrastructure and lacked good supervisors. Instead, EIS alums called career epidemiology field officers (CEFOs) were posted to such states, though they focused primarily on terrorism and emergency response.

The new bioterror money undoubtedly improved preparedness for many potential public health emergencies, but other problems were underfunded, according to EIS alum Barry Levy, editor of the 2003 book *Terrorism and Public Health*. "These bioterror initiatives have, in general, distorted public health priorities," complained Levy, "and drained human and financial resources away from addressing current public health problems, including tobacco- and alcohol-related diseases, gun-related injuries and deaths, HIV/AIDS, and mental health disorders."

---

*In July 2008 military scientist Bruce Ivins, who worked with anthrax at Fort Detrick, Maryland, committed suicide as the FBI was amassing circumstantial evidence that he had sent the anthrax letters. Some critics remain unconvinced of his guilt.

21
INTO THE TWENTY-FIRST CENTURY

THE NEW CENTURY was scarred by 9/11, an event second only to Pearl Harbor in shaking America's sense of security, followed by the random terror of the anthrax letters a few weeks later. Other portentous events and outbreaks subsequently have grabbed headlines both in the United States and abroad. These threats mobilized EIS officers for investigations around the globe.

• In 2002 and 2003 West Nile virus exploded across the United States, infecting more than a million people; 548 died. The virus also killed millions of birds and animals. Many EIS officers helped track the new invader. John Watson, for instance, had barely arrived at his assignment at the Chicago Department of Public Health when West Nile struck. "It was just like a wave breaking over us," he recalled, with 761 cases and 48 deaths in Illinois by year's end.

• In the fall of 2002 EIS officers traced a multistate listeriosis outbreak to turkey deli products produced by Pilgrim's Pride Corporation in Franconia, Pennsylvania. On October 12 the plant was shut down, and 27.4 million pounds of product were recalled. Then the same bacteria were also traced to deli turkey produced by a New Jersey plant. A total of eight victims died, and three pregnant women miscarried. EIS officer Sami Gottlieb was somewhat nervous about appearing on television's *60 Minutes* to discuss the outbreak, but she was even more concerned when she discovered, two months into the investigation, that she was pregnant with her first child. *Listeria* bacteria are deadly to fetuses, and she had taken contaminated turkey products directly from people's refrigerators and had toured the Pilgrim's Pride facility. Fortunately for her and her husband, fellow EIS officer Scott Filler, she later gave birth to Maia, a healthy baby girl.

• In February 2003 an eight-year-old Hong Kong girl vacationing in China died, soon followed to the grave by her father. The nine-year-old son survived, but lab tests identified the H5N1 flu virus in his sputum, then in his father's remains — the first cases of avian influenza since the terrifying outbreak of 1997.* The World Health Organization issued a global alert on February 19. Two days later a Chinese doctor and his wife checked into the Hotel Metropole in Hong Kong. The physician had a high fever and dry cough. Though the couple stayed only one night, he infected at least sixteen other hotel guests and visitors, thus seeding an epidemic that would spread to thirty countries, affecting more than eight thousand people and killing nearly one thousand. The epidemic demonstrated how quickly an infectious disease could spread around the world in the jet age.

At first it appeared that the much-feared avian flu pandemic had commenced, but the labs could find no flu virus in the victims. The mysterious new killer, which had apparently originated in the Guangdong province of China, was dubbed severe acute respiratory syndrome, or SARS, caused by a coronavirus that looked like a spoked gear under the electron microscope. The common cold is also caused by a coronavirus, but this variant was far more lethal.

Dozens of EIS officers worked on SARS in the United States as well as in Vietnam, Thailand, Taiwan, China, and Cambodia. EIS officer David Wong was dispatched to his native Taiwan in mid-April, where only seventeen confirmed cases (mostly travelers from China) had been found. On April 22, however, a SARS epidemic erupted in the main city hospital, which was then locked down with police guarding the entrance.

---

*See pages 309–311.

Wong was allowed to enter to help with isolation efforts. "I didn't feel like I knew enough about SARS and how it was being transmitted to protect myself," the frightened officer said. "So I just put on the mask and did what I had to do. I didn't go to the bathroom, didn't get a drink of water. And when I took off my clothes at night, I doused myself with alcohol."

Only eight SARS cases were identified in the United States, all of whom had traveled to Asia or Toronto, and none died, in contrast to Canada, where Toronto hospitals inadvertently helped spread SARS. Of the 251 probable Canadian cases, 41 died.

By the end of 2003 SARS had disappeared as mysteriously as it had appeared. Though civet cats were a suspected reservoir, they were probably simply victims. Bats appear to be the likely carriers, as they may be for Ebola, Marburg, and Nipah viruses. Thus far, no more human SARS cases have arisen.

• In late 2003 the avian flu virus H5N1 resurfaced in Vietnam and Thailand in poultry and people. Over the next three years, it killed birds in forty-five countries in Asia, Europe, and Africa. It jumped to humans infrequently, infecting 440 people as of August 2009, of whom 262 died, a 60 percent case fatality rate.

If the virus mutates within a human (or animal) so that it remains lethal but becomes easily transmissible, then a dreadful worldwide flu pandemic will become a reality. Consider that the 1918 flu pandemic killed more than 20 million people, a mere 2.5 percent of those infected, and then ponder what H5N1 might do. At the 2004 EIS conference EIS alum Keiji Fukuda said that it was not a matter of *if*, but *when* the next flu pandemic hit. "Are we sliding into another pandemic now, watching it develop in slow motion?" he asked. Since then, Fukuda moved to Geneva to spearhead the World Health Organization's efforts to track and combat influenza. EIS officers have helped with pandemic flu preparedness and surveillance around the world.

• In May 2003, as EIS officers were still reeling from the SARS scare, another exotic disease was identified in a Wisconsin child who had been bitten by a pet prairie dog. She had contracted monkeypox, the African disease traced to giant Gambian rats and native squirrels.

Mark Sotir, the EIS officer assigned to Wisconsin, soon became an expert on the exotic pet industry. An Illinois distributor had housed the prairie dogs with Gambian giant rats imported from Ghana. By July EIS officers working with state epidemiologists had found seventy-one monkeypox cases in six states. No one died. Many victims were veterinarians treating sick prairie dogs. The investigation led to a ban on the importation of African rodents.

• In Bangladesh, giant flying foxes spread the Nipah virus. Of the thirty-six people who became ill in April 2004, twenty-seven died. EIS officers documented that person-to-person transmission had probably also occurred.

• Following a poor harvest in Kenya, in the spring of 2004 many people stored corn on the dirt floor inside their homes to make sure it was not stolen. In the warm, windowless environment, the fungus *Aspergillus* grew in the corn, producing deadly aflatoxin that killed 125 people. EIS officers investigated and documented frequent coinfection with hepatitis B, adding to the danger of liver cancer.

• In October 2004 dozens of children developed bloody diarrhea after playing with the cute little goats and lambs at a petting zoo at the North Carolina State Fair. The animals' manure contained *E. coli* O157:H7. Fifteen toddlers contracted the life-threatening hemolytic uremic syndrome, though with aggressive care, none died. North Carolina–based EIS officer Brant Goode and two EIS colleagues conducted the investigation, which resulted in state legislation to limit direct contact with animals and assure availability of soap and water. The following year similar petting zoo outbreaks occurred in Florida and Arizona.

• "Something big is going to happen during your two years here," Doug Hamilton told EIS trainees in July 2005. His prediction was quickly fulfilled. At the end of August Hurricane Katrina devastated the Gulf Coast, flooding New Orleans when the levees broke. EIS officer Peter Vranken, based in New Orleans, had to evacuate to Baton Rouge, where he called Hamilton to say that the state epidemiologist wanted to request help. The CDC Director's Emergency Operations Center (DEOC), an impressive new facility, was supposed to handle all deployments, so Hamilton transferred the call. "It seems that the CDC DEOC had been unable to get in touch with the State Epi," Hamilton wrote in a mass e-mail on Saturday, September 3, 2005, "and it took a simple phone call from the EIS officer. . . . Once again the EIS Officer cuts through the red tape and gets the job done."

Despite Hamilton's best intentions, however, the overall government response to Katrina was slow and disorganized, and EIS officers had no power to change that. "It looks like the log jam is beginning to break up and EISO are starting to join other CDC and HHS staff in the field," Hamilton wrote on September 4, and within two days eighteen officers had been sent to Gulf Coast states to help with disease surveillance and other needs. But Eric Sergienko reported that his needs-assessment assignment had "largely evaporated," so he hooked up with another Public Health Service field team. Then Beth Melius called from a Mississippi National Guard station, where a 750-bed field hospital had been set up. "They have all the equipment they need for now," Hamilton observed, "they just don't have any patients (this of course makes the epi job of collecting disease surveillance information quite easy)."

Hamilton's mass e-mails chronicled an inept DEOC's "poor communication and frequent screw-ups" (they lost Peter Vranken's request for help and could find no contact information for teams in the field). "But enough DEOC bashing (it's wayyy too easy)," Hamilton wrote. He reported the sick joke then in circulation, that the new motto would be: "CDC — At least we're not FEMA."

Eventually ninety-five EIS officers were sent out in the hurricane response, but as with most natural disasters, the much-feared infectious disease outbreaks did not materialize. What people needed were housing, shelter, and medication for their chronic illnesses. EIS officers frequently had to shift for themselves. Rob Bossarte reported that he worked fourteen-hour days on average. "So far I have been housed in a tent city, Navy ship, downtown hotel (without potable water, blankets, or working television), the gymnasium floor in a Baptist church, and a leased home without a functioning hot water heater," he reported.

On a mental health survey team, Stephanie Rutledge wrote: "We heard many horror stories of accidental deaths, rape, and theft. But many experienced considerable help and hospitality." Sandy Schumacher summarized her experience: "I think we've learned a lot about poverty in the U.S. — there is a LOT of work to be done on our own home front. Connecting people to medications and medical/mental health assistance has been a continuing theme."

• In June 2006 workers in a state office building in Bennington, Vermont, were found to have contracted sarcoidosis. The building was closed. Despite an EIS investigation, the disease's etiology is still unknown.*

• In September 2006 a nationwide *E. coli* O157:H7 outbreak was traced by the EIS to California-grown organic spinach.

• In Panama in October 2006, EIS officers traced forty-six children's deaths to a liquid expectorant cold medicine contaminated with diethylene glycol sold by a Chinese firm as harmless glycerine.†

• Rift Valley fever once again struck in northeastern Kenya, in November 2006. EIS officers flew to investigate.

• In the last few years tuberculosis had gone beyond multiply drug resistant to *extensively* drug resistant (XDR-TB), making such cases virtually untreatable. When an American with diagnosed XDR-TB flew to Europe on his honeymoon, EIS officers helped track him down, though he turned out not to have such a virulent form of TB after all.

• In July 2007 the EIS found that improperly canned Hot Dog Chili Sauce Original made by Castleberry's caused botulism.

• Though endemic measles was finally eliminated in the United States, an infected Japanese boy attending an August 2007 Pennsylvania sporting event spread the illness to three states. EIS officers helped track and contain the outbreak.

• A bizarre neurological illness in Minnesota slaughterhouse workers was traced in November 2007 by EIS officers to aerosolized pig brains.

---

*See pages 15–16.
†See pages 300–302.

• In 2007 the Marburg virus struck in Uganda, while Ebola killed in the Democratic Republic of the Congo, then hit Uganda. Monkeypox simultaneously struck in the Congo. EIS officers investigated all of the outbreaks.

• Children across the United States played the "choking game," in which they nearly strangled themselves to experience a brief euphoria caused by cerebral anoxia. An EIS officer documented eighty-two resulting deaths.

• From April through August 2008, a nationwide *Salmonella saintpaul* epidemic sickened over fourteen hundred people in the United States. In multiple states, EIS officers knocked on doors, asking people to recall what they ate, and conducting seven case-control studies. Though tomatoes were initially implicated, jalapeño and serrano peppers imported from Mexico appeared to be at fault.

• In April 2009 a completely new H1N1 influenza strain with genetic components from swine, birds, and humans emerged in the United States and Mexico. The media called it "swine flu." Over the next few months, it spread throughout the world, creating a new pandemic — ironic, since the avian flu (H5N1) had been the much-feared strain the previous few years. More than one hundred EIS officers and thousands of other public health staff, including many EIS alums, responded. Elderly people were relatively spared from any illness caused by this strain, perhaps because of pre-existing immunity from similar viruses that circulated prior to the shift to H2N2 in the 1957 pandemic. Although the 2009-H1N1 was not as deadly as the 1918-H1N1 pandemic strain, it too could kill otherwise healthy young people.

EIS alum Anne Schuchat appeared on TV's *60 Minutes* on October 18, 2009, as this book was going to press. "This is one of the really tragic parts of this epidemic," she said, "that people who are in the prime of their life, totally healthy, can suddenly become so sick." She observed that doctor visits for influenza-like illness were increasing steeply and, at a time when the flu season was supposed to be just beginning, flu-related hospitalizations and deaths were already rising alarmingly across the United States. "It's only October," she said, "and we're seeing really uncharted territory." The new swine flu had already spread to countries with avian flu. In a nightmare scenario, H1N1 and H5N1 might coinfect someone, reassorting to create a far deadlier pandemic.

And that is just a selection of recent EIS challenges. Most Epi-Aids involved infectious diseases, which remain serious problems in the United States and throughout the world.

The End of Polio?

Thus far, smallpox is the only infectious disease that has been eradicated, due to an international effort in which EIS officers and alums played an important role. Another scourge is tantalizingly close to being banished as well: poliomyelitis, a disease that has occupied the Epidemic Intelligence Service since the organization's inception in 1951.[*]

By early 2005 worldwide polio cases had declined over 99 percent from the level in 1988, the year the eradication campaign had commenced, and the disease remained endemic in only six countries: Niger, Egypt, India, Pakistan, Afghanistan, and Nigeria. On February 1, 2006, WHO declared Niger and Egypt polio-free. EIS alum David Heymann, who headed the WHO eradication effort, told a reporter: "The finish line is in sight."

Despite his encouraging prediction, Heymann knew the remaining cases would be difficult to tackle. He had taken on the polio job in the summer of 2003, just as rumors — *the polio drops are sterilizing our children and giving them AIDS!* — among Nigerian Muslims in one northern province had shut down the immunization effort there for nearly a year. During that time, polio cases spread directly or indirectly to twenty other African and Asian countries. (Most reinfected countries doused the outbreaks.)

A veteran of the smallpox eradication campaign, Heymann hoped to banish polio forever, though he acknowledged the challenges. It had long been known that oral polio vaccine caused vaccine-associated

---

[*]Guinea worm disease (dracunculiasis) has also nearly been eradicated, aided by EIS officers and alums.

polio in a few people per million and might spread to direct contacts. In 2000, however, an outbreak in Hispaniola was traced to vaccine-*derived* polio, a newly recognized entity in which the attenuated vaccine virus combines with another gut virus. Over the next few years vaccine-derived outbreaks occurred in several countries.

In the event that the entire world is declared free of wild polio for three years, WHO has an endgame plan. All countries will simultaneously cease giving oral polio vaccine. Those that can afford to do so, such as the United States, will continue to administer inactivated polio vaccine shots. WHO is trying to make IPV affordable for any developing country that wants to use it. Intense surveillance will continue. A vaccine-derived outbreak likely will occur somewhere within that first year, but it can probably be stopped with local mass vaccination.

In the summer of 2008, though, that endgame receded: northern Nigeria erupted with more than four hundred cases, and over the next year polio spilled back across the borders of fifteen other African countries. India, Pakistan, and Afghanistan still harbored the virus. EIS officers continued to help with eradication efforts.

Regardless of the ultimate outcome, Heymann hoped that the polio surveillance system would outlast the program, broadened to keep an eye on many infectious diseases. "If we succeed in that, it would leave a good legacy, along with a new generation of public health leaders. You name the major figures today in public health, and they all worked on smallpox eradication. The same will be true for the polio warriors."*

The Bigger Picture

Humanity's worst problems are self-inflicted. Why do members of *Homo sapiens* self-destruct? According to WHO, the top two global killers, accounting for nearly a third of all mortality, are ischaemic heart disease (blocked arteries) and cerebrovascular disease (insuf-

---

*Heymann left WHO in 2009 to head other public health efforts in London, but the polio eradication effort continues.

ficient blood to the brain, strokes), both of which are often caused by smoking, obesity and poor diet, and lack of exercise.

In 2004 four authors (including EIS alum Jim Marks) estimated recent "actual causes of death" in the United States — i.e., the underlying behavior or agent responsible for human demise. The top culprit was tobacco, accounting for 18.1 percent of all U.S. deaths, followed by obesity and poor diet (15.2 percent), with excessive alcohol consumption third (3.5 percent).

EIS officers and alums over the years have tackled smoking, weight gain, physical inactivity, and alcohol abuse. In 2001, for instance, EIS veteran Bob Brewer returned to the CDC to found the Alcohol Team, which snared a few EIS officers to document the appalling extent of binge drinking.

How could EIS officers motivate people to modify their drinking habits and diets, get more exercise, and quit smoking? They could provide important surveillance data and studies, but ultimately, argued EIS alum Tom Farley in his coauthored 2005 book, *Prescription for a Healthy Nation,* the cure would involve modifying our environment to make it easier and more appealing to walk, run, bike, and buy or grow healthy foods. "Health is political," he wrote, advising that "it will take fighting in Congress to get the booze ads off television, arguing in the town council to build sidewalks or fix the recreation equipment in the park, or calling state legislators to ban smoking in all restaurants."

Stripped to its essentials, the epidemiologic methodology means identifying problems, then using data to compare the efficacy of different solutions and convincing people to act on them despite obstacles, including pressure from entrenched special interest groups. Guns kill about thirty thousand people every year in the United States, for instance. Yet the CDC remains hamstrung by Congress, forbidden to endorse gun control.

In *War and Public Health* (2000), EIS alum and former CDC director Bill Foege proposed that epidemiologists should "systematically study conflict in the same way that we now study violence." But EIS alum Etienne Krug of WHO points out that less than 20 percent of the 1.6 million annual global death toll from violence is directly due to war. Most violent deaths are caused by suicide and homicide.* "That is why most of our effort is still going to violence on the individual level," he said, with even more staff devoted to road traffic deaths, 1.3 million a year, mostly in developing countries with horrendous roads and few restraints such as enforced traffic laws.

And so EIS officers continue to engage with such problems, confirming that poverty, social injustice, and frustration are at the root of many health issues. Those who are most vulnerable are the underprivileged, the malnourished, the unvaccinated, refugees.

Despite spending more for health care than any other country, the United States fails to achieve better outcomes than other major industrialized countries, in part because public health is underfunded. In 2007 CDC director Julie Gerberding asked an intriguing question. What if President Kennedy had issued a challenge not to land a man on the moon but to improve health care? In this hypothetical, tweaked speech of May 25, 1961, JFK would have said: "I believe that this nation should commit itself to achieving the goal, before this decade is out, of becoming 'A Healthiest Nation' and leading the way so that every Nation on Earth can share in this endeavor."

Public health intervention is usually invisible, since few people recognize that their lives have been saved. Yet the problems with the way we deal with private and public health care extend further than underappreciation. "Our health system is fragmented, too expensive, and with no real safety net," EIS veteran John Neff said. "The health system will not be able to handle the aging population and the burden and costs of chronic disease that will follow, or any significant bioterrorism or natural disaster that might occur."

Looming over all other problems is global warming. Experts project that by the year 2050, water may rise to cover low-lying areas such as Bangladesh, while sub-Saharan Africa could turn to desert. Millions of species may become extinct.

In 2008 EIS alum Mike St. Louis coauthored a summary article on the potential public health impacts of global warming. "The most

---

*Remarkably, there are more suicides than homicides worldwide and in the United States.

severe consequences of climate change will accrue to the poorest people in the poorest countries," he wrote, "despite their own negligible contributions to greenhouse gas emissions." Malnutrition, unsafe water, and heat waves will increase. Coastal megacities — Mumbai, Lagos, Shanghai, Dhaka, Tokyo, New York — will be vulnerable to sea-level rise and infiltration of freshwater with salt water.* Diseases carried by mosquitoes may shift to currently temperate climes. Waterborne infections such as cholera could spread. Armed conflict is likely to escalate as people fight over scarce resources or ban desperate refugees. Also, by 2050, the human population is projected to grow from its current 6.8 billion to more than 9 billion.

In the face of such overwhelming problems, it would be easy to despair. Australian EIS alum John Murray turned to writing fiction after revisiting African villages where he had worked on refugee problems to find that the adults had died of AIDS, leaving only orphans. One of his characters perhaps spoke for him: "I guess I helped some people, but I'm not sure it did much good in the long run. The whole thing was like patching a roof with bubble gum."

Nonetheless, EIS officers continue to fight one battle at a time, one outbreak at a time, adding incrementally to our knowledge base and inching toward solutions. "EIS is the emergency room of public medicine," said EIS alum Jim Buehler. "For many problems, the things you study with the tools of field epidemiology are the more superficial manifestations of things that go deeper — racism, poverty, underemployment, inadequate access to medical care. We come in to sort out what tipped the balance so that bad things happened. But we seldom deal with the underlying causes." Yet Epidemic Intelligence Service officers can shine a spotlight and suggest solutions.

The Troubled Gerberding Years

CDC morale suffered during the tenure of CDC director Julie Gerberding, from 2002 to 2009. Addressing the freshman EIS class in July

---

*As EIS alum Lee Riley wrote in 2007, 1 billion people (15 percent of the world's population) live in urban slums in appalling conditions, many of them in coastal cities.

2005, she stressed the need for excellence in the "interface between CDC and our customers, our stakeholders." To do this, "government systems need to be modernized," she said, "with the same efficiency as businesses."

Gerberding frequently used business terminology, referring to the CDC as a "strong brand," and she reorganized the CDC in a process she named the Futures Initiative, which upset many CDC veterans.* As part of the shake-up, Gerberding renamed venerable divisions such as the Epidemiology Program Office, which contained the EIS. Now it sounded more like a corporate human resources department: the Office of Workforce and Career Development.

A litany of complaints echoed in CDC offices: *I don't even know who I'm supposed to report to. We have these endless committee meetings. There's just another layer of bureaucracy on top of everything.* Yet few identified examples of specific obstruction of key public health approaches.

It was difficult to distinguish Gerberding's decisions from policies forced on her by higher authorities. The Bush administration and conservative politicians leaned on Gerberding and the CDC to comply with a value-laden agenda, so, for example, those working on AIDS were ordered not to push condoms or use sexually explicit language.† Disaffected longtime CDC leaders were choosing early retirement.

Most physicians entering the EIS had simultaneously joined the U.S. Public Health Service Commissioned Corps, a uniformed service that offered good benefits and a retirement option after twenty years. Ever since C. Everett Koop had insisted on it in 1987, EIS officers in the Commissioned Corps had grudgingly worn their uniforms on Wednesdays. Now there were requirements to perform push-ups and sit-ups, and in July 2008 officers would be forced to wear their uniforms every day.‡

---

*When Bill Foege reorganized the CDC in 1980, he faced similar criticism.

†George W. Bush must be given credit, however, for vastly increased funding for AIDS and malaria.

‡The April 2005 skit satirized the "transformation" of the Commissioned Corps. "Where can they insist you pretend you're military, / When you're just a bunch of science geeks?" the EIS officers sang. "All your independence, / Free thinking and good sense / They will all erode away."

In the aftermath of Hurricane Katrina, in which dozens of EIS officers performed health surveillance and pitched in wherever they could, EIS officers sent pointed queries to the director. "It seems as though nobody in the government really was prepared to handle a disaster of this magnitude," wrote one officer. "How did it come to pass that CDC appeared so uncoordinated in its response?" Gerberding did not address their questions.

Three congressional committees probed CDC's performance. In April 2007 five former CDC directors went public with their ongoing concerns. "There's a perception now that politics trumps science and truth," Bill Foege said, adding that it was hard to retain topflight epidemiologists when "people debate the efficacy of condoms or the need for vaccinations."

Jeff Koplan echoed Foege. "During the Nixon, Reagan, and Bush One administrations, the government had a conservative cast," he said, "but the level of pushdown stopped at the CDC director. Bush Two moved down levels of an organization, trying to reconfigure it to serve political ends." Koplan dismissed the transformation of the Commissioned Corps as "applying superficial trappings of the military to a group that has nothing to do with the military. The last thing you want is for the EIS to turn into a Green Beret troop."

Some officers joked that EIS stood for "Everyday I Sit," since there were more deskbound, computerized activities than ever before. With increased state and local epidemiological expertise (often provided by EIS grads) there were fewer calls for domestic Epi-Aids.

Yet the CDC remained the world's premier public health and preventive medicine organization. EIS alum Don Francis stated that, in order to insulate the CDC and the EIS from political pressure, the entire Public Health Service should be revamped as a quasi-governmental body similar to the Federal Reserve.

It is unlikely that the CDC and EIS will be insulated from politics any time soon. Legislation can have a positive impact on public health — cigarette taxes; warning labels on aspirin and tampons for, respectively, Reye's syndrome and toxic shock syndrome; removal of lead from paint and gasoline; better food inspection and consumer information; seat belt laws; bike paths; and much more. On the other hand, politicians have blocked gun control advocacy, voted for large appropriations for bioterror while cutting other budget items, and protected herbal medicines from regulation.

Congress also determines direct funding for public health. "The budget is a constant battle," EIS director Doug Hamilton wrote in July 2008, "because we have a small core allocation and all the rest is scrounged together each year." Yet the EIS produces the frontline troops of public health as well as the replenishing lifeblood of the CDC and of state and local health departments, WHO, the Bill & Melinda Gates Foundation, schools of public health, and more, bringing idealistic young professionals into the battle against the world's threats to health.

The EIS is still a vital institution, as is its parent organization, and with Barack Obama in the White House, there is clearly more support for global public health efforts without conservative ideological restrictions. Obama asked for Gerberding's resignation as of his inauguration. As interim director, EIS alum Rich Besser began to restore morale and got high marks for his clear communications during the onset of an apparent swine flu pandemic in 2009. Then in May 2009 Obama took the unusual step of personally choosing EIS alum Tom Frieden, then the New York City health commissioner, as the permanent new CDC director.

22

L'EXPERIENCE FAIT LA DIFFERENCE

JANUARY 25, 2006, *Niger, West Africa*. After sleeping in a tiny mud hut, covered by my bednet, I arose and used the toilet—a four-square-inch hole in the floor. Then I watched the village stir and come to life. Children drove donkey carts. A goat excreted by the dirt roadside. Women laughed and greeted one another as they got cook fires started in front of their adobe homes. A barefoot man in a blue satin robe and a white pillbox hat sat on a bench next to another whose head was swathed in a bright yellow turban. I was in the town of Téra, the middle of nowhere, but which, in comparison to the more remote villages, seemed like the Big City, with its gas station, cell phone tower, Coca-Cola poster, and single restaurant.

After two years of research and hundreds of interviews, I was finally out in the field, following second-year EIS officers Natasha Hochberg and Melto "Jamie" Eliades in Niger, the world's poorest country by United Nations criteria. The prior month public health personnel had attempted to distribute insecticide-treated bednets to every household in the country with a child under five, along with vitamin A and oral polio vaccine drops. Hochberg and Eliades were training and directing a team of locally hired "enumerators" who would visit randomly selected villages throughout the country to assess how successful the distribution had been. I would tag along for the first week of the project, then fly to Kenya to follow another EIS officer.

The hanging bednets, which can repel insects within a thirty-meter radius, were intended to prevent malarial mosquitoes from biting children and their families. This program had a very personal meaning for me. During a brief visit to Niger in August 2003, my friend Liz Lasser, who worked for an international health organization, had been bitten by a mosquito carrying the *Plasmodium falciparum* parasite. She hadn't bothered to take antimalarial medication. A vibrant, idealistic woman of forty-nine, she developed fever, chills, and body aches. Her lungs filled with fluid, and she died of pulmonary edema shortly after entering a hospital near her home in England.

Each year more than 500 million people become infected with malaria, for which there is (as yet) no effective vaccine. Nearly 3 million die, most of them young children in sub-Saharan Africa. Almost everyone in Niger has contracted malaria repeatedly. Having developed partial resistance, those who survive to adulthood usually have milder—but still painful—symptoms. The Niger villages I visited were in the southern part, compounds of mud huts with thatched or pueblo-style roofs set on an arid plain surrounded by millet stubble and scrub bush, reachable by red dirt tracks or brown sand.

Trim and nearly six feet tall, Natasha, thirty-one, was a Harvard graduate who had gone on to medical school. She had worked in clinics in Peru and Honduras, then had been matched with the CDC Parasitic Diseases Branch in July 2004. Her father, Fred Hochberg, had served as an EIS officer in the early 1970s.

Natasha was the lead EIS officer in Niger, keeping track of nine teams, getting enough gas, and dealing with money problems, glitches with the PalmPilots with built-in Global Positioning System (GPS), and more. An intense perfectionist and worrier, she drove herself hard.

Jamie Eliades worked in the CDC Malaria Branch. In Téra the night before, he and I had eaten at the Restaurant Lamitie (*sic,* Friendship Restaurant), a shack of sticks with woven mats for roof and walls.

We enjoyed our chicken and couscous, though I didn't drink the water. (Natasha opted out of the meal, having once contracted typhoid from African fare.)

At six foot six, with a relaxed manner and easy smile, Jamie, thirty-seven, was a "gentle giant," according to Natasha. After a residency in emergency medicine, he had earned a master's degree in public health and eventually applied for the CDC program. By the time I met him, Jaime had been to fifty-five countries. He had helped with the first national bednet distribution and assessment in Togo, later volunteering for Niger as well.

He was a calming influence. "It's good to have opposite personalities on a team," he explained, finishing his meal. As we left the restaurant, I took a photo of its misspelled sign announcing SPECIALITE AFRO-EROPENNE, L'EXPERIENCE FAIT LA DIFFERENCE. Yes. *Experience Makes the Difference* could be the motto of my trip, or for that matter, of the EIS.

That day, after hours of rough driving, we had visited the village of Zoribi. As the interviewing team was choosing random huts and conducting the survey in Djerma, the local tribal language, a young mother carrying her daughter had approached Natasha to ask for help, pointing at the child's grotesquely swollen heel. Natasha gently examined it and answered her apologetically in French. She advised her to go to the nearest health clinic to get antibiotics, since we didn't carry any.

Why can't someone give this poor little girl some medicine? I later wrote in my journal. *I know that the argument is that we are doing public health, doing a bednet and polio vaccine survey, not primary health care. And if we get involved with trying to take care of everyone, we will go nuts and be diverted. But . . .*

Later I gave Natasha a small amount of money and asked her to get it to the local health clinic for treatment of the girl's foot. She thanked me and said, "You know, I get so wrapped up in our program, and so stressed out, sometimes I need a reminder that we can stop and help just one person." One out of every four children in Niger dies before the age of five. It is through public health programs such as immuni-

zation, clean water, proper nutrition and vitamins, and bednet distribution that most of those deaths might be averted.

Since I would have been a distraction if I had gone into the huts
during surveys, I stayed outside in the villages, where the children
crowded round me. Most of the girls wore head scarves, bracelets,
and traditional clothes, while the boys wore drab cast-off Western
T-shirts and shorts. Most children smiled and laughed, pushing
closer; a few shy kids hung back. They were beautiful. Intelligence
and curiosity shone from their eyes. *Over a quarter of the children die
here,* I thought.

To engage them, I sang "If You're Happy and You Know It." They
began to clap their hands. Then I gestured to them encouragingly,
asking for a *chanson,* and after some hesitation one little girl sang in
Djerma. Two children began to dance, stomping their feet, leaning in
and circling each other, as the others sang and clapped around them.
Finally, a man shouted at them, and they left, apparently ordered back
to work, fetching water or carrying firewood.

One woman invited me into her hut. Like most of the women,
she wore a startlingly bright traditional dress of white, yellow, blue,
and red, a shiny purple head scarf, two necklaces of tiny shells, and
big hoop earrings. Though she had no visible bednet, she proudly
showed me the filter she used to keep guinea worm copepods* out of
the water that she stored in carefully stacked clay pots.

At every village, Natasha and Jamie first visited the village elder.
Because both of them towered over everyone, they usually squatted
respectfully, explaining their mission. I was impressed with their ability to organize and train the teams (in sessions back in the capital of
Niamey), plan this difficult survey of a vast and sparsely populated
country, and maintain a sense of humor.

"Jamie and I made a great team," Natasha told me after the sur-

---

*Guinea worm disease (dracunculiasis) involves a life cycle in which worm larvae are in-
gested by freshwater copepods. When a person drinks water with guinea worm copepods,
female worms grow up to three feet long, emerging with painful ruptures. The worm releases
her larvae into water, and the cycle begins anew. In 1985 the CDC/EIS joined a worldwide
effort to eradicate the disease.

vey was completed. "I tend to be compulsive; that's how to get work done. He'd tell me it was okay to give the teams a day off." There had been multiple flat tires, gas crises, cell phone inaccessibility, disgusting lodging, and software problems, but the teams actually finished ahead of time.

The effort revealed that 87 percent of the surveyed children under five had received polio vaccinations during the December 2005 campaign, and that 64 percent of the households with young children had received a bednet. Yet only 15.4 percent of the children had slept under an insecticide-treated bednet the previous night, presumably because the January–February survey took place during the dry season, when mosquitoes are not a big problem.

In September 2006 EIS officer Julie Thwing led teams that repeated the random assessment during the rainy season, finding that 55.5 percent of children under five had slept under an insecticide-treated bednet the previous night. Though not the official 80 percent goal, this was a dramatic improvement. From 2006 through 2009, ten other African countries have conducted similar bednet distribution campaigns in conjunction with immunization drives.

The bednet surveillance project in Niger is typical of the unsung work of EIS officers. It would have received little notice if I had not tagged along.

Making a Difference in Kenya

January 31, 2006, Homa Bay, Kenya. After Niger, I traveled to Kenya, where I visited three rural elementary schools with Ciara O'Reilly. A five-foot, one-hundred-pound blonde Irish native, the thirty-one-year-old EIS officer presented quite a contrast to the Africans she served. After earning a Ph.D. in food microbiology, Ciara began with the CDC Foodborne and Diarrheal Diseases Branch in August 2004. Just before I met her in Kenya, she had spent two days aboard a cruise ship in the Caribbean, where norovirus was spread by passengers' vomitus.

The transition from the luxurious cruise ship to African poverty was jarring, but Ciara had been to Kenya the previous year to set up a diarrhea study, so she knew what to expect. "Kenyans are better able to appreciate small things than we are," she told me. "If something good happens, they have such joy."

At one of the schools we visited, children stood on the barren school grounds to sing songs and recite poems they had written for their safe water club. Though many were barefoot, they wore the school uniform — boys in white shirts and blue shorts, girls in blue dresses with white collars — and there was indeed joy on their faces, even though a storm had recently ripped the corrugated roof from their school building, built from bricks they had made themselves. Many of them were also AIDS orphans.

Ciara and Matt Freeman, a young epidemiologist with the Center for Global Safe Water at Emory University, were there to assess the impact of the Safe Water System (SWS), which had been implemented by CARE (with funding from Coca-Cola) the previous summer in forty-five primary schools in Nyanza Province in western Kenya. Ciara and Matt had trained local enumerators to administer questionnaires to randomly selected students and their parents or guardians.

Diarrhea from polluted water kills over 2 million people annually, mostly children in developing countries. The SWS teaches people to treat their drinking water with diluted bleach and to dispense it from spigots in narrow-topped containers too small for hands to reach in.[*]

This school had two sources of water. The better one was a river down the dirt road, a half hour away. The other was a ten-minute walk, but it was foul and stagnant. We were looking at the latter when an old man told us that people who drank this water went loco and got diseases. As he spoke, several emaciated cows ambled up and waded in to drink.

At the schools, I watched children stop at a handwashing station after leaving latrines, as they had been taught. They drew water to drink from brown narrow-topped clay pots with metal spigots, and they demonstrated how they added a capful of WaterGuard, the diluted bleach solution, to treat new water.

---

[*]See page 272.

The next day I walked through the dry scrub with Elvis, a Luo-speaking enumerator, as he visited parents or guardians in their small mud homes, questioning them about their knowledge of WaterGuard and the Safe Water System. The third house was very small, with a bare double-bed foam mattress leaning against the wall. The woman in the house was a recent AIDS widow with seven children. Her husband had had three wives, but one of them, with six children, had also died. The third remaining wife was childless. So these two women had thirteen children to care for and were very poor. Yet this woman still managed to buy WaterGuard for their water.

Over the next few days I helped Ciara and Matt enter data from the questionnaires into laptops. "Now you know what being an EIS officer is really like," Ciara told me, referring to the tedious job in oppressive heat. Some of the surveys were heartrending: an eighty-six-year-old woman caring for three AIDS-orphaned grandchildren; two adults, eleven children, all sleeping in one room. An enumerator's comment on the last situation: "The family is very desperate and I really wondered how they manage their daily bread."

As I walked the single paved street of Homa Bay every morning and evening, I encountered women carrying twenty-liter plastic buckets of water on their heads — water retrieved from a pool, ditch, or rivulet. Children riding bicycles carried jerry cans of water. All polluted. Ciara told me about a local control school she had visited that did not have the SWS program. "A teacher showed me a bucket of water they drank. Scum floated on top of the brown water, and sediment coated the bottom," she said. With most people earning less than a dollar a day, even the pennies needed for WaterGuard were hard to come by.

When the data from Ciara's survey were tabulated, they told a positive story. Student absenteeism in the intervention schools had dropped by 35 percent, while in nonproject control schools it had risen by 5 percent. More parents had heard about WaterGuard than those interviewed during a baseline survey, though only a few more actually used it at home.

My final day in Kenya, I drove with Ciara over terrible, dusty roads one more time, to visit hospitals and clinics where she was conducting a baseline study of what caused diarrhea in another area of Nyanza Province. One hospital was located in Siaya, hometown of Barack Obama's father.* Stool samples from the hospital were tested twice a week at the CDC lab in Kisumu to determine what had caused diarrhea and what sort of drug resistance had developed. In Bondo District Hospital, the drinking water was not treated with WaterGuard, and about fifteen children a month died there.

Ciara's study found that in children under five, three bacteria together — Shigella, Campylobacter, and Salmonella — accounted for about half of the pathogens identified. The other half was caused by rotavirus, which is impervious to WaterGuard.† Ciara also found that the bacteria were highly resistant to three common antibiotics, but responded to others.

Since the time I followed Ciara in Kenya, she has graduated from the EIS but stayed on as a staff member in the same branch. She helped to launch the Global Enterics Multi-Center Study (GEMS), which will expand the Kenyan diarrhea project to eight locations worldwide in an unprecedented prospective case-control study to determine what diarrheal pathogens are killing children under five, and to what drugs they are susceptible.

And CARE (with funding from many public and private organizations) has begun to implement the Safe Water System in an additional two hundred schools in Nyanza Province. Some schools will also get latrines, while others will, in addition, get a borehole well or rainwater harvesting. The idea is to see which interventions are cost-effective and sustainable. It is a three-year project, and there are plans to expand it to fifteen hundred more schools.

The programs were nearly derailed by ethnic violence in Kenya following the disputed presidential election of December 27, 2007.

---

*Six months later, in August 2006, then-Senator Barack Obama came to Siaya to visit his grandmother. At the CDC outpost in Kisumu, at the request of EIS alum Kayla Laserson, Obama and his wife, Michelle, publicly submitted to HIV testing to encourage locals to do the same.

†Later in 2006, two oral rotavirus vaccines were found to be safe and effective, though getting them to poor children around the world is another matter.

"Kisumu looks different these days," Ciara e-mailed, "with many buildings burnt to the ground." Still, she had managed to train staff for the prospective diarrhea study and was preparing to launch it. A power-sharing agreement between the incumbent Mwai Kibaki and his opponent Raila Odinga was hammered out in late February, and Kenya settled back into an uneasy peace.

That February 2008 EIS officer Sapna Bamrah, thirty-four, arrived in Kenya to assess the impact of the violence on AIDS and tuberculosis health clinics, where 180,000 people had been taking antiretroviral drugs. As an EIS officer, Sapna had already ventured to Azerbaijan to look at mortality surveillance from land mines; to Vietnam to study the impact of Pur, a water treatment product made by Procter & Gamble; to Nepal to assess the nutritional status of Bhutanese refugees; and to Swaziland to conduct a randomized survey of rape and molestation of young girls. Now in Kenya, she found that while many health clinics had been temporarily closed or abandoned, the system was beginning to recover more quickly than had been feared.

I interviewed her in August 2008, a month after she completed her EIS service and remained with the CDC. She acknowledged that "sitting on committees, wearing a uniform, and following rules and regulations has little to do with public health," and that politics sometimes subverted science. But Sapna concluded: "For every moment I am frustrated, I am continually inspired and amazed at what people in the EIS and in this agency are doing. The average American has no idea the amount of energy spent in the United States and the world by people who really believe in protecting the public."

EPILOGUE:
THE EIS LEGACY

IN SOME FIVE HUNDRED INTERVIEWS, EIS officers told me surprisingly similar stories about their experience: *The EIS changed my life, shaped my career, gave me a worldview. Those were the best two years of my life.* Of course, not every former officer felt that way, but for the overwhelming majority, the Epidemic Intelligence Service was transformative.

"An enormous amount of experience was crammed into my short two years of EIS, 1976 to 1978," observed David Morens. "I remember it as intense, fly by the seat of your pants, exhilarating, collegial, with a sense of teamwork, camaraderie, and nonstop excitement. Almost everything I have done since then derives from and/or has been greatly influenced by what I did in EIS."

Similar sentiments come from recent EIS grads. "EIS is unlike any other training program," said Puneet Dewan (2001–2003). "You are given anything you can possibly handle, with supervision and guidance. It's a unique experience that permits you to work on things you would never possibly be able to do otherwise, develop expertise rapidly or fall on your face." Dewan unknowingly echoed founder Alexander Langmuir, whose approach was to "throw them overboard. See if they can swim, and if they can't, throw them a life ring, pull them out and throw them in again."

Many felt instantly at home in the CDC program. "When I came to EIS," Sue Binder recalled, "I found myself with people I would have chosen as friends. They were intelligent, active, had good politics, cared about people, wanted to make a difference." Similarly, Pia Mac-Donald called her EIS colleagues "the most interesting, neat people I ever met in my life."

Patrick Moore added: "Most EIS recruits are not run-of-the-mill people. They aren't doing it to make lots of money. We really felt we were putting ourselves at risk, selflessly facing down bad diseases to help other people."

In the early years, most physicians joined the EIS to avoid the draft, but many remained in public health once they realized that they could have such a powerful impact on thousands of lives. That same realization occurred to latter-day officers such as Scott Harper, who observed: "Working as an EIS officer in public health was exciting, important, and satisfying. Whether investigating an outbreak or writing policy for vaccines, I had the opportunity to affect many more people's lives than a clinician seeing thirty people a day."

"I'm blessed to be part of the EIS cycle," Amanda Sue Niskar said. "For every outbreak the media hears about, there are so many more that never happened because we did our job." Kay Kreiss recalled thinking, *This is the best job I'm ever going to have, with infinite backup and no administrative responsibility.*

"Being dropped into an outbreak, given the authority to investigate it and do the detective work, then apply that knowledge to curbing the current outbreak and preventing future ones — there's no better work in the world," Scott Holmberg said. "Wherever you go, everybody wants the same two things — peace and prosperity. It doesn't matter whether their lips are stretched and they are dyed blue, or whether they sit in front of a computer. They are worried about family, friends, tribe, nation."

Oh, You Did EIS

It isn't surprising that young (and not-so-young) people who join an elite, high-pressure organization bond with one another. The annual

April EIS conference begins that process. In the lecture halls, new EIS officers listen to ten-minute presentations from current officers on an array of topics. In a typical EIS conference that I attended in April 2004, freshmen listened to (among many others) talks on measles in the Marshall Islands, a multistate *Salmonella* outbreak traced to pre-cut melons, resistant syphilis in San Francisco, arsenic-laden water in Bangladesh, obese preschoolers in Missouri, the psychological response to sniper attacks in the District of Columbia, marital violence in Oregon, a new dog-tick vector for Rocky Mountain spotted fever in Arizona, enforcement of alcohol-consumption age limits in New Hampshire, monkeypox in Wisconsin, and *E. coli* O157:H7 traced to alfalfa sprouts in Colorado.

After each talk, the presenting EIS officer answered questions about the investigation, usually from EIS alums. Since Langmuir's death, others have risen to become chief gadflies during the Q&A period.

In July new officers return to Atlanta for four weeks of intense training. The course is almost entirely taught by EIS veterans. In July 2005, when I sat in, Steve Thacker began with a truncated history of the Epidemic Intelligence Service. He explained the proper approach to public health as answering four basic questions. *What is the problem?* Surveillance plays a key role here. *What is the cause of the problem?* Identify the risk factors. *What works?* Evaluate interventions. *How do you do it?* Intervene in the most effective manner.

EIS director Doug Hamilton explained how to conduct an outbreak investigation, giving examples from past EIS officers. *Verify the diagnosis. Develop a case definition. Time. Place. Person. Communicate findings.* Denise Koo emphasized the importance of "consequential epidemiology," quoting Goethe: "Knowing is not enough; we must apply."

Then the training covered cohort and case-control studies, P values, recall bias, epidemic curves, standard deviation, risk versus rates, chi-square distribution, odds ratios, confidence levels, Epi Info usage, and other esoterica vital to an epidemiologist. Anthropologist Holly Williams emphasized that culture drives behavior and that reality is always complex, subjective, and changing. "You can quantify what happened but not why," she explained, as she urged the usefulness of focus groups in refugee camps and other settings. Bruce Dan delivered his SOCO lecture on how to deal with the media: Choose a single overriding communication objective and keep repeating it, in various ways, in answer to any question.

In the afternoons officers split into small groups for case studies of real epidemics, in which they were fed information a bit at a time, discussing the conclusions that could be drawn and the best ways to generate and test hypotheses. The course ended with lectures on bioterrorism, then a field exercise on natural disasters such as heat waves and tornadoes in which officers conducted random door-to-door surveys. *If you needed to evacuate due to a disaster, where would you go? Who do you think is at greatest risk during a heat wave? If you were driving on the highway and saw a tornado approaching, what would you do?* Then the officers had to present their summary findings with commentary.

By the time the newly minted EIS officers dispersed to their assignments, they had begun to absorb some of the accumulated wisdom of EIS veterans, many of whom passed on vintage quotes from their own mentors, such as Stan Foster's maxim, "You get what you inspect, not what you expect," or Mike Gregg's favorite admonition by philosopher George Santayana: "Skepticism is the chastity of the intellect. It is shameful to surrender it too soon to the first comer."

Not all EIS graduates had undiluted affection for the institution. "EIS is a club," observed Jim Buehler. "At its best, EIS instills a spirit of dedication, pride, and can-do mentality. At its worst, EIS engenders a sense of smugness and endless capacity for self-congratulation." William Atkinson commented sardonically: "It is common knowledge that EIS officers have been known to ascend directly to heaven."

Yet most veterans of the program genuinely value the "old boy/girl network" aspect of the EIS. "I owe the EIS a lot, not only for where I am sitting right now [at WHO in Geneva], but in terms of thinking and training," Swiss native Roland Sutter said. "I have the ability to call hundreds of people with the dumbest questions, and they will be patient and answer." Kevin De Cock, a Belgian, agreed: "Inadvertently you become part of a network, a society that now reaches globally. I can meet people in Europe, Africa, the United States — *oh, you did EIS* — and you just know you have certain shared ways of communicating, of looking at problems."

Indeed, it takes a special kind of person to assume duties that will necessarily put his or her health, even life, in peril from exotic diseases, natural disasters, and warring factions. EIS officers must leave home and family at a moment's notice, work limitless hours in inhospitable circumstances, and feel energized by the experience. And whatever criticism may be leveled at the CDC, it takes a special kind of organization to select, train, and support these first responders of world health.

Public Health Giants

There are more than three thousand EIS alums whose global impact has been astonishing for a relatively small government program. One is Bill Foege, who suggested a focus on river blindness and guinea worm eradication programs at the Carter Center and went on to educate Microsoft philanthropist Bill Gates about global public health priorities at the Gates Foundation.

At WHO, EIS graduates work on malaria, polio, measles, women's reproductive health, childhood tetanus, violence, AIDS, and other sexually transmitted infections. D.A. Henderson oversaw the global eradication of smallpox, while David Heymann directed polio eradication efforts. Rafe Henderson was head of the Expanded Program on Immunization at WHO for many years. Mike Merson took on global diarrheal diseases, while the late Jonathan Mann led the fight against AIDS.

EIS grad Bill Stewart became the U.S. surgeon general. Jeff Koplan, Bill Foege, and Jim Mason headed the CDC, with Mason going on to become assistant secretary for health and acting surgeon general. Many have served as state and local epidemiologists throughout the United States. Tom Frieden became New York City's health commissioner and then CDC director.

Steve Schroeder headed the Robert Wood Johnson Foundation, a health philanthropy, while Ward Cates was president of Family Health International's research division. David Fraser became the president of Swarthmore College and wrote a landmark paper providing a critical foundation for undergraduate programs in epidemiology and public health.

Other EIS grads have been innovators. Andy Dean developed Epi Info, a software program for field epidemiologists that has been translated into fifteen languages. Ralph Paffenbarger conducted pioneering studies proving the benefits of vigorous exercise. Jim Marks fostered the Behavioral Risk Factor Surveillance System.

Others, like Marc LaForce, who directed the Meningitis Vaccine Project, developed lifesaving immunizations. Don Francis conducted the first field trial for an AIDS vaccine, though it was unsuccessful. Larry Corey worked on another possible AIDS vaccine, while Seth Berkley launched the International AIDS Vaccine Initiative. Myron (Mike) Levine founded the Center for Vaccine Development at the University of Maryland School of Medicine, where he developed an oral typhoid vaccine, among others. His son Orin Levine (also an EIS alum) worked on affordable pneumococcal vaccines. Stan Plotkin, co-editor of the classic textbook *Vaccines,* developed the rubella vaccine now used throughout the world and worked extensively on the development of other vaccines, including polio, rabies, varicella, rotavirus, and cytomegalovirus. Jim Maynard fought the drug industry to get an affordable hepatitis B vaccine produced in Indonesia.

Many other EIS grads became professors, researchers, and deans of schools of public health. For instance, Harrison Spencer served as dean at Tulane as well as the London School of Hygiene and Tropical Medicine before heading the Association of Schools of Public Health. Al Sommer followed D.A. Henderson at the helm of the Johns Hopkins School of Public Health. From his platform at Vanderbilt, Bill Schaffner recruited several generations of new EIS officers. Philip Brachman and many other EIS veterans taught at the Rollins School of Public Health at Emory University, where Gene Gangarosa helped to fund and found the Center for Global Safe Water.

Karl Western, Dale Lawrence, Roger Glass, David Morens, and

others worked in laboratories and conducted research at the National Institutes of Health. Rei Ravenholt promoted family planning around the world for USAID, then focused on tobacco-related health issues.

Ron Davis became president of the American Medical Association. Robert Thompson plied his epidemiological skills as an administrator for Group Health Cooperative, a pioneering Seattle HMO, where he drove studies on subjects as diverse as breast cancer, bicycle helmet usage, and domestic violence.

Female EIS alums, who have outnumbered males in recent classes, will be the predominant public health leaders in the coming decades. Karen Starko found the link between aspirin and Reye's syndrome. Kathy Shands led the battle against toxic shock syndrome. Helene Gayle was recruited from the Gates Foundation to serve as the executive director of CARE. Others pioneered in the field of maternal and child health. After her EIS service, midwife Judith Rooks wrote the definitive text *Midwifery and Childbirth in America* and consulted in twenty-four countries. In 2002 Linda Bartlett documented the world's highest maternal mortality rate in remote northern Afghanistan, where unattended women sometimes suffered from obstructed labor for days before dying, their babies undelivered.

Other entrepreneurial EIS grads have started businesses and non-profits. Ron O'Connor founded Management Sciences for Health, an NGO that helps to deliver medicines in forty countries in the developing world. Joel Selanikio created and directed DataDyne.org, which partners with the CDC, WHO, and other organizations to provide inexpensive mobile technical support, primarily in Africa and Asia, utilizing cell phones and an EpiSurveyor PDA that he developed. David Addiss joined the Fetzer Institute, an enterprise seeking to promote the "power of love and forgiveness in the emerging global community," where he directed the program on science and spirituality.

Many EIS graduates have remained at the CDC, becoming mentors and supervisors for new officers. Others have written, coauthored, and edited textbooks, written novels, and pursued careers in journalism.

EIS officers or alums identified new diseases such as Legionnaires' disease, Lassa fever, Ebola, AIDS, hantavirus pulmonary syndrome, and Lyme disease. Others helped find the cause of killers such as neural tube defects and eosinophilia-myalgia syndrome, thereby making it possible to prevent them. For some conditions, such as chronic fatigue syndrome or Gulf War syndrome, EIS officers have brought a healthy skepticism to their proposed causes.

The EIS program has spawned clones and imitators around the world. Canada started the first such program in 1975, and in 1980 the CDC loaned an EIS grad, David Brandling-Bennett, to Thailand as the first temporary resident advisor for a new Field Epidemiology Training Program (FETP). As of April 2009 there were thirty-six FETP or similar programs serving eighty-two countries, with plans to develop eight new programs to serve eleven additional countries.*

There are five single-country programs with no official ties to the CDC, but all have had former EIS officers contribute advice or training. EPIET, based in France, covers the twenty-seven nations in the European Union. The majority of its founders were European EIS graduates.

Footprints on the Globe

In 1951 Alexander Langmuir seized a Cold War opportunity to fund a small training program for young epidemiologists who would keep an eye out for biological warfare while responding promptly to unintentional epidemics. Today these EIS officers are the world's premier frontline disease detectives.

For an obscure government program, the Epidemic Intelligence Service has produced remarkable results. Perhaps it has done so in part by remaining relatively small, nimble, and flexible. One of the lessons of the EIS's history is the impact that one person can have.

---

*In the near future, some EIS officers will probably be given two-year assignments overseas, similar to state-based EIS positions. Not all FETP programs have endured. EIS clones in Indonesia, Hungary, and the Côte d'Ivoire folded. EIS alum Rafe Henderson spearheaded two separate efforts to initiate an EIS-like program at the World Health Organization, but both imploded without sufficient long-term support.

Put creative, intelligent, well-trained, motivated individuals into the right environment, and the outcome can save lives and lead to vital careers. EIS officers and alums have had an impact far beyond their original numbers. Today, with global public health bedeviled by substantial threats, the lifesaving work performed around the world by these shoe-leather epidemiologists is more essential than ever. The EIS program and its offspring have, in short, influenced and defined how field epidemiology and public health are practiced on our planet.

A NOTE ON SOURCES

I donated my research materials to the Manuscript, Archives, and Rare Book Library of Emory University, including material collected by Elizabeth Etheridge for her 1992 history of the CDC. The full bibliography is posted at http://marbl.library.emory.edu/, and a year after this book's publication, the original uncut manuscript with endnotes will also be available there. I can be reached at markp@nasw.org. — Mark Pendergrast

Books

There are only two other books specifically about the Epidemic Intelligence Service. *Epidemic Detectives,* by Fred Warshofsky (Scholastic Book Services, 1963), is a slim paperback, long out of print. In *Beating Back the Devil* (Free Press, 2004), Maryn McKenna wrote primarily about the exploits of the EIS class of 2002–2004, with selected historical flashbacks.

Other books document EIS officers' exploits. *Epidemic!,* by Jules Archer (Harcourt Brace Jovanovich, 1977), somewhat cursorily covers the outbreaks of the 1970s, followed by *The Disease Detectives,* by Gerald Astor (Dutton, 1983), a more satisfactory effort. Elizabeth W. Etheridge's *Sentinel for Health* (University of California Press, 1992), a history of the CDC, is an invaluable resource filled with EIS stories.

EIS officers have figured prominently in other books as well, including *Annals of Epidemiology* (Little Brown, 1967) and *The Medical Detectives* (Washington Square Press, 1980), both by the late Berton Roueché, who mastered the art of popular epidemiological narrative in his medical columns for the *New Yorker*. In *The Coming Plague* (Farrar, Straus and Giroux, 1994), Laurie Garrett included many EIS officers and alums.

Field Epidemiology, edited by Michael B. Gregg (Oxford University Press, 3rd edition, 2008), is a textbook written almost entirely by EIS alums. *Highlights in Public Health,* edited by Richard A. Goodman et al. (CDC, 1998), provides a compilation of seminal articles from the *Morbidity and Mortality Weekly Report,* mostly written by anonymous EIS officers.

Secret Agents, by Madeline Drexler (Joseph Henry Press, 2002), is an excellent compendium on emerging diseases, as is *The New Killer Diseases,* by Elinor Levy and Mark Fischetti (Crown, 2003). Both feature EIS investigations.

Other related works include *Protecting America's Health,* a history of the U.S. Food & Drug Administration by Philip J. Hilts (Knopf, 2003), as well as the more critical *FDA Follies* (Basic, 1994), by Herbert Burkholz. *Plagues and Politics,* by Fitzhugh Mullan (Basic, 1989), is the history of the U.S. Public Health Service. The history of CDC Public Health Advisors, who frequently partnered with EIS officers, is told in *Ready to Go,* by Beth E. Meyerson et al. (American Social Health Association, 2008).

Control of Communicable Diseases Manual (American Public Health Association, 2008, eighteenth edition), edited by EIS alum David L. Heymann, is a comprehensive resource on infectious diseases, while *A Field Guide to Germs* (Doubleday, 2002), by Wayne Biddle, is a more entertaining alternative for the general reader. *Emerging Infections,* edited by Joshua Lederberg et al. (National Academies Press, 1992) is the classic work on newly identified diseases.

Other books cover more specific topics, in alphabetical order:

AIDS:

Randy Shilts's *And the Band Played On* (St. Martin's Press, 1987) remains the best account of AIDS' emergence in the United States. Greg Behrman's *The Invisible People* (Free Press, 2004) covers the disastrous spread of AIDS worldwide. EIS alum Scott D. Holmberg analyzed missteps in AIDS research and treatment in *Scientific Errors and Controversies in the U.S. HIV/AIDS Epidemic* (Praeger Press, 2007). Helen Epstein's *The Invisible Cure* (Farrar, Straus and Giroux, 2007) critiques AIDS approaches in Africa.

Anthrax:

The 2001 anthrax bioterrorism is covered in Leonard A. Cole's *The Anthrax Letters* (Joseph Henry Press, 2003) and Marilyn W. Thompson's *The Killer Strain* (HarperCollins, 2003).

Bangladesh:

Disaster in Bangladesh, edited by Lincoln C. Chen (Oxford University Press, 1973), covers the 1970 cyclone, 1971 war for independence, and subsequent starvation and smallpox spread. Several chapters were written by EIS alums.

Biological and chemical warfare:

Seymour Hersh wrote an early exposé, *Chemical & Biological Warfare* (Anchor Books, 1969), while Ed Regis penned the history in *The Biology of Doom* (Henry Holt, 1999). Russian defector Ken Alibek's *Biohazard* (Random House, 1999) details the Soviet Union's program. *Toxic Terror,* edited by Jonathan B. Tucker (MIT Press, 2000), includes a chapter on the 1984 Rajneeshee salad bar contamination. Michael T. Osterholm and John Schwartz added *Living Terrors* (Delacorte Press, 2000) and Judith Miller et al., *Germs* (Simon & Schuster, 2001). W. Seth Carus wrote *Bioterrorism and Biocrimes* (Minerva Group, 2002), a detailed compendium.

Cholera and other waterborne diseases:

In *The Ghost Map* (Riverhead Books, 2006), Steven Johnson told the story of John Snow and the 1854 London cholera outbreak. *Epidemic Enteric Infections Among Prisoners of War in Korea,* edited by Albert V.

Hardy et al. (Florida State Board of Health Monograph Series, No. 4, 1963), covered the shigellosis outbreak among POWs during the Korean War. W.E. Van Heyningen and John R. Seal wrote *Cholera: The American Scientific Experience* (Westview Press, 1983), a history of the Cholera Research Laboratory in Bangladesh, including the development of oral rehydration therapy. *The Blue Death,* by Robert D. Morris (HarperCollins, 2007), included the 1993 Milwaukee *Cryptosporidium* outbreak and the 1994 cholera/shigellosis epidemic in Goma, Zaire. Philip Gourevitch's *We Wish to Inform You That Tomorrow We Will Be Killed with Our Families* (Farrar, Straus and Giroux, 1998) documented the 1994 Rwandan genocide and cholera outbreak in the Goma camps. *Bill Bryson's African Diary,* by Bill Bryson (Doubleday, 2002), is a slight book that briefly covers Homa Bay, Kenya, and the Safe Water System.

Chronic fatigue syndrome:
Hillary Johnson's *Osler's Web* (Crown, 1996) offers good background information from a "believer's" point of view. Edward Shorter's *From Paralysis to Fatigue* (Free Press, 1991) and Elaine Showalter's *Hystories* (Columbia University Press, 1997) provide skeptical coverage.

Foodborne diseases:
Spoiled, by Nicols Fox (Basic Books, 1997), gives excellent coverage of *E. coli* O157:H7 and other diseases, featuring various EIS investigations. *E. Coli O157,* by Mary Heersink (New Horizon Press, 1996), is a first-person account by a mother whose son nearly died of the infection. *Fast Food Nation,* by Eric Schlosser (Houghton Mifflin, 2001), is a well-researched popular account. *Addressing Foodborne Threats to Health,* from the Institute of Medicine (National Academies Press, 2006), includes a good summary chapter on *Cyclospora* outbreaks by EIS alum Barbara Herwaldt.

Global health and population:
The Global Burden of Disease: 2004 Update (World Health Organization, 2008) and *World Report on Violence and Health* (WHO, 2002) provide overviews. *World Population to 2300* (United Nations, 2004) contains population projections.

Gun control:

Disarmed, by Kristin A. Goss (Princeton University Press, 2006), offers summary history. *Violence in American Schools,* edited by Delbert S. Elliott et al. (Cambridge University Press, 1998), contains a chapter by EIS alums Mark Rosenberg and James Mercy.

Heat waves:

Eric Klinenberg's *Heat Wave* (University of Chicago Press, 2002) details the 1995 events in Chicago, as does *Natural Disaster Survey Report: July 1995 Heat Wave* (NOAA, December 1995).

Hemorraghic fevers:

Fever!, by John G. Fuller (Ballantine Books, 1974), recounts the 1969 discovery of Lassa fever. *Ebola,* by William T. Close (Ivy Books, 1995), provides an accurate dramatization of the first 1976 Ebola virus outbreaks, written by Mobutu's former physician. *The Hot Zone,* by Richard Preston (Random House, 1994), recounts the 1989 Ebola scare in the Reston, Virginia, monkey house. *Virus Ground Zero,* by Ed Regis (Pocket Books, 1996), is about the 1995 Ebola outbreak in Kikwit, Zaire.

Hospital infections:

Proceedings of the International Conference on Nosocomial Infections (American Hospital Association, 1971) covers the conference held in 1970 at the CDC. *Hospital Infections* (Lippincott Williams & Wilkins, 2007, fifth edition), edited by EIS alum William Jarvis and previously edited by EIS alums Philip S. Brachman and John V. Bennett, is the classic text.

Influenza:

Gina Kolata's *Flu* (Farrar, Straus and Giroux, 1999) and John M. Barry's *The Great Influenza* (Penguin, 2005) tell the story of the 1918 flu pandemic. *The Epidemic That Never Was,* by Richard E. Neustadt and Harvey Fineberg (Vintage, 1983), and *Pure Politics, Impure Science,* by Arthur Silverstein (Johns Hopkins University Press, 1981), review the troubled 1976 swine flu campaign. *Influenza: Virus, Vaccines, and Strategy* (Academic Press, 1976) offers a contemporary snapshot just before the campaign began. *Catching Cold,* by Pete Davies (Michael Joseph, 1999), covers the 1997 appearance of H5N1 in Hong Kong. *Seasonal & Pandemic Influenza,* edited by Arnold S. Monto and Richard J. Whitley (New York University, 2006), provides a good overview.

Legionnaires' disease:

Anatomy of an Epidemic (Doubleday, 1984), by Gordon Thomas and Max Morgan-Witts, is about the 1976 Legionnaires' outbreak. *Legionella,* edited by James Barbaree (American Society for Microbiology, 1993), includes a retrospective chapter by honorary EIS alum Walter Dowdle.

Polio:

David M. Oshinsky's *Polio: An American Story* (Oxford University Press, 2005) is an excellent history. Richard Carter's out-of-print *Breakthrough: The Saga of Jonas Salk* (Trident, 1966) provides important background on the politics and science behind the switch from the Salk to the Sabin vaccine, as does Peter Radetsky's *The Invisible Invaders* (Little Brown, 1991). Paul A. Offit's *The Cutter Incident* (Yale University Press, 2005) is a detailed account of what went wrong in 1955. Tim Brookes and Omar Khan wrote about the effort to eradicate polio in *The End of Polio?* (American Public Health Association, 2007).

Sick building syndrome:

Indoor Air Quality, edited by P. J. Walsh et al. (CRC Press, 1984), has a summary chapter by EIS alum Kathleen Kreiss.

Smallpox:

Donald R. Hopkins, an honorary EIS officer who took part in smallpox eradication, wrote the classic history, *The Greatest Killer: Smallpox in History* (University of Chicago Press, 2002). Three books on smallpox eradication are indispensable: *Smallpox and Its Eradication,* by Frank Fenner, D.A. Henderson, et al. (World Health Organization, 1988), also known as the Big Red Book; *Smallpox: The Death of a Disease* (Prometheus, 2009), by EIS alum D.A. Henderson, who directed the global eradication effort; and *CDC and the Smallpox Crusade,* by

Horace G. Ogden (CDC/GPO, 1987). Ogden's book is based on a more extensive unpublished manuscript by Mark LaPointe. Pascal Imperato wrote *A Wind in Africa* (Warren H. Green, 1975) about the Mali program. There is also *The Eradication of Smallpox from India,* by R.N. Basu et al. (WHO, 1979), and *The Eradication of Smallpox from Bangladesh,* by A.K. Joarder et al. (WHO, 1980). *Quest for the Killers,* by June Goodfield (Birkhauser, 1985), contains a good chapter on smallpox eradication. Two popular modern accounts that also cover the fear of smallpox being used in bioterrorism are *The Demon in the Freezer,* by Richard Preston (Ballantine Books, 2002), and *Scourge,* by Jonathan B. Tucker (Atlantic Monthly Press, 2001).

Toxic shock syndrome:
The Price of a Life, by lawyer Tom Riley (Adler & Adler, 1986), is a well-researched book chronicling one woman's death from toxic shock syndrome.

Tuberculosis:
Health of the City: Focus on Tuberculosis (New York City Department of Health, 1995) summarizes the battle against TB in New York City. Tracy Kidder's *Mountains Beyond Mountains* (Random House, 2003) discusses Paul Farmer's push to treat multiple-drug-resistant TB.

Tuskegee syphilis study:
Bad Blood, by James H. Jones (Free Press, 1993), is the classic history.

Other books by EIS alums:
With his wife, Susan Fisher-Hoch, EIS veteran Joe McCormick wrote a memoir, *Level 4* (Turner Publishing, 1996), as did C.J. Peters (not EIS, but in charge of CDC Special Pathogens and many EIS officers) in *Virus Hunter* (Anchor Books, 1997). Many other EIS alums have written or edited textbooks. John Murray turned to fiction, publishing *A Few Short Notes on Tropical Butterflies* (HarperCollins, 2003), a critically acclaimed collection of short stories, many featuring idealistic but conflicted public health scientists.

Periodicals

EIS officers usually published initial investigation results in the CDC publication, *Morbidity and Mortality Weekly Report* (*MMWR*), frequently followed by more comprehensive articles in a wide array of professional medical journals. General-interest periodicals often provided contemporary coverage. Some feature stories focused on the Epidemic Intelligence Service.

Archives and Government Documents

Archival resources: The CDC Global Health Odyssey Museum in Atlanta houses a miscellaneous collection of materials, including some boxes of reprints assembled by Alexander Langmuir and large scrapbooks of media clippings relevant to the CDC from the 1950s and 1960s. The CDC Public Health Image Library contains many historical photographs and illustrations (http://phil.cdc.gov/phil/home.asp). In offices within the CDC Office of Workforce and Career Development are Epi-Aid reports from investigations of EIS officers, abstracts from annual April EIS conferences, and back issues of the *EIS Bulletin,* previously called *Memorandum, The Bulletin,* and the *Director's Bulletin.* The CDC Division of Creative Services maintains a good collection of videotaped interviews and events related to the EIS and CDC. *Ripples in the Waters of Epidemiology,* a three-VHS set of interviews conducted by honorary EIS alum David Sencer with former EIS officers in 2001, is invaluable, as are the DVDs of the scientific sessions of EIS's fiftieth anniversary celebration in 2001.

The Countway Library of Harvard Medical School has two cartons of Epi-Aids from the 1950s and 1960s, as well as bound reprints of professional articles by EIS officers from those decades.

The Alan Mason Chesney Medical Archives at the Johns Hopkins School of Public Health in Baltimore contains the correspondence of Alexander Langmuir and some handwritten notes, mostly after 1970.

The National Archives and Records Administration, southeast region, in Morrow, Georgia, holds salvaged records of the CDC/EIS (http://www.archives.gov/southeast/). These are open to the public. In Ellenwood, Georgia, the Southeast Federal Records Center holds CDC records for ten years, then destroys all but the few that go to the NARA facility in Morrow. These records are only accessible with CDC permission.

Interviews

Interviews (in person or by phone, e-mail, or mail) were conducted by Mark Pendergrast, 2003–2008. Years listed after EIS alum names indicate their date of entry in July of that year. Those who entered in 1970, for instance, are known as the "class of 1970" rather than 1972, the year they graduated. Non–EIS interviewees are asterisked.

Eli Abrutyn (1968)
David Addiss (1985)
Mary Agocs (1988)
Russ Alexander (1955)
Larry Altman (1963)
Pamela Anderson-Mahoney (1995)
John Andrews (1975)
Fred Angulo (1993)
Paul Arguin (1997)
Robert Armstrong (1966)
Bernard Aserkoff (1967)
William Atkinson (1983)
George Baer (1961)
Bill Baine (1972)
Sapna Bamrah (2006)
Alan Barbour (1974)
Robert Barnes (1985)
Roy Baron (1977)
Jerry Barondess (1951)
Drue Barrett (1992)
Linda Bartlett (1998)
Mark Beatty (2000)

Consuelo Beck-Sagué (1985)
Jim Beecham (1976)
Ed Belongia (1988)
Elise (Jochimsen) Beltrami (1995)
Diane Bennett (1984)
John Bennett (1965)
Gary Berger (1971)
Ruth Berkelman (1980)
Seth Berkley (1984)
Richard Besser (1991)
Robin Biellik (1985)
Robert Biggar (1973)
Sue Binder (1984)
Paul Blake (1969)
Martin Blaser (1979)
Dan Blumenthal (1972)
John Boring (1955)
Philip Brachman (1954)
David Brandling-Bennett (1971)
Joel Breman (1976)
Bob Brewer (1989)
Carolyn Bridges (1996)

* Martha (Waits) Brocato
Jake Brody (1957)
John Brooks (1998)
Claire Broome (1977)
Jim Bryan (1961)
Dan Budnitz (2001)
Jim Buehler (1981)
Joanna Buffington (1990)
* Jack Bunn
Mike Bunning (1998)
John Burke (1973)
Jay Butler (1989)
Dorothy Calafiore (1954)
Glyn Caldwell (1967)
Carlos "Kent" Campbell (1972)
Matt Cartter (1983)
Ken Castro (1983)
Ward Cates (1974)
Jim Cheek (1990)
Wairimu Chege (2002)
Bob Chen (1984)
Arthur "Gene" Chin (1997)
Tom D.Y. Chin (1954)
Pamela Ching (1992)
Terry Chorba (1983)
Mitch Cohen (1976)
Tom Cole (1985)
Lyle Conrad (1965)
José Cordero (1979)
Larry Corey (1973)
Phil Craven (1971)
John Crowell (1966)
John Crump (2000)
Jim Curran (honorary 2004)
Kate Curtis (1996)

Craig Dalton (1992)
Bruce Dan (1979)
Lucy Davidson (1984)
Megan Davies (1998)
Jeff Davis (1973)
Ron Davis (1984)
Andy Dean (1974)
Kevin De Cock (1986)
Malcolm Denley (1951)
George Denniston (1961)
Catherine Dentinger (1997)
Puneet Dewan (2001)
Richard Dicker (1980)
Greg Dimijian (1962)
Tim Dondero (1977)
Sam Dooley (1988)
Irene Doto (1954)
Walt Dowdle (honorary 1991)
Scott Dowell (1993)
Jeff Duchin (1992)
Philippe Duclos (1986)
Bruce Dull (1957)
Peter Dull (2000)
Fred Dunn (1957)
Herbert DuPont (1967)
Mark Dworkin (1994)
William Dyal (1963)
Allan Ebbin (1967)
Mark Eberhardt (1983)
Brian Edlin (1989)
Tom Edwards (1976)
Bob Eelkema (1962)
Ted Eickhoff (1959)
Mickey Eisenberg (1973)
Melto "Jamie" Eliades (2004)

Bill Elsea (1960)

John Emmett (1951)

Terry England (1978)

David Erickson (1974)

* Elizabeth Etheridge

Ruth Etzel (1985)

Bruce Evatt (1968)

Gerald Faich (1970)

Henry Falk (1972)

* Odom Fanning

Tom Farley (1987)

Charles Federspiel (1952)

Danny Feikin (1996)

Roger Feldman (1968)

Marc Filstein (1977)

Mark Finch (1982)

Thea Fischer (2003)

David Fleming (1983)

Bill Flynt (1965)

Bill Foege (1962)

Bob Fontaine (1973)

Don Forthal (1984)

Stan Foster (1962)

Don Francis (1971)

David Fraser (1971)

Tom Frieden (1990)

Dara Friedman (2001)

Eli Friedman (1961)

* Alvin Friedman-Kien

Curtis Fritz (1994)

Keiji Fukuda (1990)

Jim Gale (1964)

Gene Gangarosa (1964)

Howard Garber (1966)

Julie Garner (1969)

Helene Gayle (1984)

Kathleen Gensheimer (1981)

* Julie Gerberding

Ken Gershman (1989)

Brad Gessner (1991)

Jerry Gibson (1971)

Roger Glass (1977)

(William) Paul Glezen (1957)

Tom Glick (1967)

Gary Goldbaum (1984)

Mark Goldberger (1976)

Marcia Goldoft (1985)

Brant Goode (2004)

Rick Goodman (1978)

George Grady (1962)

Don Graham (1978)

Phil Graitcer (1976)

Herman Gray (1951)

Tom Grayston (1951)

Richard Greenberg (1974)

Carolyn Greene (2001)

Sheldon Greenfield (1966)

Mike Gregg (1966)

Patty Griffin (1985)

Kevin Griffith (2001)

David Grimes (1975)

Marta Guerra (2000)

Mary Guinan (1974)

Bob Gunn (1976)

Bernie Guyer (1972)

Robert Hahn (1986)

Robert Haley (1973)

Jack Hall (1955)

Bill Halperin (1975)

Doug Hamilton (1991)

John Hamilton (1968)

Gwen Hammer (1999)

John Hanrahan (1981)

Scott Harper (2000)

Jeff Harris (1981)

John Harris (1974)

Lee Harrison (1985)

Ron Hattis (1969)

Mike Hattwick (1970)

Harry Haverkos (1981)

Jim Hayslett (2000)

Clark Heath (1960)

Katrina Hedberg (1986)

Wynn Hemmert (1973)

D.A. Henderson (1955)

Ralph "Rafe" Henderson (1965)

Tom Hennessy (1994)

John Herbert (1974)

Veronica Herrera-Moreno (1995)

Chuck Herron (1971)

Brad Hersh (1987)

David Heymann (1976)

Betsy Hilborn (1995)

Susan Hillis (2002)

* Martin Hines

Alan Hinman (1965)

Gottfried Hirnschall (1989)

John Ho (1979)

Mei-Shang Ho (1986)

Natasha Hochberg (2004)

Charles Hoge (1989)

Charles Hoke (1974)

Susan Holck (1978)

Scott Holmberg (1982)

Gary Holmes (1985)

Joe Horman (1966)

Bob Horsburgh (1987)

Marcus Horwitz (1974)

Danny Hudson (1966)

Paul Hudson (1983)

Sara Huston (1995)

Yvan Hutin (1996)

* Pascal "Pat" Imperato

Greg Istre (1980)

Dick Jackson (1975)

George Jackson (1970)

Harold Jaffe (1981)

Robert Janssen (1985)

Janine Jason (1980)

George Johnson (1961)

Donna Jones (1988)

Josh Jones (2001)

Steve Jones (1969)

Tim Jones (1997)

Hannah Jordan (2005)

Wilbert Jordan (1973)

Paul Joseph (1961)

* Suzanne Junod

Henry Kahn (1972)

Jimmy Kahn (1969)

Mary Kamb (1989)

Karen Kaplan (1987)

Adam Karpati (1997)

Dolly Katz (1995)

Arnold Kaufmann (1963)

Andy Kaunitz (1982)

Richard Keenlyside (1976)

* Hugh Kelsey

Alex Kelter (1980)

Ali Khan (1991)
Ed Kilbourne (1980)
James Kile (2002)
Peter Kilmarx (1994)
Ann Marie Kimball (1977)
Robert Kim-Farley (1981)
Herschell King (1966)
Tobias Kircher (1981)
Paul Kitsutani (1998)
Doug Klaucke (1979)
Marlin Kleckner (1956)
Don Klein (1966)
John Kobayashi (1979)
Shellie Kolavic (1996)
Denise Koo (1991)
Jeff Koplan (1972)
Kay Kreiss (1978)
Etienne Krug (1995)
Judy Kruger (2001)
Calvin Kunin (1954)
* Howard Kushner
Marc LaForce (1966)
George "Sandy" Lamb (1962)
Steve Lamm (1970)
Ed Lammer (1982)
Phil Landrigan (1970)
Mike Lane (1963)
Scott Laney (2006)
* Marc LaPointe
Kayla Laserson (1997)
Dale Lawrence (1973)
Peter Layde (1977)
Marci Layton (1992)
Lisa Lee (1988)
Charles LeMaistre (1951)

Myron "Mike" Levine (1970)
Orin Levine (1994)
Richard Levine (1972)
Ron Levine (1963)
Barry Levy (1973)
Deborah Levy (1996)
Anna Likos (2003)
Scott Lillibridge (1990)
Matt Loewenstein (1969)
Carlos Lopez (1976)
Andrew Luk (1992)
Don Lyman (1970)
* Francesca Lyman
(George) Marshall Lyon (1998)
Pia MacDonald (2000)
Tom Mack (1964)
Bill Mac Kenzie (1991)
Dennis Maki (1969)
Polly Marchbanks (1985)
Ed Marcuse (1969)
Jim Marks (1976)
Mike Martin (2000)
Arthur Marx (1995)
Laurene Mascola (1982)
Jim Mason (1959)
Tim Mastro (1988)
* Gene Matthews
Jim Maynard (1960)
Joe McCormick (1973)
* Joe McDade
Angie McGowan (2002)
John McGowan (1969)
Cam McIntyre (1976)
Peter McPhedran (1966)
Bob Mellins (1953)

Jim Mercy (1982)

Mike Merson (1972)

* Okech John Migele

Don Millar (1961)

David Miller (1960)

Eric Mintz (1989)

Joel Montgomery (2002)

Ron Moolenaar (1992)

Anne Moore (1991)

Pat Moore (1987)

Roscoe Moore (1971)

John Morawetz (1983)

* Mary Moreman

Leo Morris (1959)

Dale Morse (1976)

Wiley Henry Mosley (1961)

Joe Mulinare (1981)

Ben Muneta (1989)

Kristy Murray (1999)

* Shiva Murugasampillay

Stan Music (1971)

Ira Myers (1951)

Andy Nahmias (1958)

Tim Naimi (1998)

Denis Nash (1999)

Neal Nathanson (1955)

John Neff (1963)

Amanda Sue Niskar (1996)

Harold Nitowsky (1951)

Joel Nitzkin (1967)

Al Noonan (1970)

Alvin Novack (1959)

Mark Oberle (1975)

Kate O'Brien (1995)

Rick O'Brien (1975)

Patrick O'Carroll (1985)

Ron O'Connor (1967)

* Paul Offit

Ciara O'Reilly (2004)

Kevin O'Reilly (1981)

Walt Orenstein (1974)

Howard Ory (1971)

* Mike Osterholm

Steve Ostroff (1986)

Ralph Paffenbarger (1951)

Malcolm Page (1957)

Allen Paris (1977)

Boris Pavlin (2004)

Fred Payne (1953)

* Mary Pendergast

* Ambrose Pendergrast

Brad Perkins (1989)

Norm Petersen (1955)

Bert Peterson (1979)

Rossanne Philen (1988)

Michael Phillips (2000)

Steven Phillips (1979)

Stanley Plotkin (1957)

Lou Polish (1989)

Marjorie Pollack (1977)

Ken Powell (1974)

Dana Quade (1960)

Lynn Quenemoen (1992)

Linda Quick (1995)

Rob Quick (1990)

Kenneth Quist (1955)

Rei Ravenholt (1952)

John Redd (2000)

Jennita Reefhuis (2001)

* Ed Regis

Art Reingold (1979)
Barth Reller (1968)
Pat Remington (1982)
Robert Remis (1981)
Henry Retailliau (1976)
José Rigau (1977)
Lee Riley (1981)
Ron Roberto (1962)
Les Roberts (1992)
Roger Rochat (1968)
Martha Rogers (1981)
Judith Bourne Rooks (1971)
Mark Rosenberg (1974)
Michael Rosenberg (1978)
Richard Rothenberg (1968)
Diane Rowley (1980)
* Jean Roy
Jeff Sacks (1979)
Cathy Samples (1976)
Julia Samuelson (1998)
Sanjeeb Sapkota (2003)
* David Satcher
Bill Schaffner (1966)
Peter Schantz (1974)
Wally Schlech (1980)
Donald Schliessmann (1951)
George Schmid (1979)
Steve Schoenbaum (1967)
Larry Schonberger (1971)
Peter Schrag (1966)
Steve Schroeder (1966)
Anne Schuchat (1988)
Myron "Mike" Schultz (1963)
Ira Schwartz (1981)
Richard Seibert (1954)

Jim Sejvar (2000)
Joel Selanikio (1995)
Jan Semenza (1995)
David Sencer (honorary 1975)
Dan Sexton (1972)
Wayne Shandera (1980)
Roger Shapiro (1996)
Don Sharp (1992)
Mike Shasby (1975)
Colin Shepard (2001)
Henry Shinefield (1951)
Mike Siegel (1993)
Dean Sienko (1984)
Tom Sinks (1985)
Kirk Smith (1996)
David Sokal (1978)
Al Sommer (1969)
Harold Sours (1977)
Harrison Spencer (1972)
Walter Stamm (1973)
Sally Stansfield (1980)
Karen Starko (1978)
Jim Steele (honorary 1975)
Allen Steere (1973)
* Claudia Stein
Gail Stennies (1994)
Mike St. Louis (1985)
Charlie Stoltenow (1991)
Raymond Strikas (1983)
Scott Stryker (1978)
Dennis Stubblefield (1966)
John Sullivan-Bolyai (1976)
Roland Sutter (1987)
David Swerdlow (1989)
Tina Tan (2000)

Rob Tauxe (1983)

Steve Teutsch (1977)

Steve Thacker (1976)

Polly Thomas (1981)

Robert "Tom" Thompson (1967)

Doug Thoroughman (1996)

Michael Thun (1980)

Bruce Tierney (2001)

Tom Török (1984)

Marc Traeger (2000)

Sue Trock (1987)

Rick Trowbridge (1971)

Marvin Turck (1960)

Jessica Tuttle (1991)

Carl Tyler (1966)

Tim Uyeki (1998)

Jim Veazey (1974)

Andy Vernon (1978)

Tom Vernon (1966)

Ron Waldman (1979)

John Ward (1984)

Rita Washko (1993)

Bill Watson (honorary 1983)

David Wegman (1967)

Jason Weisfeld (1973)

Edie Welty (1982)

Tom Welty (1982)

Bruce Weniger (1980)

Karl Western (1967)

Mark White (1975)

Andy Wiesenthal (1978)

Holly Ann Williams (1996)

(Richard) Joel Williams (1995)

Walt Williams (1981)

David Williamson (1985)

Brad Winterton (2000)

Kevin Winthrop (2000)

Bob Winton (1973)

Celia Woodfill (1993)

Brad "Woody" Woodruff (1987)

Chris Woods (1997)

Nick Wright (1963)

Milford Wyman (1955)

Fujie Xu (1998)

Lorraine Yeung (2002)

* James Harvey Young

Lynn Zanardi (Blevins) (1998)

Gabe Zatlin (1962)

Stephanie Zaza (1991)

Patrick Zuber (1994)

Jelka Zupan (1990)

ACKNOWLEDGMENTS

EIS alum Andy Vernon, one of my best high school friends, first told me about the Epidemic Intelligence Service and suggested that I write its history. He also served as a critical, helpful reader.

I owe a tremendous debt to nearly five hundred EIS alums who provided information, including interviews, EIS memoirs, published papers, diaries, letters, speeches, and photos. Several EIS veterans whom I interviewed have died, including Eli Abrutyn, Russ Alexander, Ron Davis, Mike Gregg, EIS administrator Mary Moreman, Ira Myers, Ralph Paffenbarger, Donald Schliessmann, and Walter Stamm. Thanks also to non-EIS public health experts, who gave me a different perspective, and to Susan, Lynn, and Paul Langmuir for sharing memories of their father.

EIS officers always act as part of a team, but with so many characters, I could not do justice to everyone involved. Laboratory scientists, CDC supervisors, Public Health Advisors, state, local, and international health officials, and many others provided vital support for investigations and deserve more acknowledgment than they generally receive.

My local librarian, Susan Overfield, cheerfully filled my numerous interlibrary loan requests at the tiny town library in Essex, Vermont. At the southeast region of the National Archives and Records Administration in Morrow, Georgia, Charlie Reeves (now retired) and Andre Wilkerson were extremely helpful. EIS alum Lyle Conrad, always available and supportive, escorted me to the Federal Records Center, then in East Point, Georgia, providing essential comments on the material we found. FDA historians Suzanne White Junod and John Swan helped with appropriate material. Thanks to archivists at the Countway Library of Harvard Medical School, at the Johns Hopkins School of Public Health, and at the National Library of Medicine, and the staff at the CDC Library.

Many people within the CDC helped with this project, but Steve Thacker, director of the Office of Workforce and Career Development, stands out for always being willing to answer my questions or refer me to others who could, and Larry Schonberger was equally responsive. Hugh Kelsey, then head of the CDC Public Health Image Library, and Mary Hilpertshauser of the CDC Global Health Odyssey Museum were also extremely helpful.

Philip Brachman, who succeeded Alexander Langmuir as the EIS chief, generously shared his knowledge, library, and time. Former CDC director David Sencer, an honorary EIS officer, provided insight and suggestions. Elizabeth Etheridge, who wrote *Sentinel for Health* (1992), a history of the CDC, shared her research material, including interview transcripts.

I was fortunate to have scientific and lay readers who caught factual errors and suggested stylistic improvements, including Carolyn Barnes, Philip Brachman, Lyle Conrad, Marylen Grigas, Ilze Henderson, Rafe Henderson, Alan Hinman, Scott Holmberg, Steve Jones, Jill MacGlaflin, David Morens, Britt Pendergrast, John Pendergrast, Nan Pendergrast, David Sencer, Steve Thacker, and Andy Vernon. I am solely responsible for the final product, however.

Grants from the Josiah Macy Jr. Foundation (administered by the Task Force for Child Survival) and the CDC Foundation (a nongovernmental organization) made it possible for me to hire part-time researchers, including Osarobo Adeghe, Imad Al-Akkak, Ryan Austin, Albert Barskey, Steve Cormier, Christie Emch, Ryan Estaris, John Ishaq, Matthew Koch, Beth Leftwich, Purvi Patel, Michael Phillips,

Laura Robinson, Brenda Thompson, Evan Tiderington, Kelley Urry, and Sarah Wiegel. My father, Britt Pendergrast, also conducted archival research, but he refused payment.

Diane Meyerhoff transcribed some taped interviews and presentations. Anne Exler created a digital index of my research material. My neighbor Laura McVey brought order to my files.

In Seattle, Rei and Susan Ravenholt provided a guest room, as did Bernard Nahlen in his home near the World Health Organization in Geneva. In Niamey, Niger, Jamie Eliades graciously shared his hotel room.

Many thanks to Lisa Bankoff, my longtime ICM agent, for her advocacy and for finding Andrea Schulz, my editor at Houghton Mifflin Harcourt, who loved the idea of a book on disease detectives, championed its acquisition, and honed it, along with coeditors Lindsey Smith and Tom Bouman. As with my previous two books, freelance editor Regina Hersey helped to prune and shape the original manuscript without interfering with my voice or style. Line editors David Hough and Dan Janeck meticulously checked punctuation, usage, and facts.

Finally, to my wife, Betty Molnar, I owe a large debt for this book, and not just for her love, support, and patience when I had to travel. A nurse who has served every type of patient from pediatrics to hospice, she also spent time as an infection control practitioner. With this breadth of knowledge, she was a careful, critical reader.

INDEX